D0812211

Clinical Management of Stuttering in Older Children and Adults

Richard E. Ham, Ph.D.
Professor of Speech/Language Pathology
Florida State University
Professor Emeritus, Hearing and Speech Sciences
Ohio University

AN ASPEN PUBLICATION®
Aspen Publishers, Inc.
Gaithersburg, Maryland
1999

Library of Congress Cataloging-in-Publication Data

Ham, Richard, 1931–
Clinical management of stuttering in older children and adults / Richard E. Ham.
p. cm.
Includes bibliographical references and index.
ISBN 0-8342-1117-3 (alk. paper)
1. Stuttering—Treatment. I. Title.
RC424.H229   1999
616.85'5406—dc21
98-46351
CIP

Copyright © 1999 by Aspen Publishers, Inc.
All rights reserved.

Aspen Publishers, Inc., grants permission for photocopying for limited personal or internal use.
This consent does not extend to other kinds of copying, such as copying for general distribution,
for advertising or promotional purposes, for creating new collective works, or for resale.
For information, address Aspen Publishers, Inc., Permissions Department,
200 Orchard Ridge Drive, Suite 200, Gaithersburg, Maryland 20878.

Orders: (800) 638-8437
Customer Service: (800) 234-1660

About Aspen Publishers • For more than 35 years, Aspen has been a leading professional
publisher in a variety of disciplines. Aspen's vast information resources are available in both
print and electronic formats. We are committed to providing the highest quality information
available in the most appropriate format for our customers. Visit Aspen's Internet site for
more information resources, directories, articles, and a searchable version of Aspen's full
catalog, including the most recent publications: **http://www.aspenpublishers.com**
Aspen Publishers, Inc. • The hallmark of quality in publishing
Member of the worldwide Wolters Kluwer group.

Editorial Services: Nora Fitzpatrick
Library of Congress Catalog Card Number: 98-46351
ISBN: 0-8342-1117-3

Printed in the United States of America

1 2 3 4 5

*To the founders who built new roads for us to follow.
They so often were stutterers themselves and lived with
the structures they built. As researchers, teachers, and,
most of all, clinicians, they set standards for us all.*

CONTENTS

PREFACE

BACKGROUND

This book took some time to develop—about 48 years. It started in 1951 when I was a college junior and changed my major from theater to "speech correction." I started immediately with a child client with an articulation problem. However, my interest blossomed when I observed Clyde Rousey work with a female teenaged stutterer and saw Bob Hejna apply Rogerian nondirective therapy with an adult male stutterer. My initial interest was confirmed the next quarter when, as a member of Charles Elliot's undergraduate stuttering class, I went through Hahn's (1943) *Stuttering: Significant Theories and Therapies*. I was hooked, and I remain so today.

As I grew in knowledge and evolved, nearly all the techniques I learned involved observation and application of the old medical model—see one, do one, teach one. Very rarely was there an in-print model for me to follow. In fact, a residuum of the 1930s and 1940s attitude of "don't let anyone find out what your secret therapy methods are" still existed. Thank goodness things have changed in terms of attitude. In terms of application, however, the problem of learning exactly what is involved in Clinician X's or Dr. Y's methods remains. Today, there is a tendency to charge a hefty fee for a seminar so one can secure knowledge and earn continuing education credits at the same time.

Another problem with special methods and techniques is that they often bypass (or just fail to mention) the importance of the early steps in therapy that prepared the client for whatever special approach is being discussed. Moreover, minimal attention is paid to transition practices, transfer of therapy skills, and conduct of maintenance programs. This problem often was balanced by the fact that early therapy could easily go on for several years, and many of the foregoing needs were met (somewhat) along the way. However, as we moved into behavior modification and fluency induction we also saw more and more "fast track" therapy that tended to leave a semi-fluent client, rather quickly, on his or her own resources to survive after dismissal. I therefore felt a growing need to review therapy procedures in some detail, from first to last.

Another problem area involves student preparation, in particular, the texts used in academic coursework. Most of these works have been or are excellent classroom texts about stuttering, and I have written my share. However, the key words of the previous sentence are "about stuttering." They were, and are, texts about the entire area of stuttering—definition, history, research, theory, philosophy, and overviews of current therapies. I have no problems with that. Such an approach is needed to teach. However, to a certain extent, students in training need access to more specific information about management procedures (at least, those I supervise do). To a major extent, clinicians employed in various settings have expressed a need for a resource that delineates specific procedures.

STRUCTURE OF THE BOOK

This book is not "about" stuttering. It is about management techniques in diagnosis, evaluation, and therapy for stuttering and other communication problems. In teaching introductory and advanced courses for more than 40 years, I have used some wonderful classroom texts. Yet every semester when the lectures reached management procedures I heard student statements such as "But how do you do that?" or "The book gives the rationale, but not the procedures for. . . ." Progressively, I developed a syllabus of class projects in various evaluation and management procedures. They were assigned as point-producing projects. As the number of projects and points grew, at some point "Eureka!" struck, and I started work to construct this resource book.

Although its procedures are structured to refer to fluency disorders, all the techniques apply to a wide range of communication problems. Rate reduction is an excellent approach for many dysarthrias; relaxation benefits hypertense vocal function and spastic conditions in general; Easy Onset facilitates many apraxic and hypertense problems among others. I hope that all who use this resource will find its contents applicable to a wide range of communication disorders.

This book and the techniques included lean toward older stutterers, those about 8 to 9 years of age and older. There are some young-child orientations in certain sections. However, young children are not discussed extensively for a number of reasons.

- Family involvement and family counseling programs alone would require an entire book.
- Schools, teachers, and group structures would fill another book.
- There is a trend to use packaged programs for the very young. Although some of these programs are excellent, some are lamentable. This book provides almost no coverage of commercial programs. They are numerous and constantly growing in number. Further, I do not wish to limit myself to writing "about" therapy by listing therapy programs.
- The political split between working with "stuttering" and working with children who are "fluency challenged." Techniques in this book basically are presented as for stuttering and stutterers. It is a hair-splitting, but real, difference of opinion.

For these and other reasons, child coverage is curtailed.

OTHER FRAMES OF REFERENCE

Many readers of this book may find themselves saying, "That's not the way I learned it!" In quite a few instances, the procedures are not presented the way *I* learned them. Over years of use and adaptation, some techniques have changed significantly. When readers are aware of major differences (not "right" and "wrong," but "other ways"), I would be glad to hear from them and enrich my knowledge. Other readers may say, "Ham didn't even mention the XYZ approach." In some instances, procedures are left out due to my ignorance about them or my unfamiliarity with them. Most of the procedures in this book are those that I know and have used. In some instances, space considerations clipped my coverage. In general, I did not include procedures where

- A specialized training program or seminar is required for basic acquisition.
- Expensive, scarce, or complex equipment or procedures are required.

- Commercially packaged programs or software is required.
- Assistants, technicians, and support staff of various types are needed.

COVERAGE DEPTH

Depth of coverage is variable across topics. Space limitations are part of the reason. However, I also tried to apply common sense and reduce coverage where a speech-language pathologist with general experience and adequate intelligence could take and apply procedure X. On the other hand, procedure Y is offered in a detailed, step-by-step process. At times, I will say, "For this step, use the same word lists that are provided for procedure W." I believe there is enough similarity among certain areas of information, structures, and examples to provide adequate clues on how to do this. At any rate, the structural parts or steps are always laid out as suggestions, not mandates. I want readers to use their experience and their insight into a particular client to revise or add to any procedures discussed in the book.

TERMINOLOGY

In reading publications, I often come across a word and wonder, "What did the author mean by that?" To try and minimize that difficulty, I will define terms as I go along. Most definitions are general in use and typical. However, all definitions are offered within *my frame of reference*. I make minimal use of general dictionaries or American Speech-Language-Hearing Association (ASLHA) lists of preferred terms. Although I have studied the recent definitions report from the fluency Special Interest Group of ASLHA (1998), I decided to use the terms with which I am comfortable.

SUMMARY

This book was a pleasure to write. I frowned over a few procedures that I have used but did not like a whole lot, yet even then enjoyed trying to express myself clearly.

A problem stemming from over 40 years of experience is trying to remember to include "little points"—those vital actions that are almost automatic to experienced users of a technique. If there are omissions, please let me know. I hope all graduated, certified, and licensed professionals will use this book for many years. Enjoy!

REFERENCES

American Speech-Language-Hearing Association. (1998). *Terminology pertaining to fluency and fluency disorders*. Unpublished manuscript.

Hahn, E.F. (1943). *Stuttering: Significant theories and therapies*. Stanford, CA: Stanford University Press.

CHAPTER 1

Diagnosis and Evaluation of Stuttering

- Overview
- Terms and Definitions
- Tests, Forms, and Procedures in Evaluation
- Prediction
- Laterality Measures
- Tests and Forms
- General Assessment and Interview Concerns
- Special Issues
- Summary

OVERVIEW

Chapter 1 addresses the topics of when disfluency is called dysfluency, the adequacy of listeners as judges, the appropriateness and accuracy of our measuring devices, the political correctness of certain labels, the values and dangers of early intervention, and on and on. As I reviewed my own beliefs and information, and those of others, I became more exasperated and frustrated, and finally realized I was becoming sidetracked. The goal of this book is to communicate procedures I know about or have used that I want to lay out for consideration. The emphasis is on "lay outs" that are usable, rather than those that are "about" things. However, in this chapter I deliberately introduced a number of outside sources to a degree not matched in other chapters. This decision was made to offer the reader additional sources for specific tests, measures, and procedures. Generally, I tried to use the original publication detailing the items and its development. In several instances, my most appropriate resource was the pub-

1

lisher, although I generally tried to avoid that less informative type of referral. A number of recent texts have printed copies of some of the measures (Conture, 1990; Culatta & Goldberg, 1995; Curlee & Siegel, 1997; Ham, 1986, 1989; Kent, 1996; Peters & Guitar, 1991; Shipley & McAfee, 1998; Silverman, 1996; Wall & Myers, 1995). Some are highly organized with a form on every other page; others are less specific but provide worthwhile discussions about areas of diagnosis and evaluation. In this book I will cite some specific forms, but generally I will adhere to those outlines or forms or procedures that I have used.

Age Factors

Age or maturation complicates any overview of diagnosis and assessment, because it has a significant relationship to stuttering. Many years ago the field developed the terms primary and secondary stuttering to indicate the basic separation between so-called childhood and adult stuttering. *Primary* referred to the supposed easy, effortless, rhythmic repetitive dysfluencies, with little or no awareness on the part of the speaker. *Secondary* stuttering referred to the aware, tense, disrhythmic, distorted patterns of older stutterers, usually involving avoidances and attitude problems. Recognizing that the shift between the two stages is too abrupt and not reflective of reality, the term *transitional* stuttering was invented to cover children who had started to show advanced symptoms but still retained some of the simpler characteristics as well. The term also was meant to apply to older stutterers who, for whatever reasons, had retained much of their younger, simpler syndrome aspects. The primary stutterers generally were thought to function mainly during the time from onset of stuttering to 5 or 6 years of age; transitional stuttering was meant to cover the time period from 5 or 6 years up to 8 or 9 years (it used to be until adolescence for some authorities); and secondary stuttering covered the stutterer exhibiting a general pattern of advanced stuttering characteristics. The three labels were clumsy to define and failed to encompass many individuals who presented with patterns of speech that did not jibe with the definitions or age groupings.

Originally I planned to divide evaluation into age groups, as I have done before (Ham, 1989). However, to minimize confusion and simplify presentation I ultimately decided to organize by diagnostic and evaluation categories. Some of them apply equally, no matter what the age; some are almost totally child related; and some are pretty much adult oriented. I believe this organizational approach will be of greater use to the clinician who does not want prescriptions for a complete diagnostic workup (I did that in both previous books), but needs help, suggestions, or explanations concerning specific problems or measures.

Diagnostic Goals

The goals of any diagnosis are to determine whether or not a problem exists, and to append a label to any problem discovered. Corollary to the discovery/label aspects is the factor of *evaluation*, where the precipitation or onset, development, and related factors are explored. Finally, most diagnoses will attempt to recommend resolution(s) for the problem, preferred modes of approach, and some sort of prognostic estimate. Embedded in the procedures of this chapter are resources to attempt to achieve those various goals.

Applications

I hope this chapter will be a repository of methods and procedures relating directly to the diagnosis and evaluation of stuttering. It does not contain anything about articulation tests and little about language evaluation, because I assume that readers are competent in those broad areas. There is, however, information on both areas as they relate to stuttering. This also is true of respiration and phonation.

This chapter also tries to strike a balance between "old" procedures, some of which are not available in current textbooks, and newer, more popular approaches. A factor involved here is "procedure popularity." For instance, right now (and rightly so) so-called speech naturalness in stuttering is popular (see chapter 3). Certain politically correct approaches to labels and intervention are current. By the same token, certain procedures have fallen out of use for reasons not much better than those that supported some of the recent additions to our resources and practices.

TERMS AND DEFINITIONS

Overview

I think it is important to provide a number of terms and definitions concerning stuttering that will be used in this chapter and throughout the book. In later chapters, some terms will be redefined for particular purposes. First, I will provide basic terminology to define different forms of core stuttering spasms, followed by an indication of the usual elements involved in core struggles. Next, the possible or probable overflow struggles to the rest of the body will be identified. Some of the struggle and overflow phenomena also can be classified as part of the associated behaviors group, which subdivide into spasm-specific avoidances and communication-general avoidances in overall speech. First of all, however, I need to consider the definition of three terms: stuttering, dysfluency, and spasm.

Special Terms: Stuttering, Dysfluency, and Spasm

The communication disorder called stuttering suffers from a combination of problems ranging from confusion about its very definition to politically correct objections to certain labels, to difficulties differentiating between fluency disruptions that are normal and abnormal. Regarding definitions, I can say simply that either there are too many definitions of stuttering, or none at all. The Special Interest Division #4 (fluency disorders) of the American Speech-Language-Hearing Association (ASLHA) generated a working paper titled *Terminology Pertaining to Fluency and Fluency Disorders* (ASLHA, 1998). The direct definition of stuttering (section 2.5) takes approximately four single-spaced typed pages to discuss. Even though the effort was excellent, the real definition of stuttering remains uncertain. I therefore will assume that readers know what they mean when they use the word "stuttering."

Another problem is the use of the label "stutterer." In all of its publications, ASLHA has adopted the "person first" frame of references; thus there are no longer "stutterers"; but only "persons who stutter." I wonder if we as professionals should call ourselves speech-language pathologists or, because the majority of the time we do not practice speech-language pathology, we should be called "persons who practice speech-language pathology as a profession." Clumsy? People call me a "teacher," not a person who teaches. The Special Interest Division working paper (ASLHA, 1998) states that some persons who practice speech-language pathology as a profession now refer to people who stutter by the acronym, PWSs. Is becoming an acronym less, or more, demeaning than becoming a label, especially when the label defines the communication problem experienced by the individual and the acronym may be a mystery to some?

Another problem in nomenclature (or semantics) is the question of *dis*fluency versus *dys*fluency. The special interest division working paper provides an excellent discussion of this problem (items 2.3, 2.4 on pages 3 through 5) and its confusions (ASLHA, 1998). It appropriately notes that *dis* and *dys* are used interchangeably by some and that different definition sources may define both prefixes in conflicting ways. In this book I will use the following frames of reference:

> **Dysfluency**—a basic synonym for stuttering that may extend beyond stuttering to include problem areas such as cluttering, neurogenic stuttering, and so on. It also covers the occasional *dis*fluencies that are not subject to ordinary levels of control by the speaker.
>
> **Disfluency**—production continuity losses or errors (linguistic or motor) that could be controlled by the speaker if he or she expended ordinary attention and effort.

Those are not good definitions, and they can be distorted as speakers and parameters change. In general, this book will discuss disfluencies as what "everybody does" and dysfluencies as what the PWS does when speech is labeled "stuttering."

I use the word *spasm* to indicate stuttering moments. I fell into this usage because the old term, "block," was used by some to refer to a stoppage (what some call a silent pause), while others used it to refer to any stuttering event. The terms "stuttering event," "dysfluent occurrence," and "moment of dysfluency" all sound vague and pompous. One could say "stutter," as in "He produced a stutter," but I usually avoid subverting a verb into a noun. On the other hand, the term "spasm" has certain values. A *spasm* is a sudden, strong contraction or series of such contractions of a muscle or muscle group, usually without conscious control. This definition seems to describe any "moment of stuttering." It separates from attitudes, eye contact, and avoidance behaviors and obviously refers to the core spasm–related struggles. I find the term applicable and use it often.

Spasm Categories or Types

The Core Spasm

The core spasm, as previously defined, subdivides into three primary plus two mixed categories: repetition (clonic), prolongation (tonic), and stoppage (tonic). The prolongation is sometimes called a tense pause or a tense pause–audible, and the stoppage is sometimes called a tense pause or a tense pause–inaudible. The other two categories are mixes of the two basic, clonic and tonic, types of spasms: clonotonic (starts clonic and ends tonic) and tonoclonic (starts tonic and ends clonic). The child stutterer is usually nearly all clonic, with repetitions that are easy, rhythmic, and limited in number. As time and awareness progress, efforts to overcome the mild spasms intensify and disrupt the ease and rhythmicity of the repetition pattern. The spasms may develop the indicated tonic or mixed forms.

Spasm Struggles and Overflow

The struggle during a stuttering spasm reflects what the speaker is trying to do to overcome the spasm. In effect, as noted many years ago, most of stuttering can be what is done by the speaker in an effort not to stutter. Struggles divide into three levels or areas:

1. Spasm struggle
2. Proximal struggle
3. Distal struggle

Spasm struggle goes beyond the core spasm (repetition, prolongation, stoppage), although it becomes an integral part of the core behavior. The struggle is a reflection of the intensity of the effort to fight through the spasm. An easy, rhythmic repetition is far removed from the multiple repetitions emitted with increased loudness, force, broken rhythm, and so forth. Spasm struggles come in many forms: lip licking, tongue protrusion, jaw jerks, jaws agape, laryngeal elevation and closure, glottal shocks, and so on.

Proximal struggle is linked to the spasm struggle. Without the spasm, the proximal struggle is not likely to occur. It includes muscles of facial tension and expression, forehead corrugators, optic sphincters, nasal dilators and contractors, strap muscles of the neck, and shoulder girdle muscles. For some mature stutterers, their behaviors do not extend beyond this level; others show extended struggle.

Distal struggle involves the rest of the body and can be almost any major or minor part thereof. Behaviors I have seen include extensive whole-body tension; rhythmic or jerky movements of arms, hands, fingers, legs, and feet that may be "in space" or against the body, floor, chair, or wall; finger snapping; and postural extensions or crouching. These and other behaviors can occur as part of the struggle of a specific stuttering spasm. However, they also can function in the general avoidance aspects of associated behaviors (see discussion that follows) whether in the word-specific or communication-general categories.

Associated Behaviors

For many years, associated behaviors were called "secondaries" because they developed as secondary responses to the primary stuttering spasm (or were part of the more intense "secondary level of stuttering"). Confusion occurred over the use of the term, mainly because some used "secondaries" to refer to behaviors of lesser importance. For a number of years I used the term associated behaviors to label those behaviors that occur because of stuttering and are, therefore, associated with it. I have problems with my own usage because every associated behavior in stuttering can be used by persons who do not stutter (PWDNSs?) for varied reasons. When I thought about it I was reminded that every nonstuttering person (NSP) produces repetitions, prolongations, and stoppages under the label of *dis*fluency. Yet, these behaviors are separated from the stuttering label. Feeling no wiser, but obscurely comforted, I have retained the category of associated behaviors.

Word-Specific Avoidances

Readers who are well versed in stutterer behaviors should skip this section.

Associated behaviors properly divide into behaviors that are keyed to a specific word where stuttering is anticipated, or has begun. The anticipation of stuttering can be keyed to specific words (such as the person's name), to the particular locus of a word (e.g., clause boundary), and so on. Some stutterers use associated behaviors selectively, whereas others seem to "shotgun" their avoidances without definition of the target word.

> **Postponement**—any physical or vocal behavior intended to delay the attempt on a phoneme, syllable, or word in an effort to avoid anticipated stuttering.
>
> My name is uh . . . Richard.
> My name is, well now . . . it's . . . Richard.
> My name is . . . Richard.
> What did you say?
> My name is [stop, scratch head, sigh] is Richard Ham.

Starter—any physical or vocal behavior intended to initiate breathstream release, vocal fold movement, and/or articulator movement contiguously with (as a part of) the anticipated phoneme, syllable, or word.

My name is uh Richard.
My name is [snap fingers] Richard.

Retrial—the behavior in which the speaker manifests audible and/or visible dysfluency or struggle in an effort to produce a phoneme, syllable, or word; then gives the effort up (stops trying); and then starts a new effort.

My name is . . . My name is . . . My name is . . .
My name is Ri-ri-ri . . . My name is . . .
My name is Rrrrrr . . . My name is . . .

Retrials should not be confused with an extended, prolonged stuttering spasm. Sometimes it is hard to discern when the spasm is slowed down and reduced, but not really stopped, and then builds up again.

My name is Rrrrr [freezes into stoppage, still trying, then] ri-ri-ri . . . .

The speaker in the example above started with a prolongation, went into a silent stoppage, began to suddenly push harder, and jerked into a repetition.

Revision—can be part of a retrial, or it can be regarded as an aspect of substitution or circumlocution.

Retrial/revision: My name is Ri-ri . . . . Just call me . . . .
Retrial/substitution: My name is Ri-ri . . . . Dick.

There is a term that has floated around for at least the last 50 years (maybe 2,000) used to refer to feared words that "always" cause trouble for the stutterer. This term is "Jonah" words. It covers words such as personal names, addresses, telephone numbers, must-use words, and so on. There can be Jonah people and Jonah situations as well. Words, numbers, terms, names—all can result in the avoidances mentioned previously, but particularly seem to relate to the next two specific avoidance behaviors.

Substitution—replacement of an intended-use word by a synonym, or near synonym. It may occur before the Jonah term ever is tried, or it may occur as a retrial substitution.
Circumlocution—replacement of an intended-use word by a phrase or sentence. For example, the stutterer may replace "Hello, may I speak with Dorothy?" with "Hello, may I speak with your older sister?"

There are five other avoidances that can be word specific.

Mutism—a word-specific or communication-general avoidance. It may be limited, as in, "Would you give me a _____, please?" [pointing to the item desired]. It also can move toward situation avoidance by saying "I dunno" every time a question is asked.

Release—any behavior to affect escape from spasm as part of the struggle sequence in the spasm. It is referred to here because some persons use interjections (sounds, words, movements) to try and release out of a stuttering spasm.

Eye contact—the speaker with otherwise good eye contact looks away when she or he stutters, trying to reduce perceived communication pressure and avoid presumed negative expressions on auditors' faces. One can argue whether this behavior is part of the spasm or a response to the occurrence of the spasm. It happens frequently.

Distorted preparatory sets—very stylized and unusual (sometimes grotesque) articulatory postures preliminary to making a production attempt on a phoneme, syllable, or word. See chapter 8 for a discussion of prepatory sets.

Respiratory anomalies—too deep or too shallow inhalation, excessive exhalation prior to sound initiation, or trying to talk too long on a single breath. The respiratory evaluation section later in this chapter discusses overall respiratory concerns.

Communication-General Avoidances

The behaviors just described concern efforts to fight specific stutterings or anticipated stutterings. This general avoidance category covers those behaviors intended to reduce, overall, the probability that *any* stuttering will occur on *any* word.

Mutism—(or semimutism) the speaker talks much less often and in shorter amounts than otherwise equivalent nonstuttering persons. Some stutterers reduce verbal output by over 90% based on the "If I don't talk, I don't stutter" truism. At other times, persons demonstrate the "yup/ nope" pattern. An example from a later-cited crisis of a clinician with only three pages of questions for her first therapy session, had this type of behavior:

How long have you stuttered?
Years.
How has it changed over the past 4 or 5 years?
Hasn't.

Have you ever had therapy before, when you were younger?
Yep.
Did you find the therapy a lot of help at that time?
Nope.
Why do you think the therapy didn't provide very much help for you?
[shoulder shrug]

Altered speech production—the speaker habitually speaks in a mode or pattern that alters typical speech parameters.
* Rate (fast/slow)
* Volume (loud/soft)
* Pitch (high/low)
* Inflection (monotone, stereotyped, excess)
* Stress (reduced, increased [and usually equalized])
* Dialect, accent (anything from a regional departure from general American to strong foreign accent imitations)
* Implied attitude (challenging, belligerent, meek, sarcastic, humorous, or comedic)
* Physical (may take word-specific behaviors and use them broadly on most productions: rhythmic movements, elaborate and/or constant gestures, physically turning away from auditor, or advancing to invade auditor's personal zone)

Respiratory—the speaker may typically speak very breathily with air wastage and frequent inhalations; may talk extremely long on one breath, trying not to stop and therefore decrease risk of stuttering. See the respiratory evaluation section later in this chapter for various respiratory abnormalities.

Summary

Making a list of associated behaviors is useful in diagnosis and evaluation. Usually, its compilation should be done openly with the help of the client. The client should help detect both word-specific and communication-general avoidances (see chapter 3 on self-analysis). The list of behaviors should help focus attention in evaluation. In addition, some other sources might be helpful. Cooper (1982) suggested 20 characteristics of dysfluency that could relate to management intervention modes. Twenty suggestions (of behaviors) are offered, and the different elements are keyed to management procedures such as Easy Onset, breathstream management, and so forth. Shipley and McAfee (1998) provide a four-page form, cueing its users to look for motor behaviors in 14 areas including the nose and forehead. Each area has two to six subcategories indicating the kinds of behaviors for which to look. An older, but useful, list of stuttering behaviors is found in Darley and Spriestersbach's (1978) Checklist of Stuttering Behaviors. It contains 26 behaviors, from repetitions to dilating nostrils, gasping for air, head movements, and so on; it also has blanks for added behaviors. Peters and Guitar (1991) reproduce Woolf's (1967) Perception of Stuttering Inventory. (I list both sources because Woolf's original publication is in a foreign journal and may not be easily accessible for some.) The inventory has 60 behavior categories, where about 15 items are behavioral or personal avoidances, about 20 concern actual struggle with stuttering spasms, and 19 items involve anti-expectancy behaviors. I disagreed with Woolf's categorizations for the remaining five or six items. Also, Ham (1986) presents a 27-item list of behaviors, with blanks for additions. The list starts with repetitions-prolongations and moves through the various avoidance, struggle, and overflow behaviors.

TESTS, FORMS, AND PROCEDURES IN EVALUATION

The following discussion covers a variety of areas, and "hops around" somewhat. Essentially, the section is intended to supply the "how to" or "what is" information areas for evaluating fluency disorders. In many instances the examiner is required either to identify or label behaviors or to evaluate aspects of these behaviors. Over the years I have found that identifying or labeling of behaviors serves us fairly well, but our adequacy in more complex or subtle areas of judgment is questionable. For instance, Kent (1996) reviewed perceptual assessments of speech and voice disorders and found that general agreement among judges and observers is extremely poor. Very specific data (occurrence of repetitions, prolongations, and so on) may be reported with greater accuracy. However, more subjective or subtle aspects of speech judgments do not show high interjudge correlations. Thus, it often seems to come to a variation of the old saw, rephrased here, "I may not know what stuttering is; but I know it when I hear it!" I hope so.

Dysfluency Categories

Dysfluencies previously were categorized by the form of the spasm. That description is expanded here. Spasms also can be described more specifically, as follows:

PR = phrase repetition
WWR = whole-word repetition
PWR = part-word repetition
P = prolongation
S = stoppage

The easiest way to track these behaviors is to have the client read (if able) aloud and then speak on a chosen topic (describing a picture, telling a story, etc.). The preceding categories will be set out for counting and evaluation in the discussion of spasm frequency.

Associated Behaviors—Word Specific

These behaviors were detailed previously. They will be used again within the discussion of spasm severity. At present, I will provide an outline in Exhibit 1–1 for identifying word-specific avoidances. The evaluator should have the client read aloud and provide a spontaneous speech sample until a level of at least 100 words in each category (some prefer as high as 300 words) is attained. The easiest way to track these behaviors is to record the productions and play back the tape to count or evaluate. The number of stuttering spasms is counted and, on each spasm, a determination is made whether any avoidances occurred and, if they occurred, what they were. These data will be used again in severity measurement.

Establishing a baseline for specific avoidances is useful in fluency therapy (if the therapy is effective, the avoidances will disappear or be significantly reduced) and of greater importance in symptom therapy where avoidances often are under direct attack. The data compiled in Exhibit 1–1 should be subjectively reviewed, asking the following three questions:

1. How effective are the behaviors relative to stuttering?
2. How aware does the client seem to be of the behaviors?
3. What relationship, if any, does there seem to be between intensity of struggle, duration of spasm, and the number of avoidances or the number of times the same avoidance is used?

Associated Behaviors—Communication General

This behavior cannot be accurately assessed until the evaluator has worked with a client for some weeks. However, the "What do you do when . . .?" questions are covered in a later discussion of the tests and forms.

Exhibit 1–1 Avoidance behaviors

Total Words Uttered _____   Total Stuttered Words _____

Avoidance Behavior	*Not Observed*	*Rare*	*Occasional*	*Frequent*	*Very Frequent*
Postponement					
Starter					
Retrial					
Revision					
Substitution					
Circumlocution					
Mutism (gave up)					
Release					
Poor Eye Contact					
Preparatory Set Distorted					
Respiratory Anomaly					

Of the total spasms, how many had avoidances totaling ___0 ___1 ___2 ___3 ___ 4 or more?

Generally, I save those for management home assignments and use a briefer form, such as the one in Exhibit 1–2. The client is asked to read each item and quickly respond (avoid "It depends . . ." judgments, and move to the next item). The information provides insight as to whether the person is so generally avoidant that therapy transfer will be difficult, whether counseling is indicated, whether fluency therapy would be an easier approach, or whether symptom therapy avoidance reduction might be valuable.

562

Exhibit 1–2 Avoidances in use in general speech

For each general behavior below, mark 1, 2, or 3 (1 = never, 2 = occasionally, and 3 = often). For each item, the question is, "Do you talk this way to avoid ALL stuttering, not just stuttering on a specific word?"

Behavior	With Family	With Friends	With Strangers
	1 2 3	1 2 3	1 2 3
Change my rate of speech			
Change how loudly I talk			
Change the pitch of my voice			
Talk in a monotone			
Change my eye contact			
Talk with fake accent, dialect			
Make special physical movements			
Breathe differently			
Have a special attitude, behavior			

Attitude Measures

Attitudes toward speaking and stuttering are important, possibly as important as the frequency, severity, and other aspects of the stuttering spasms themselves. Most of the attitude measures are presented later, in the section titled "Tests and Forms." However, a few general points can be made. Exhibit 1–3 presents 10 questions for the clinician. Depending on location, the client's age, and other factors, questions can be added or dropped. Each question is phrased so that a "yes" answer suggests a poor attitude toward speech or stuttering. The contributions to management decisions are obvious.

Fear Hierarchy

Development of a fear hierarchy is covered in detail in several different chapters. Also, the factors involved in the gradations between or within a fear hierarchy are suggested in some of the checklists and inventories summarized in the section "Tests and Forms." Basically, a fear hierarchy identifies the communication situations a particular client meets (or should

---

Exhibit 1–3 Attitude considerations

> After adequate observation of the client, attempt to answer the following questions:
>
> - Does the client seem to avoid calling himself or herself a "stutterer"?
> - If there has been prior therapy that failed, or succeeded but relapsed, does the client blame the therapy or herself or himself?
> - Considering age, sex, and socioeconomic status, does the client appear to lack appropriate contacts with friends, coworkers, interest groups, social or civic groups, and so forth?
> - Does the client have a large number of different avoidance behaviors?
> - Does the client typically use more than one kind of avoidance behavior per spasm?
> - Does the client seem to project an overtly noncommittal, hostile, uncaring, or subservient attitude about his or her stuttering?
> - Is the client's overall stuttering spasm pattern "wide open and overt" or "hidden and covert"?
> - Does the client generally fail to maintain good eye contact, just fail to maintain good eye contact when stuttering, or possess good eye contact even when stuttering?
> - Does the stutterer express or imply that outside pressure brought him or her to you, or is the referral self-generated?
> - Does the client seem to be overly concerned with "making a good impression," steering away from unpleasant topics?

meet). The situations are then rank ordered in terms of the amount of stress (or stuttering) they seem to cause. In Exhibit 1–4 (for early evaluation purposes only), a few questions are asked. The responses can provide useful direction for later, more detailed investigations.

Exhibit 1–4 Preliminary fear hierarchy

For each communication category or communication situation below, rate the probable amount of stuttering you think you might experience.

Situation	Little Trouble	Average Trouble	Above Average	Much Trouble	Try to Avoid
Telephone, family					
Telephone, friends					
Telephone, business					
Telephone, strangers					
Talking with family					
Talking with friends					
Talking with coworkers					
Talking with strangers					
Making a speech to					
A known group					
A business group					
A group of strangers					

Spasm Frequency

Counting spasms is one of the most common forms of baseline measures, and it is dear to the hearts of fluency therapists. Sometimes, frequency determines acceptance for therapy. Often, especially in fluency programs, it determines (or is) the dismissal criterion. Generally, it is expressed in one or more of the following forms:

sw/m	stuttered words per minute
ss/m	stuttered syllables per minute
%sw	percent stuttered words
%ss	percent stuttered syllables

In order to calculate the above values, two (or three) measures are needed: total talking time (TTT; T3), the total number of words uttered (TWU), or the total number of syllables uttered (TSU). The total stuttered words (TSW) and the total stuttered syllables (TSS) also must be counted.

$$\text{sw/m} = \frac{\text{TSW}}{\text{T3}} = \_\_\_\_ \times 60 = \text{sw/m}$$

$$\text{ss/m} = \frac{\text{TSS}}{\text{T3}} = \_\_\_\_ \times 60 = \text{ss/m}$$

$$\text{\%sw} = \frac{\text{TWS}}{\text{TWU}} = \_\_\_\_ \times 100 = \text{\%sw}$$

$$\text{\%ss} = \frac{\text{TSS}}{\text{TSU}} = \_\_\_\_ \times 100 = \text{\%ss}$$

It is preferable to test the client in reading aloud, as well as in spontaneous speech. The figures will probably differ between the two modes because the rate for reading and talking usually differ. Also, some stutterers feel that reading is better because they can break eye contact with the auditor, reduce or alter their prosody, do not have to worry about word selection, and can look ahead to see what is coming. Of course, some persons have more trouble with reading because they lose auditor support, cannot select words, cannot substitute or circumlocute, and can look ahead and see danger coming.

In Exhibit 1–5, at least 100 words (if possible) of free speech should be collected. The evaluator should record them for playback. On playback, T3 is measured and converted to seconds. Each stuttering spasm is counted only once.

Exhibit 1–5 Talking time, words uttered, and words stuttered

Have the client read aloud for at least 100 words (300 preferable); have the client speak with you until you can be sure of at least 100 countable words (300 preferable). Record and analyze.

Measure	*Reading*	*Talking*
Total talking time (TTT, T3), in seconds	____	____
Total words uttered (TWU)	____	____
Total stuttered words (TSW)	____	____
Total syllables uttered (TSU)	____	____
Total stuttered syllables (TSS)	____	____
Total spasm time (TST)	____	____
Fluent speaking time (T3 – TST = fluent speaking time)	____	____

Other measures

Words per minute (wpm) $\dfrac{TWU}{T3}$ = ____ × 60 = wpm

Syllables per minute (spm) $\dfrac{TSU}{T3}$ = ____ × 60 = spm

Percent stuttered words (%sw) $\dfrac{TSW}{TWU}$ = ____ × 100 = %sw

Percent stuttered syllables (%ss) $\dfrac{TSS}{TSU}$ = ____ × 100 = %ss

> My name is Ri-ri-ri. . . .
> My name is Ri-ri, it's Rrrrr, my name is Ri. . . .

The first example is obviously one spasm. So is the second example. It does not matter how many times the speaker tries the same word (same location)—it is all one spasm.

> What is your name?
> It's Riiiii, uh Ri-ri. It's Richard.
> I'm sorry, I didn't catch that. What did you say?
> It's Rrrrrrrichard!

This example presents two stuttering spasms, because the last spasm on "Richard" is a new response to a different stimulus. Also, in counting words, the words that are repeated in the stuttering spasm, or are part of a revision attempt, are not counted. It is easy to spot in reading. If a prewritten sentence should be "I have never been able to find a rainbow," but it comes out "Iiii, well I have ne-ne-ne I've neeee, never b-b-b-b- I've never been able to fiii, that is to find a raaaa, a raaaa, a rainbow," both sentences have the same TWU score, and a 5 TSW score. This result is achieved because all the repeated or extra words are directly associated with stuttering spasms.

These somewhat confusing rules are necessary in order to have stable and accurate counts to use in calculating frequency and severity scores. The evaluator also will calculate overall speaking rate based on words per minute (wpm) or syllables per minute (spm). These measures are calculated with the word count exclusions previously cited. A third rate that may be calculated is wpm or spm *exclusive of spasm time*. It may be done scientifically or approximately by listening to the tape and adding together the various spasm times and subtracting that amount from T3. This figure can significantly alter rate and frequency measures (also makes a very good baseline measure). Very often, stutterers appear to have a slow overall speaking rate (T3) but, when the spasm time is eliminated, the person actually is talking faster than many fluent speakers.

One of the truisms of stuttering is that stuttering increases as language complexity increases. In working with children, language assessment should be a standard part of the evaluation, with methods such as the Stocker Probe (Stocker, 1980) applied. Apparently, the language effect is not completely stable, as Silverman and Ratner (1997) failed to find this distinction in a group of seven stutterers, ages 10 to 18 years. As language complexity was increased, accuracy of text repeating decreased and *dis*fluencies increased, but there was no significant correlation between complexity and *dys*fluencies. However, in a cautionary note, Martin, Parlour, and Haroldson (1990) suggested that if the dysfluency count was expressed in %sw instead of yes/no on dysfluencies, the strength of the relationship is reduced. I would like to see the study repeated on children ages 4 to 10 years, rather than 10 to 18. Wilkenfeld and Curlee (1997) did note that the length of a child's response was significantly related to stuttering occurrence (preschool males). They were testing to see if there was a stuttering difference in response to questions, to requests, and to comments. They found no consistent relationship. In a different direction, Howell and Au-Yeung (1995) reported that they could find no relationship between children's stuttering and phonological category of the stuttered words. This finding was true across the age group (2 to 12 years), the stuttering severity, or the word types.

Spasm Severity

Severity relates to frequency; the more stuttering events there are, the greater the perception of severity. However, simple occurrence does not seem to be as significant as what the speaker actually does when he or she is stuttering. Struggle seems to be very important. Armson and colleagues (1997) had 29 judges evaluate 10 preschool children. Some evaluated only in terms of yes/no for stuttering on words, and other judges rated the perceived degree of struggle on each stuttering. They found that high agreements on yes/no correlated significantly with the judgments of perceived struggle. Severity evaluation is included in the items listed in a later section titled "Tests and Forms." Severity, since the Iowa severity scale days (Sherman, 1952), has been evaluated on a number of factors, including

> **Frequency**—the higher the %sw, the greater the severity
> **Spasm duration**—longer durations equal higher severity
> **Visible struggle**—severity increases as direct struggles increase
> **Overflow**—severity perception increases as spasms overflow into the body

In addition, some severity forms include an average measure of the longest stuttering spasm. They also may include a count of how many spasms were accompanied by observable avoidance behaviors. In Riley's (1972) stuttering severity instrument (SSI), only spasm frequency, longest spasm duration average, and overflow concomitants are used. The tool also provides a weighted, standardized scoring system. Other scales (not really tests) use a 5-, 7-, or 9-point rating scale to equate with certain criterion levels. The adequacy of judgments by listeners has been mentioned earlier and has been strongly criticized over the years. However, to a degree, some of this criticism should face the question, "When does a difference make a difference?" Statistical significance must be balanced by functional utility.

Martin, Haroldson, and Woessner (1988) evaluated perceptual scaling of stuttering severity, using a 7-point scale (least severe = 1) and found that observers could reliably judge severity of stuttering on either a moment-by-moment basis, or during spontaneous speech accumulation. Their research also suggested that when comparing the severity judgments of two speech-language pathologists (SLPs), both should use (and be comfortable with) the same scale.

Martin, Haroldson, and Woessner (1988) also examined counted frequency of stutters and judgments of severity and found them to be related. However, it is a complex relationship and the SLP should not dispense with one or the other. If the intervention mode is fluency reinforcement and the target is the near-mythical zero stuttering point, then diagnostic frequency counts are best for a baseline criterion. On the other hand, if symptom modification is preferred, the judged severity of spasms may be a better pretherapy baseline. I have difficulty with the separation just expressed. Because most fluency programs leave a residual dysfluency (or some semirelapse occurs), then I would like to know that any stuttering "hanging around" is less severe than before therapy started. By the same token, in symptom therapy, I expect the frequency of spasm to go down as the client learns to control and reduce the severity of any particular spasm.

The severity scale I developed for my own use is offered in Exhibit 1–6. I have found it to be both useful for evaluation, as well as productive for therapy baselines and management planning. In Exhibit 1–6, the formula for %sw was provided in the previous discussion. I have split struggle-overflow into two categories, proximal and distal, because the latter usually responds much more quickly to reduction or elimination efforts in therapy. The category of average spasm duration can be calculated spasm by spasm, or approximated. The longest spasm duration can be set by timing the three longest durations, adding their values, and dividing by 3. Actually, I am flexible here. Some clients may have many durations that are quite similar. Some may average 2 or 3 seconds on almost everything, but have one spasm that runs 8 to 10 seconds. In that case I use the one, longer time, because averaging three spasms would give me a figure of 4 to 5 seconds, obscuring the fact that the client could have a much higher duration. On the avoidance category, I use a yes/no system (i.e., Was there or was there not an avoidance?). The number or forms of avoidances per spasm create more data than I can score reliably early in diagnosis. The process provides good baseline data. For therapy use I also will draw lines to connect the data points, so both the client and I can see changes as therapy progresses.

Exhibit 1–6 Severity evaluation of stuttering

Fill in the "o" under the appropriate rating scale number. See severity ratings below.

	Rating		Rating	
Measure	*1 2 3 4 5*		*1 2 3 4 5*	
Percent stuttered words	o o o o o		o o o o o	
Struggle/overflow: Proximal	o o o o o		o o o o o	
Struggle/overflow: Distal	o o o o o		o o o o o	
Average spasm duration	o o o o o		o o o o o	
Longest spasm duration	o o o o o		o o o o o	
Avoidance presence	o o o o o		o o o o o	

Severity score equals the sum of all the ratings above, divided by 6, or by the number of items rated.

%sw rating: 1 = less than 2%; 2 = 2%–5%; 3 = 5.1%–10%; 4 = 10.1%–20%; 5 = over 20%

Proximal struggle (face, head, neck, shoulders): 1 = little or none; 2 = just noticeable; 3 = obvious; 4 = distracting; 5 = extreme, gross

Distal struggle (body, hands, limbs): 1–5 categories, same as for proximal struggle

Average spasm duration: 1 = about 1 second or less; 2 = 1–2 seconds; 3 = 3–5 seconds; 4 = 6–10 seconds; 5 = over 10 seconds

Longest spasm: 1 = 1 second or less; 2 = 1–5 seconds; 3 = 6–10 seconds; 4 = 11–20 seconds; 5 = over 20 seconds

Avoidance presence: 1 = few or none; 2 = up to 20% of spasms; 3 = 21%–40%; 4 = 41%–60%; 5 = over 60% of spasms

Adaptation

Adaptation is a measure of the recurrence of unreinforced behavior. If a stutterer is not penalized for stuttering during a first rendition, spasms tend to reduce in subsequent readings (same situation, same material, same time period). This consecutive reduction in stuttering spasms is called adaptation. It has been a topic of interest in fluency disorders for over 50 years. Shipley and McAfee (1998) state that some SLPs "still" measure adaptation (and consistency). If this statement is true, I regret the reduction in interest for reasons that will become clear.

The standard measurement method for adaptation is to have a client read aloud the same passage five consecutive times, in serial order. First, the clinician ensures that the client is familiar with all words in the passage and then follows on his or her own copy as the client reads aloud. On the first reading a "1" is written over each stuttered word. On the second reading a "2" is placed over each stuttering, and so on through readings 3, 4, and 5. The terms used in adaptation measures are the familiar TSW, plus Rx (the earlier reading of the five consecutive readings) and Ry (the later reading of the five consecutive readings). Note that Rx simply occurred before the later reading. If the second reading (Ry) was the fifth one (R5), then Rx could be the first, second, third, or fourth reading (R1, R2, R3, R4). If Ry was actually R2, then Rx would have to be R1. To measure adaptation between readings there are many precise, lengthy formulas. I have found the one that follows to be useful:

$$\frac{(\text{TSW in Rx}) - (\text{TSW in Ry})}{\text{TSW in Rx}} = \underline{\hspace{1cm}} \times 100 = \text{adaptation \% for RxRy}$$

For example, a client's five readings yielded stuttering spasms per reading of 27, 17, 15, 12, and 8, respectively. In order to measure adaptation from the first reading (R1) to the second reading (R2), the calculation would be:

$$\frac{(\text{TSW for R1}) - (\text{TSW for R2})}{\text{TSW in R1}} = \frac{27 - 17}{27} = \frac{10}{27} = 0.37 \times 100 = 37\% \text{ for R1–R2}$$

A measure of adaptation across all five readings (R1–R5) would be:

$$\frac{(\text{TSW for R1}) - (\text{TSW for R5})}{\text{TSW in R1}} = \frac{27 - 8}{27} = \frac{19}{27} = 0.70 \times 100 = 70\% \text{ for R1–R5}$$

In general, the largest reduction between two adjacent readings usually occurs between R1 and R2. Two factors may be responsible: acquired familiarity with the repeated material and diminished anxiety. There are several possible interpretations of adaptation scores, which are generally untested and unverified. These interpretations, or assumptions, include:

- An extreme R1 to R5 reduction, or even extinction (zero), may indicate a "suggestible" stutterer who will show rapid initial progress in therapy, will not be a good candidate for symptom therapy, and will be a high-risk relapse client unless transfer and maintenance are planned and executed carefully.

- A client who extinguishes (zeroes out) by R3 may be so mild a stutterer as to make therapy questionable, or the client may later exhibit the "flight to fluency" supposedly to escape the negative pressures of the situation.

- A very slowly falling curve from R1 to R5 (low adaptation) may suggest candidacy for symptom modification therapy.

- Almost no adaptation from R1 to R5 might suggest a basic neurogenic dysfluency problem where tension and anxiety are of less significance than a flawed neuromotor timing and coordination capacity.

- A rising curve in which successive readings show an increase in dysfluencies from R1 to R5 may suggest one of two problems. First, stuttering for this person has such an emotional basis that the "failures" in each reading progressively increase the anxiety and tension and, hence, the stuttering. This finding may indicate a need for early and vigorous desensitization, or even for outside counseling prior to speech management. Second, *cluttering*, not stuttering, may be the problem. Presumably R1 was most fluent due to closer attention to new material, and subsequent Rs kept slipping as less and less attention was paid each time.

I wish to emphasize that these five interpretations have always been speculative, but they are interesting.

There are other ways to measure adaptation. Some of them are "unscientific," but still can be useful in management. These measures are as follows:

- Have the stutterer monologue for about 3 minutes, which will generate six 30-second speech intervals. Record the effort and play back, counting the spasms in each 30-second interval. In place of R1, the first reading, use I1, the first 30-second unit. Adaptation can be calculated across I1, I2, and so on through I6. One also could use 15-second intervals and pull 15 consecutive seconds out of each 30 seconds, or other combinations.

- Over the first five management sessions, arrange for the client to start each session with a 1-minute monologue on a set topic. Record each monologue and count the total stutterings in each 60 seconds. Use the five sessions to measure situation adaptation.
- Prewrite a telephone call to a place of business (e.g., a grocery store) with at least 30 or 40 words in it. Have the client call five different grocery stores, recording his or her side of each call. Count the spasms in each of the five calls for a different measure of situation adaptation.

Adaptation can also be measured in terms of spasm durations (whether they get shorter over time or with repeats). Spasms and avoidances also could be counted and combined to see if, over repeats, the number of avoidances per spasm and/or the overall percentage of avoidances drops. Overall, adaptation is not an earth-shaking measure in either assessment or management. However, it is easy to do, quick to calculate, and a helpful "add on" to material collected in frequency and severity analyses.

Consistency

As indicated earlier, Shipley and McAfee (1998) contend the measurement of consistency is not common. I think this finding is more regrettable than any slippage from adaptation. There are several formulas available for consistency. Probably the best one, with the most reliable expression of consistency, is the formula described by Wingate (1984). It requires some care to use, but it is very useful. In more general terms, consistency can be calculated fairly simply using the following formula:

$$\frac{\text{Ry stuttered words also stuttered in Rx}}{\text{TSW in Rx}} = \underline{\quad} \times 100 = \% \text{ consistency}$$

To apply this formula, I would use a reading passage and have the client read it aloud five times, marking each stuttering as described for adaptation. An example is provided below:

12345 2	135	1234	12	45	12345	1		1234
There is	no truth	to the rumor	that	I am	selling	my		business
3	1235	1	12345	15		12345		
and will	leave	town.	I think	my enemies	are after	me.		

Consistency is usually measured between the first reading (R1) and the last reading (R5), but comparisons can be done between R1 and R2, and so on. On the five readings, the TSW totals were R1 = 12, R2 = 9, R3 = 9, R4 = 7, and R5 = 8. The raw consistency scores were:

Readings Compared	Number of Same-Word Stutters
R1/R5	7
R1/R4	6
R1/R3	8
R1/R2	8
R4/R5	5

As is evident, the apparent similarity in scores is misleading, and the Wingate formula would compensate for this problem. In the simpler form, consistency would be calculated:

$$\frac{\text{R5 stutterers that occurred on same words in R1}}{\text{TSW in R1}} = \frac{7}{12} = 0.58 \times 100 = 58\%$$

Consistency measures can be of value. Clients who are well below 50% in consistency may be served better by fluency reinforcement programs, as opposed to symptom modification approaches. Because the latter approach targets specific moments of stuttering, lower consistency scores portend greater difficulty in predicting when symptom controls will be needed. Low consistency scores can call for therapy attention to self-monitoring improvement to try and compensate for stuttering locus variability.

Respiration and Phonation

Respiratory evaluation of stutterers is not a topic that many diagnosticians pursue because the old idea that stuttering was caused by, or exacerbated by, improper breathing habits is no longer accepted as a blanket theory or fact. Most stutterers appear to present respiratory anomalies in speech associated with the actual moment of stuttering, but usually present few or no anomalies associated with their periods of fluent speech or vegetative breathing. However, respiratory anomalies can (and do) occur among some stutterers in the areas of vegetative breathing, fluent speech, and stuttered speech. For that reason, basic information about respiration, including some basic measures and observations is presented.

A number of anomalies can occur prior to and during stuttering spasms. One can argue that the philosophy of classical fluency reinforcement therapy negates the need to pay attention to dysfluency-related respiratory anomalies because therapy will remove the cause of the anomalies, stuttering spasms. As pointed out previously, this targeted 100% correction rarely occurs, and if there is some danger of relapse (there usually is, except for very young children), then there is a problem if there are anomalies of any type associated with stuttering. This does not mean that a fluency program must stop or delay while a sidetrack program on respiration is implemented. Indeed, many fluency programs operate on the primary basis of shaping and shifting the breathstream management of the speaker.

In preparing to evaluate respiration, there are a few normative terms that require definition. Extended information can be found in *Speech and Hearing Science, Anatomy and Physiology* (Zemlin, 1998).

> **Vital capacity**—the maximum amount of air, following a maximum exhalation, that can be inhaled.
> **Tidal air**—the amount of air inhaled and exhaled during a normal breathing cycle (no maximum efforts).
> **Inspiratory reserve**—the additional amount of air that can be inhaled after the end of a normal inhalation.
> **Expiratory reserve**—the additional amount of air that can be exhaled after the end of a normal exhalation.

There are many ways of evaluating respiration for speech. Soft speech, loud speech, male/female and age factors, and so forth, all contribute to normal variations.

Measurement Devices and Procedures

Respiration evaluation can be complex, time consuming, and expensive. Spirometers (wet and dry); manometric pressure devices; airflow analyzers; pneumotachometers, pneumographs, and electromyographs can be used to measure respiration (Boone & McFarlane, 1988). However, in most instances single measures and accurate observation will suffice. Of course, accurate observations include the detection of respiratory anomalies that may require some of the sophisticated evaluation systems just listed.

Basic Testing and Observation Procedures

Each client must be evaluated as an individual, and the bottom line will be determined by what the client sounds like in terms of respiratory support. When the client speaks with no observable stuttering, do you hear or see

- Excessive breathiness on (fluent) utterances?
- Inappropriately frequent inhalations?
- Too loud or too soft voice (both waste air)?
- Noticeable air release just prior to speaking?
- Too frequent or too hard glottal attacks?
- Strained, breathless quality?

The clinician should watch body movements during respiration to determine the predominant respiratory pattern. The results can be recorded in Exhibit 1–7.

> **Thoracic**—expansion of the central thoracic area. It is the most common respiratory pattern.
> **Diaphragmatic-abdominal**—expansion of the lower thorax and upper abdominal areas. It is the most efficient method if heavy demands are made on the respiratory system.

In reading and monologue, determine whether the client is able to:

- Display a slow, quiet inhalation?
- Exhibit an easy, fairly quiet exhalation?
- Demonstrate the ability to maintain a quiet, sustained "aaah" for at least 10 seconds?
- Show the ability to count quietly out loud from 1 to 10 on one breath?

Exhibit 1–7 Respiratory predominance

Without calling attention to the observation, watch the client's breating multiple times. When confident with observations on vegetative breathing, complete the information below.

Clavicular breathing	___absent	___occasional	___extreme
Breathing posture	___adequate	___poor	___pathological
Vocal stridor	___absent	___minimal	___obvious
Cycle depth	___adequate	___low	___high
Cycle frequency	___adequate	___low	___high

Comments about observations:

Changes (if any) that occur during speech:

Additional questions concerning general respiration and speech respiration are presented in Exhibit 1–8.

Measurement of the s/z Ratio

A student once told me, "If the s/z ratio wasn't there, somebody would have had to invent it." The s/z ratio is a measure of the maximum duration of production of the phonemes /s/ and /z/ by the client. Voiced fricatives typically use less air than voiceless fricatives; because more air is needed to create an audible sound for the voiceless productions, it is useful to establish and interpret the voiceless/voiced production time ratio in diagnostic evaluation. Control and release of air can be evaluated by the reliable s/z ratio, so long as it is used appropriately. This procedure must be modeled (start to finish) several times by the clinician, and efforts produced with inadequate attention to directions should be rejected and not used in calculating s/z scores. With younger children, it may take 10 to 15 tries, with rest breaks to avoid hyperventilation. The clinician should always watch for hyperventilation, at all ages. With the client standing erect (not "braced") and relaxed, the clinician gives the following instructions:

Exhibit 1–8 Overall respiratory function: Observations of speech breathing

Depth of cycles
  Fluent speech   ___adequate ___shallow   ___deep, prolonged
  Dysfluent speech   ___adequate ___shallow   ___deep, prolonged
Frequency of cycles
  Fluent speech   ___adequate ___too frequent ___too few
  Dysfluent speech   ___adequate ___too frequent ___too few
Exhalation interrupted by inhalation
  Fluent speech   ___none   ___occasional   ___frequent
  Dysfluent speech   ___none   ___occasional   ___frequent
Spasms started or interrupted by inhalation
  Fluent speech   ___none   ___occasional   ___frequent
  Dysfluent speech   ___none   ___occasional   ___frequent
Spasm started (too heavily) or interrupted by exhalation
  Fluent speech   ___none   ___occasional   ___frequent
  Dysfluent speech   ___none   ___occasional   ___frequent
Utterances generally breathy, wasting air
  Fluent speech   ___none   ___occasional   ___frequent
  Dysfluent speech   ___none   ___occasional   ___frequent

Are there particular phonemes or syllables that seem to be associated with any respiratory anomalies? ___no ___yes Describe:_____

Result of Hixson "5 × 5" respiratory force test
  ___adequate (5 seconds @ 5 cm) ___inadequate Explain:_____

I want you to take as deep a breath as possible, and hold it until I signal, like this. [Model a very strong "vital capacity" inhalation, obviously hold it, then signal with your hand, and let the air out.] Notice, I did not just let it come out fast; I let it out slowly. What I want you to do is let it out while you produce a very gentle /s/. You must try and produce the /sssss/ as long as you can, until you have absolutely no air left. Like this. [Model another maximum inhalation, a hand signal, and then a properly prolonged /s/.] Okay, now you try it.

It may work the first time, or inhalation may be too shallow, release to breathy, and so on. The procedure should be repeated as needed until the client produces three /sss/ productions that are acceptable. Each effort is timed (in seconds) from moment of first release to final "collapse." The three times are recorded, with the longest one circled. The clinician then says to the client:

> That was excellent. Now I want to do it all over again, almost exactly as before, with only one change. Instead of releasing the air with a quiet /sssss/, I want you to let the air out with a quiet /z/, like this. [Model and produce a /zzzzz/.] Ready?

Exhibit 1–9 provides a structure to record the /s/ and /z/ productions and calculate the ratio.

The clinician secures and times three acceptable productions, as with /s/. All three times are recorded and the longest one is circled. Typically, the /z/ measures will be longer than the /s/ measures. Overall duration times will be around 10 seconds for young children, whereas adult measures will be about 20 to 25 seconds. Now the s/z ratio is calculated by taking the longest /z/ time and dividing it into the longest /s/ time. In general, the resulting (normal) ratio will be at or a little less than 1.0. Two possible concerns are:

1. Is the /s/ or the /z/ time duration below 10 seconds for children, or below 15 to 20 seconds for adults?

Exhibit 1–9 Respiratory applications

1. Able to sustain a clear, gentle vowel production for _____ seconds
2. Can produce 10 clear, separate /ah-ah-ah/ series in one breath
   ___Yes ___No
3. s/z ratio evaluation

/s/ Trial No.	Seconds Duration	/z/ Trial No.	Seconds Duration
1	_____	1	_____
2	_____	2	_____
3	_____	3	_____

4. Longest /s/ divided by longest /z/ equals: $\dfrac{s}{z} =$ _____

5. Recommendations: ___No ___Yes   Explain: _____

2. Is the s/z ratio approximately 1.2 or higher? If so, after rest, the entire measure should be repeated with instructions emphasized and several models given. If similar results are obtained, attention should be directed toward more thorough analysis of respiration capacity and use.

Measurement of Air Pressure

A simple measure of air pressure availability can be used when a stutterer appears to speak with an abnormal lack of force or air supply. This simple measure was described by Hixson, Hawley, and Wilson (1982). The equipment needs include a straight-sided, smooth, clear water glass that will hold at least 12 cm of liquid; white tape to put on the glass (one vertical strip, from top to bottom); a centimeter ruler; a marking pen; a flexible plastic straw; and a large-size (1¾") paper clip. The clinician marks the glass into centimeter divisions, inserts the straw (held in place by paper clip), and has the client "blow bubbles" against the water pressure.

Measurement of Laryngeal Tension

Although fluent speech is the area being addressed, it may be informative to make observations during moments when the client is stuttering and compare them to those during fluent speech. The procedure is as follows:

- Have the client phonate, read aloud, or talk freely. Observe for unusual elevation of the shoulders, and atypical rigidity of the head and neck.
- Listen for audible evidence of laryngeal tension, as indicated by loudness and possible glottal shocks.
- Look for visible evidence of tension. Where the sternocleidomastoid muscle originates near the manubrium sterni and nearby clavicle, an upside-down V is formed with sucked-in soft tissue inside the V. In excess tension the sucking effect is very pronounced. Remember that vocal attacks may be breathy (air release before vocal folds approximate), glottal (hard vocal fold closure before any air release), or simultaneous (air release and vocal fold closure occur together).
- Have the client stand normally and phonate a prolonged /i/ vowel and place the flat of your palm firmly against the upper abdomen, just above the navel. Normally during /i/ production, a "pulsing" will be

felt against your hand as the /i/ is sustained. The lower the degree of pulsing felt (or absence of), the greater the amount of tension there will be in vocal fold function (Boone & McFarlane, 1988).

Articulator Coordination

Diadochokinesis

In the history of stuttering, the articulators have been targeted for props, cushions, pads, cutting, burning with hot irons, and so on. Various studies have suggested that at least some stutterers lack oromotor coordination skills. Howell, Sackin, and Rustin (1995) evaluated stutterers aged 7 to 12 years (compared with fluent controls). They reported that the stutterers had longer voiced onsets in plosive production, were less effective in lower lip movements in a tracking task, and had larger minimal movements of the articulators when these movements were made without the support of visual feedback. Of course, by even the lower end of their age range, it is possible to suggest that these behaviors result from stuttering and not vice versa. This finding reinforces the idea that certain young fluency problems may need speech-motor coordination improvement before any attention is paid directly to dysfluent utterances. Riley and Riley (1983) found some "stuttering children" could be dismissed from therapy once oromotor training brought them to adequacy levels (i.e., there was no need for direct work on stuttering). Today, oromotor variation among adult stutterers usually is not evaluated, but a basic check on diadochokinetic and rhythmokinetic patterns is advised. The younger the client, the more advisable the review becomes.

In this context (fluency) articulation coordination is limited to consideration of diadochokinetic and rhythmokinetic patterns in a limited sampling process. Diadochokinesis is measured at labial, lingua-alveolar, and lingua-velar contact points, using the consonant-vowel (CV) pairs /puh/, /tuh/, and /kuh/. Five-second samples of each are recommended. Fletcher (1972) established that children 6 to 9 years of age could produce about 20 single syllables in less than 5 seconds (about 3.5 to 5.0 seconds). Riley and Riley (1983) stated that children 4 to 5 years of age could produce 20 syllables during 5 seconds. In production of the trisyllabic /puhtuhkuh/, Fletcher indicated that about five productions sets in 5 seconds would be typical for children around 6 years of age. Children 12 to 13 years of age could produce approximately nine trisyllable sets in 5 seconds. Riley and Riley reported that their 5-year-old subjects averaged a little less than five trisyllables in 5 seconds, and they felt 4-year-olds were not up to this complex task. Exhibit 1–10 is intended for use in evaluation of articulator coordination, including measurement of diadochokinesis.

To test diadochokinesis, the clinician slowly models production of the /puh/, /tuh/, and /kuh/ CV pairs. Then he or she models the rapid production of one, /puh/, for 5 seconds. Next, the client is instructed as follows:

> I want you to say puh-puh-puh, as fast as you can until I say "stop." Like this. [Model again.] Take a deep breath, hold it, and then start as fast as you can when I signal, and go until I say "stop."

Several practice efforts may be necessary for the person to find a comfortable speed and settle down to it. The client repeats the process for the other two CV pairs. Then the client tries /puhtuhkuh/ for 5 seconds. I skip two CV pairs over the age of 6 years and use them in place of the triad below the age of 6 years. When testing children, "pattycake" can be used in place of /puhtuhkuh/.

Rhythmokinesis

Rhythmokinesis involves uttering a CV pair while producing a modeled rhythm pattern. Inflection patterns such as "How *are* you?" and "Shave and a haircut, two bits!" can be used. In fact, any rhythm and any CV pair can be used. Refrains from popular songs, television jingles, theme music, and so on are possible examples. Several efforts may be needed because motor ability, not perceptual skills, is being tested. I do not score rhythmokinesis, but describe the client's capacity to generate a rhythmic pattern.

PREDICTION

Overview

The consistency measures discussed earlier in this chapter may be sufficient predictors at an early stage. Nevertheless, prediction of stutter-

Exhibit 1–10 Articulator coordination

Articulator movements (speed, accuracy, range of motion, etc.) ____
could not understand directions

Lingual
  protusion   __ poor __ variable __ adequate, slow __adequate
  Side-to-side   __ poor __ variable __ adequate, slow __adequate
  Resistance   __ good __ variable __ one side weak   __weak bilaterally
Facial
  movements __ good __ variable __ one side weak   __weak bilaterally
Jaw
  movements __ good __ variable __ one side weak   __weak bilaterally
Palatal
  movements __ good __ variable __ one side weak   __weak bilaterally

Diadochokinetic rate (per 5 seconds). Check all characteristics that apply.

Syllables	Number Produced	Slow, Labored	Weak	Irregular	Errors
/puh/	_____	__	__	__	__
/tuh/	_____	__	__	__	__
/kuh/	_____	__	__	__	__
/puhtuh/	_____	__	__	__	__
/puhtuhkuh/	_____	__	__	__	__

Rhythmokinesis (following a rhythm pattern)

___ adequate ___ lacking ___slow, labored ___ jerky, irregular

Perception of touch on various areas (client's eyes closed)

Facial
  areas __ good __ right side poor __ left side poor __ poor bilaterally
Upper
  lip   __ good __ right side poor __ left side poor __ poor bilaterally
Lower
  lip   __ good __ right side poor __ left side poor __ poor bilaterally
  Lingual __ good __ right side poor __ left side poor __ poor bilaterally
  Palatal __ good __ right side poor __ left side poor __ poor bilaterally

ing is significant for stuttering management, regardless of the form of the intervention. Very few clients ever are willing to use fluency reinforcement 100% of the time (and, generally, clinicians do not want them to), so some prediction capacity is significant for decisions of when to use it. In the same way, prediction is valuable for several symptom edification procedures, especially preparatory sets. The following material provides methods for evaluating prediction capacity.

Explanation

Some clients can predict when they will stutter; some cannot. Predicting the specific occurrence of a moment of stuttering can be long term or short term; usually it is the latter. The argument can be made that predictions are self-fulfilling (i.e., you stuttered because you predicted you would stutter). That point is irrelevant. A correct prediction is its own verification. Self-fulfillment factors may be important later in therapy, but early in therapy, prediction is a factor to build on. It can occur in both reading and free speech. In reading aloud, the stutterer can look ahead to anticipate problems with particular words. The stutterer also can look ahead in spontaneous speech. Again, self-fulfillment notwithstanding, prediction is a variable to investigate. In the earlier discussion of stuttering loci it was noted that loci can provide the initial keys to prediction. Stuttering is more likely to occur on

Jonah words	Words previously stuttered on
Initial phonemes	Proximity to a previously stuttered word
Longer words	Unfamiliar words (especially in reading)
Longer sentences	Stressed syllables in polysyllabic words
Significant words	Nouns, verbs, adjectives, adverbs
Anything the individual stutterer has come to focus attention on	

One way to start a discussion of consistency and prediction is to direct the client's attention in that direction with a series of related questions. The list provided in Exhibit 1–11 is not exhaustive and it can be supplemented with a clinician's own items. The questions should be open ended because every client will display different prediction possibilities.

Exhibit 1–11 Loci of stuttering (client evaluation)

Read each speech production act below and decide how often you probably stutter there. Check the appropriate column. Column labels are: rare, less than 10% of the time; occasional, 11% to 30% of the time; often, up to 60% of the time; and very often, over 60% of the time. If you cannot make any estimate at all, leave the line blank.

Speech Item	Probability Stuttering Will Occur			
	Rare	*Occasional*	*Often*	*Very Often*
Your name				
Your address				
Your telephone number				
Other specific numbers				
Friends' names				
Strangers' names				
Words over three syllables				
First letter(s) of word				
Stressed word in a phrase				
After a breath				
First word in a phrase				
Word near a stuttering				
Second or third word in a phrase				
Hard to pronounce words				
Specific speech sounds				

continues

Exhibit 1–11 continued

Stressed syllable in word
Very important words

The client's answers will provide some insight about stuttering loci that can be compared with the clinician's observations. The client's information may be limited and unreliable at first, but it is a start. Moreover, the process helps the client view stuttering from a new standpoint—something to be studied and understood, rather than avoided.

Word Prediction

Another way to probe prediction and consistency factors is to provide the client with an extended word list. The client is asked to read each word, silently, and indicate the words he or she thinks would have a high stuttering probability if he or she were reading the list aloud (see Exhibit 1–12). This task can be done at home or in the clinic. The client then gives the list to the clinician and receives a "clean" list in return. The client is asked to read the list aloud while the clinician follows on the marked copy. The clinician marks each stuttered word. Often, it is useful to have the client do the marking at home, return the sheet, and then let it sit for a while before reading it aloud. When the client reads aloud, the session should be recorded for later analysis of spasm types, durations, and other factors.

Sentence Prediction

Following word prediction, where the words are isolated, the clinician can move to prediction and consistency measurement on structured sen-

Exhibit 1–12 Word predictions of stuttering

Look over each word below, knowing that later you will be asked to read the list aloud. If any words are unfamiliar, tell the clinician. Put a check by each word where you think there is a better-than-average chance that you will stutter. When you are finished, give this sheet to the clinician.

hopeful	under	entire	aster	dig	topple	luster
oats	bundle	kick	end	knobby	war	middle
rebel	zipper	lad	own	bed	purple	when
set	thirty	no	me	waggle	rat	tap
cat	gurgle	hero	cat	pack	hero	skip
ash	three	dancer	satin	tailor	older	go
corny	east	waste	neither	muppet	rascal	zero
lady	pillow	bite	us	extra	apple	dip
zip	cap	shepherd	bitter	goodbye	thorny	knee
window	more	robe	tray	lost	east	shuttle
washer	pour	ebb	noodle	wig	mother	river
zebra	soap	old	back	paddle	hunter	shoo
third	ask	dealer	turtle	lover	gosh	owner
costly	who	up	enter	ample	do	nest
cake	seating	backer	shameful	whistle	there	nest
mat	webbing	run	ten	leave	gabble	pet
enter	hate	upper	good	copper	stump	cradle
klaxon	over	thin	ant	double	zeal	seven
woe	help	shame	flay			

tences. As before, the client is asked to mark any words or word spaces where he or she thinks stuttering is highly probable. The clinician takes the marked copy and provides a clean copy to the client, preferably after a time delay. The initial sentences should be short and contain all one-syllable words. Later, sentences should reflect increases in word length and sentence length. About six personal questions should be mixed among the 15-item total.

1. My name is _____ _____.
2. How old are your cats?
3. I was born in the year _____.
4. My dad's first name is _____.
5. There is no way that I can see that car.
6. How can you make a big mess like that so fast?

7. Have you seen the big blue book that my aunt gave me?
8. This is just as far as I can go when I don't really know who you are.
9. My full street address is _____.
10. Television reduces emotional content to embarrassing inadequacy.
11. You may call me Saturday night at my residential telephone number.
12. Considerable anguish was felt by the multitude of citizens who clustered near the Senator. His filibusters in Congress were famous.
13. I was about _____ years of age when I started to stutter, but I don't really remember very much about it.
14. The family member who gave me the most criticism and the least help with my stuttering was _____.
15. Some people seem to think that any person who is a politician is not very reliable and cannot be relied upon to tell the truth.

Additional prediction activities include paragraph reading, marking words in advance (returning sheet for a clean copy); making a series of prewritten telephone calls with advanced markings on predicted stutterings; and asking "live" memorized questions of strangers on the street or in stores, predicting what words will be stuttered.

Work on prediction and consistency factors usually improves self-monitoring and self-analysis and also facilitates desensitization. As the client continues to work on all related areas (production, monitoring, analysis), each area strengthens the others. The client builds up a store of information, learns to observe accurately and objectively, and comes to recognize the factors most associated with his or her stuttering occurrences.

LATERALITY MEASURES

Overview

Under the old Travis-Orton theory (Bloodstein, 1993, 1995), laterality was a major factor in stuttering theory and treatment. Handedness was viewed as an outward expression of either normal or confused brain hemispheric dominance. When I graduated from college I was equipped with numerous tests for manual, visual, and foot-leg laterality and dexterity. Over the years, enthusiasm for laterality diminished sharply. Over the past decade or so, with greater sophistication in instrumentation, some researchers have expressed renewed interest in lateral brain hemisphere dominance for processing and organizing communication. Pool et al. (1991) reported blood flow asymmetry changes as stuttering severity increased. Ingham, Fox, and Ingham (1994) indicated that stutterer subjects showed increased neuron activity in supplementary cortical motor areas during solo reading aloud, but extra activity was reduced or absent during unison speech (choral reading). In a test of dichotic listening (simultaneous, competing messages are fed to the ears, one to each ear), Blood and Blood (1989) found that males tended to higher right-ear (left hemisphere) preference, but overall male and female subjects were not significantly different in terms of ear or hemisphere dominance in listening. They did note that female subjects with a left-ear (right hemisphere) preference tended to be severe (not moderate or mild) in their level of stuttering. Curlee and Siegel (1997) present complete review of laterality and neurological function.

Applications

Most research in laterality is being done in technical, time-consuming, and expensive ways. Laterality inventories are not used widely. In fact, interest in laterality is limited to young children who may show laterality confusion as part of a potential or actual generalized problem of subclinical neuromotor discoordination. When questions arise in a diagnosis, information from Exhibit 1–13 can be used, and referrals made if in-depth laterality testing is desired.

TESTS AND FORMS

Exhibit 1–14 lists the sources where the tests or forms mentioned can be found. Most are journal publications that are widely available. This list complements an earlier summary of sources for tests and forms. Some overlap exists between the two lists.

Exhibit 1–13 Reviewing laterality

Age: ____ years ____ months   Sex: ____ male ____ female

*Answer the following questions by marking R if the person uses the right
hand most of the time, L if the person uses the left hand most of the time, or
R/L if the person is inconsistent most of the time. If there has been "no
opportunity" for the client to perform the act, leave the item blank.*

	Laterality		
Action	R	L	R/L
Which hand typically is used to			
Hold a knife, fork, or spoon?			
Use a pencil, crayon, etc.?			
Throw a ball, etc.?			
Grasp a door knob, handle, etc.?			
Turn a dial?			
Pull on a drawer knob?			
Move buttons or zippers on garments?			
Cut with scissors?			
Scratch nose, etc.?			
Comb hair?			

GENERAL ASSESSMENT AND INTERVIEW CONCERNS

Overview

In this penultimate section, there are several things to accomplish. I want
to provide some context for diagnosis and evaluation activities. Then I
want to turn major attention to interview and case history material for the
component parts emphasized here. The component outline could have

Exhibit 1–14 Resources for tests and forms

A-19 Scale. A 19-item, yes/no measure of children's perception of and attitude toward their own speech. (Andre and Guitar; in Peters & Guitar, 1991)

C.A.T. (Children's Attitudes Toward Talking) Revised. Similar to the Erickson S-24 Scale. Children respond true/false to 32 statements about their speech. (DeNil & Brutten, 1991)

Check List of Stuttering Behaviors. A checklist of 27 categories of spasm, struggle, and associated behavior characteristics, with extra blanks to add items. Examiner rates each stuttering event across all 27 (+) items. (Darley & Spriestersbach, 1978)

Cluttering Checklist. A rating scale of 33 potential indicators of a person who clutters, rather than stutters. More extensive information, evaluation and management information concerning cluttering can be found elsewhere. (Daly, 1993; Daly & Burnett, 1996)

Inventory of Communication Attitudes. The inventory contains 39 statements identifying speech situations, divided into triads of 13 generic situations (e.g., three on telephone use, three on formal presentations, three on argument/conflict with a friends, etc.). The 39 situations are rated four times, each time on a 7-point scale: self-enjoyment of each situation, own speech skills in each, others' enjoyment of each situations, and others' speech skills in each. (Watson, Gregory, & Kistler, 1987)

Iowa Scale of Severity of Stuttering. A fairly simple 7-point scale that covers %sw, tension degree, spasm duration, disfluency pattern, and associated body movements. Each category is rated on the 1 to 7 scale. (Sherman, 1952)

Perception of Self. Essentially a 25-item bipolar adjective checklist, rating bipolar qualities (nervous/calm, quiet/loud, etc.). Can be taken by client, can be filled in by others (about client), or can be filled in by client (about others). One statement is pegged at "1" and its bipolar opposite is pegged at "9," with seven degrees of strength between. (Kalinowski, Lerman, & Watt, 1987)

Physician's Screening Procedure for Children Who May Stutter. A very broad, general form for physicians, teachers, or others. It is divided into six categories: dysfluency type, frequency, child reactions, etc. Depending on occurrence or characteristic, behaviors are categorized in four levels from "normal" to "very abnormal." (Riley & Riley, 1989)

S-24, Erickson Scale. In the revised form, 24 statements about speech and speech attitudes are rated on a true/false basis. Adult norms for stutterers and nonstutterers are provided. (Andrews & Cutter, 1974)

---

continues

Exhibit 1–14 continued

> **Stuttering Problem Profile**. A list of 86 statements concerning feelings, actions, and behaviors associated with stutterers. All are stated in a positive form, or as a rejection of negative attitudes. The statements are intended to help the client and the clinician select target goals in therapy planning. (Silverman, 1980)
>
> **Stutterers' Self-Ratings of Reactions to Speech Situations**. A list of 40 speaking situations. The 40 items are rated on a 5-point scale for situation avoidance, for enjoyment of each situation, for stuttering probability in each, and for the frequency with which each situation is encountered. (Darley & Spriestersbach, 1978)
>
> **Stuttering Severity Instrument (SSI)**. A standardized measure of severity for children and adults, readers and nonreaders. It provides separate scores for spasm frequency, average of longest spasm duration, and the effects on listeners of struggle or overflow behaviors. The three scores, added, convert to an age-adjusted severity score. (Riley, 1972)

been placed in the first paragraph of this chapter. However, I am more concerned with having the needs of a particular evaluation procedure dictate what components should be utilized than in setting up a rigid model that insists on a particular structure and sequence for every diagnosis.

Basic Diagnostic Outline

The organization of a diagnostic session is subject to many mandates and personnel preferences. Many training programs routinely take 2 to 5 hours for evaluation procedures, whereas some school clinicians are lucky to have 20 minutes. The proposed session assumes that participants are enthusiastic, organized, reliable, and informed and that the time schedule is convenient for everybody.

> **Appropriate history form**—preferably mailed out 2 weeks before appointment, and preferably returned by mail 2 to 3 days before the appointment.
>
> **Interview**—based on an already-completed case history or (often) to fill out a case history form. Client should be recorded (videotaped if possible). If the client is a child, I prefer at least 15 minutes' observation of child with caregiver before I join them to conduct the interview. Upon

my entrance, the child leaves the room and either waits outside or starts diagnostic activities with my assistant.

Speech sample—obtained by whatever means. Any activity that elicits discourse from a child or free speech from an older person can be used. If a person can read, five consecutive readings of the same material can be used. The odds indicate I will secure my most dysfluent speech samples immediately, with the client improving as she or he adapts to the situation (presumably this is reversed for clutterers). The parenthetical statement is meant professionally. My purpose is not to "give the client a hard time," but to sample speech when there might be stress and compare it to later speech samples.

Speech/language tests (formal)—administered if indicated by the age of the client.

Hearing screen—99% are a waste of time, but the 1% of value make it ethically appropriate and needed for every client.

Oral-peripheral examination—a general examination, paying particular attention to sensory awareness, range of motion, strength, accuracy, speed, and diadochokinesis.

Other special tests—administered as indicated. Relevant tests include the C.A.T. (Children's Attitudes Toward Talking) Revised; the S-24, Erickson Scale; and so forth.

Fluency induction—as available, and as desired. I generally try for four modes drawn from delayed auditory feedback (about a 200-ms delay), unison speech masking (about 85–95 dB), metronome (about 60 beats per minute), Easy Onset, pitch shift, loud speech, and so forth.

Staffing—results and impressions discussed; initial recommendations and arrangements formulated.

The foregoing must respond to the reality of time. I have been forced to accomplish the above steps in four or five sessions because of the institution, or because the young child was viable for about 20 minutes before he or she started screaming. Another time, the client refused to do anything at all unless his (fluent) twin brother was present and did every test (separately) that he performed. Clinicians need to be flexible.

Preliminary Contact

In instances where a child is to be evaluated, I prefer to collect initial information and then decide whether or not have that child in at all. If I opt to see the child, whether it is for a full-scale evaluation, whether to talk face-to-face, or to speak by telephone, I project the following information and attitude to the caregiver when prospective clients are quite young:

> I am glad you contacted me because I can appreciate your concern. Do you have about 30 minutes to talk now, or should we schedule a specific time? There is a charge of ___ for this preliminary interview, but it could save you a larger amount if we decide a complete evaluation is not needed. . . .

If the person has time at this first contact, the clinician can go ahead and get started. If the interview has to be delayed, I have a prepared list of questions on hand for when we do make contact. Also, I can mail the questions and either ask for a mail return, or for the person to be ready to answer them when I call. In general, the questions are summarized in Exhibit 1–15. It takes a little practice to keep this method under time control. For reasons of time and money, the contact should be kept to 30 minutes, approximately. If the client discourses extensively on every question, the clinician should encourage brevity. If unsuccessful, the clinician can say, "Oh, we're running over the allowed time. If we run much past the half-hour I will have to charge for another 30 minutes of consulting time."

During the discussion the clinician takes notes to help reach one of the following decisions:

- Need to reassure the informant, refer to an information source, and arrange a recheck. Call if indicated.
- Need to tell the informant that a longer, in-person session with him or her and any other concerned adults (no child). Make assignments for information, audiotape, and so forth, to be prepared and brought in.
- Arrange to schedule a full evaluation with the child present. Stipulate all records, recordings, and so on, that should be brought along.

Interview Questions

A series of interview question sets, or forms, for particular applications follows. They can be reduced or supplemented as the situation dictates.

Exhibit 1–15 Initial interview (concerning child)

Clinician: _____ Informant: _____

Client: _____ Age:___ Years ___ Months Sex: ____

Date: _____

[Insert any other geographic or demographic information desired.]

When (date if possible) was the problem first noticed? _____

Who first noticed? _____

Have others noticed? ___ Yes ___ No ___ Not sure

Does anyone disagree that there may be a problem? ___ No ___ Yes.
If yes, explain: _____

_____

Describe what caught your attention when you first noticed. _____

_____

Is the problem changed from when it was first noticed? ___ No ___ Yes.
If yes, explain: _____

_____

When the child has trouble now, which of the following do you hear?
Answer None, Some, or Lots.

Behavior	Frequency		
	None	*Some*	*Lots*
Phrase repetitions			
Word repetitions			
Part-word repetitions			
Prolongations			
Gets stuck (stoppages)			
Talks louder			
Stops talking			
Shows emotional reactions			

continues

Exhibit 1–15 continued

Talks about a "problem"

What has been done to try and reduce or stop the problem? _____

Overall, are people a little concerned, concerned, or very concerned? ___

Does any other family member or near relative have this problem? ____

When do the child's problems seem most often to occur?

___ Any time ___ When excited or upset ___ When competing for attention ___ When "X" is around ___ After disciplining ___ Other

How many times a day does the child have trouble?

___ Almost every time he or she talks ___ Very, very often ___ Frequently ___ Every once in a while ___ Not very often

---

Conventional case history forms are available in nearly all stuttering texts, and the usual history questions about development, health, nutrition, education, and all the other areas can be added. History forms should be changed as situation parameters change. For instance, for very young children, more questions should address early and ongoing speech-language development and problems; for older children, questions on social interaction and school are needed. Some of the questions repeat queries from the earlier initial interview. Under appropriate circumstances, the two can be merged.

To start, friendly and courteous introductory and rapport remarks, including reinforcement for having come, are in order. Then the following questions shold be asked:

- What referral or information source sent you to me?
- What are the reasons or concerns that brought you to me?
- At what point in time did you become aware of a fluency problem, and what were the circumstances?
- Who noticed first? Who else noticed? Any disagreements?
- Do you have any ideas as to why the problem happened, and why it happened at this particular time?
- Since your first contact with me, has there been any noticeable change in speech or in behavior?
- Since the very first time you noticed the problem, has it changed? How?

- As of right now, what is the best way to describe the child's speech? [help with cues, models]
  - Forms: repetitions, prolongations, stoppages
  - Rhythm, energy, struggle
  - PR, WWR, PWR, and so on
  - Child's efforts to struggle or control?
  - Can you imitate what the problem sounds like at various times?
  - Frequency of occurrence (by the clock, by the calendar, by the situation, and so on)
  - Any specific situations, people, words, emotions, involved ?
  - How long does any one trouble moment last? How long did the longest one you can remember last?
  (PR = phrase repetition, WWR = whole word repetition, PWR = part-word repetition)
- What are the child's emotional reactions when there is trouble (ignores, obviously ignores, shows awareness, is irritated, is angry, is frustrated, cries, uses words of distress)? (*Note:* Ambrose and Yairi [1994] found no significant relationship between differences in stuttering severity and child awareness of stuttering. However, significant differences were found concerning awareness and age. In other words, early on, children who stuttered were aware of the problem and this awareness increased with age. I cannot believe, ever, that awareness does not influence behavior. The difficulty is finding out what behavioral variable to measure and how to measure it accurately. Vanryckeghem and Brutten [1996] found, for instance, that C.A.T. scores of child stutterers were negatively affected by awareness as early as 6 years of age.)
- Since the problem started, has there been a reduction in talking, a change of attitude toward communication?
- How have the various adults tried to help?
- What have been the child's reactions to the attempted help?
- Fluency aside, what has the child's overall speech and language progress been, and what is it like now, compared with other children?
- Has the child had any continuing medical problems?
- Does the disfluency show any variations over time?
- What is a typical day for the child, from getting up to going to bed?

- Do you have ideas as to what caused the problem? (Very strong reactions are possible here if there are guilt feelings, or if there is anger directed at another adult.)
- How would you judge the child's fluency (good, poor, or terrible) when talking to each of the following people:
  - You?
  - Sibling 1?
  - Teacher?
  - Specific peer?
  - Specific relatives?
  - Spouse?
  - Other siblings?
  - Peers?
  - Strangers?
  - Others?
- Currently, how willing is the child to talk? Is willingness greater or less than a month ago?
- How have other people reacted to the child's problems?
- Drawing on the previous question, what persons have been most supportive? Who has been least supportive?
- Has the child experienced any overt acts of teasing, rejection, imitation, scolding, punishment, and so on, because of his or her speech?
- If appropriate, ask questions concerning school:
  - What is the grade level versus age?
  - Any school reports about speech?
  - Any remedial work in any studies?
  - Any problems with school peers?
  - What are the overall reports about school work?
  - Any SLP attention in school?
  - What is the teacher's role, attitude, support?
  - What is child's attitude toward school?
- Does any other person in the immediate family have this problem, or has had it in the past?
- On either side of the family, are there past problems of fluency?
- Cover related areas of rest, nutrition, and general behavior, family life, etc.
- If therapy is recommended, what is your preference among the options available?

Then, the clinician explains what else is scheduled, where the child will be going, about final staffing and recommendations, timelines or waiting lists, and so on. The caregiver should understand that the first issue is to determine whether or not there is a fluency problem that requires direct attention. If there seems to be a real problem, the clinician needs to explain what information is necessary and what treatment options are available. Finally, the informant should be encouraged to ask questions about stuttering in general or the problem in particular.

Child Interview Questions

The information obtained from questions posed to a child, any child, will depend on the child's age, social maturity, attitude toward the current situation and adults in general, and the clinician's skills. Some professionals rigorously avoid providing any suggestion to a child concerning why he or she is in this strange, unfamiliar place. Generally speaking, that attitude is dangerous nonsense. Children are far more astute than most adults realize, and they figure things out quickly. I recall when one of my child clients was seen by several neurological specialists concerning fine motor coordination. When I asked her why she thought she was seeing all those doctors, she replied, "Because I'm going blind." Her reasoning was that, because the very first thing every physician did was shine a little flashlight in her eyes, they must be checking if she could see the light, so she must be going blind. The response was logical, in a way. With rare exceptions, I argue for a fully informed child.

The following questions are to be rephrased and rearranged as desired. It may take 5 minutes to use all of them, or they can be scattered over an hour or more of activities. The questions assume an age from "precocious 4" on up.

- What were you told was the reason for coming here today?
- Do you have trouble sometimes when you talk?
- What happens when there is trouble?
- How do you feel then? What do you do?
- What do your [siblings] say when you have trouble?
- What does your mom say when you have trouble?
- What does your dad say when you have trouble?
- What do your friends around home say when you have trouble?
- What do your friends at ___ [school, day care, etc.] say when you have trouble?
- Does anybody try to help you when you have trouble talking?
- How do they try and help? Does it really help or does it make things worse?

- Have you figured out anything that helps? Does it work?
- Do you have trouble with your speech all the time, some of the time, or rarely?
- When do you have the most trouble with your speech?
- When you get stuck, do you quit there, go around it, or fight through it?
- What people have been the biggest help? What have they done?
- Why do you think you have this speech problem?

A procedure I often use with younger children is one that resembles that described by Silverman (1996). He explains his "Three Wishes Task," where the child's fairy godmother will grant the child three wishes, and the child must express those wishes. Retries are arranged, becoming more specific, if the child's wishes do not relate to fluency. In years past I have used a "big, invisible magician" and over the last 10 to 15 years I have proposed a wonderful space creature who will make one change in each of the following areas: the child's face, speech, clothes, and friends. On each aspect, I provide general suggestions and see if the child responds, or if there is avoidance of change. If the child indicates desired changes, then the clinician has entry to discuss them, specify, consider reasons, and so on.

Adolescent Questions

On my first day in student teaching, as a first-quarter senior, the school SLP sat me down in a group of five adolescent stutterers. She then disappeared to another part of the building to work with /r/, /s/, and /l/ problems, and I did not see her again until lunch. I rapidly (almost immediately) gained an appreciation of the complexities and challenges of therapy management of adolescent fluency problems. With patience and open qualities (plus a thick skin and a stern will), question approaches can be used quite effectively with adolescents. Many feel their information and opinions are ignored by adults, and the idea that an adult really wants them to talk may take a while to accept.

After introductions and explanations for the meeting, the clinician might consider some of the following questions:

- Why are you here, or why has ___ sent you here?
- Do you agree with this referral? Why?

- Generally, tell me what is your "problem with your problem"?
- What is the history of your fluency problem? When did it start? What was it like at ages 6, 8, 10, 12, etc.?
- What was the family's attitude at onset and at ages 6, 8, 10, 12, etc.? [Take your time and go through each family member at each age.]
- What was/is your response to those various attitudes?
- When you don't stutter, what is rest of your speech like?
- Does your dysfluency show variations in terms of
  - Time of day?   - Particular class?
  - At home or school?   - Day of week?
  - With boys or girls?   - With friends or strangers?
  - Reading versus talking?   - Topic of speech?
  - How people act?
- How much teasing, imitation, rejection, or other negative responses have you had in
  - Preschool?   - Grades 1–3?
  - Grades 4–6?   - Grades 7–9?
  - Grades 10–12?
- Do you have any ideas about what originally caused your problems?
- What people, specifically, make your speech better or worse?
  - None   - Siblings x, y, z
  - Specific relatives   - Specific teachers
  - Father   - Mother
  - Specific fellow students   - Others
- Compared with your peer group, how much time do you spend talking?
- When you stutter, what emotions do you feel just before, during, just after, and later?
- Do you have special problems with the telephone? Why? Describe.
- Do you avoid volunteering in class, or avoid answering when asked a question?
- Do you use any of the following behaviors to try and control stuttering? How often? [Model and describe each one.]

– Postponement	– Retrial
– Substitution	– Starter
– Revision	– Circumlocution
– Mutism	– Break eye contact
– Other	

- In fighting stuttering, is there anything you do "most of the time," stuttering or not, when you talk? [Model and describe each.]

– Talk quickly	– Talk slowly
– Talk loudly	– Talk softly
– Use monotone	– Change your pitch
– Use an accent	– Be a funnyman
– Make lots of gestures	– Other

- What is your eye contact like when you talk? What about when you stutter? If your answer is "good," describe the reactions of people when you stutter.
- Do you sometimes find that stuttering is a convenient excuse, an alibi, or that others may "let you off" because of stuttering?
- Can you look ahead and see a stuttering coming up? Discuss.
- What are all of the professional efforts to date to help you? Medical? SLP? Counseling? [Probe for specific details (i.e., dates, durations, frequency, and intensity), ask questions, make notes for future reviews, etc.]
- Do you presently have any concerns about your health? Are you taking any medications, under a physician's direction, receiving treatments, etc.?
- Overall, what do you think of school now? Like it? Hate it? Why?
- If you did not stutter, would your opinions change?
- Right now, what is your attitude toward coming in for therapy?
- If you enter therapy, what would you see as your goal(s)?
- If you enter therapy, would you prefer fluency reinforcement therapy or symptom modification therapy? (Fluency—a drastic change in speech, initially in the clinic, and then shaped as a different speech pattern to be used as often as needed. Symptom—learning how to try to control and change the characteristics of stuttering to a level that is acceptable and under control.)

- What commitments are you willing to make to therapy?
  - Regular attendance
  - Read reasonable bibliotherapy
  - Willing to work in a group
  - Complete reasonable, regular outside assignments
  - Work with classroom teachers
  - Talk to peers about your therapy
  - Talk to family about your therapy

Teacher Questions

Adult questions might logically follow child and adolescent inquiries. However, I felt the education setting tied in with a number of interest areas. Generally speaking, school work with fluency disorders can be calamitous. For every balanced, appropriate therapy program I hear of in schools, I am apprised of other programs where "I can see a stutterer twice a week for 20 minutes each time, in a group of five kids, and none of the other four stutters." Whether a school's arrangements favor or hinder fluency disorders management, classroom teachers can contribute significantly and should be interviewed and involved. This philosophy has been intensifying as SLPs are drawn more and more into the classroom itself to provide interactive intervention for communication problems in educational settings. Rather than relist questions already asked, I will present teacher information in Exhibit 1–16, in a form that can be used as an interview resource, or given to the teacher to fill out and return, or a mix. My personal recommendation is that the SLP decide how to use it on a teacher-by-teacher basis. Some teachers will bristle or sag at the idea of "one more form," whereas others will prefer it because they can schedule, at their preference, when to fill it out.

Adult Listening

To save space here, I suggest selective use of the questions that were listed for adolescents. If school questions are not appropriate, they can be rephrased for vocational settings. A few of the following questions may, or may not, be applicable:

- What is your spouse's attitude toward stuttering? Has it changed over time?

Exhibit 1–16 Information form—Educational settings

Clinician: _____   Informant: _____
Student: _____   Date: _____

General Information
Child's Age: _____ Grade: _____ Sex: ____ M ____ F
How long has child been in this school? _____ this grade? _____
Were any siblings ever at this school? ____ Yes ____ No
If answer is yes, were/are there any communication problems among
them? _____

When did you first notice the fluency problem? _____
Since your first awareness has the problem seemed to:
____ Stay about the same severity? ____ Get worse? ____ Get better?
Have other school personnel noticed the problem? ____ Yes ____ No
(If "yes," explain): _____

Have the child's parents communicated with you about a concern they
have? ____ Yes ____ No

Speech Performance
When there are fluency breaks, what are they like?

Speech Behavior	Frequency			
	Very Often	Often	Occasional	Never
Repeats phrases or phrase parts				
Repeats words				
Repeats syllables or sounds				
Repetitions are not easy and rhythmic				
Prolongs sounds of syllables inappropriately				
Gets stuck or "frozen" on some sounds				

continues

Exhibit 1–16 continued

In fluency breaks, does the child tend to replace the correct vowel with an "uh," such as "Suh-suh-circle"? ____ Never ____ Sometimes ____ Often ____ Nearly always

When there are fluency breaks does the child show any of the following behaviors?

	Frequency			
Speech Behavior	*Very Often*	*Often*	*Occasional*	*Never*
Facial grimaces				
Head jerks, movements				
Hand or limb movements				
Postural changes				
Vocal pitch changes				
Loudness changes				

In fluency breaks, what is the child's eye contact like?

From other children is there: ____ Teasing? ____ Ridicule? ____ Imitation? ____ Rejection?

What are the child's reactions when she or he has difficulty?

Comment briefly on the other aspects of the child's speech and language.

Comment briefly on the child's general level of class performance in various class areas.

Comment briefly on child's interaction with other students.

Comment briefly on child's apparent awareness of problem and feelings about it.

- How often does she or he carry on communication for you?
- Have any of your children stuttered? Any who do now?
- What restrictions do you see in your future if you continue to stutter as you do now?
- What, if any, time frame or limits have you put on therapy?
- Are you willing to involve your spouse in therapy, and is she or he willing?
- Are you able and willing to work on your speech in your employment setting?
- Are you able and willing to work on your speech in social settings?
- Do you feel that real success in therapy would affect or allow any changes in your life? Discuss in detail.
- Looking at your own past history, and considering only that aspect, what prognosis do you see for yourself? What changes are needed most to support a favorable prognosis?

SPECIAL ISSUES

Early Intervention

When I was a student, daily (direct) intervention with stutterers was a moot point for discussion. It generally did not occur. Parents could be counseled, but children were not scheduled for therapy. If scheduled at all, it tended to be for "communication can be fun" sessions. This type of enrollment involved one of those ridiculous child-adult conspiracies where each side knows why a certain thing is done or is happening (or not), but each party is expected to behave as if neither knows. I must pretend the client does not know, and the client must pretend that he or she does not know, and also does not know that I do know. Unfortunately, even today, there are SLPs who stoutly say, "I never tell them why they're coming to therapy. It might upset them." What can I say?

Interestingly, I have observed an increase in the number of professionals expressing concern over whether there are significant dangers in enrolling *dis*fluent children under the assumption that they are *dys*fluent. I find myself on both sides of the issue. Curlee and Yairi (1997) found not much in favor of early intervention (enrollment for therapy), but they suggested that professionally organized early intervention was not likely to harm a child or to increase any problems. Silverman (1996) leans to the conservative view, frankly labeling himself as being "diagnosogenic" for many young children. That is, he leans to the early Iowa (Wendell Johnson) philosophy that, to some degree (usually a major one), what we call stuttering actually started out as normal disfluencies that were misinterpreted and responded to by adults. Although this can and does happen, I do not see it as a major cause of stuttering. I will lean toward "if-in-doubt-enroll," especially if the speech struggles are overt, if out-clinic observations or recordings show stutters not seen on an in-clinic basis, and if the child's awareness and concern level are present, consistent, and strong.

Curlee and Yairi (1997) evaluated both sides of the intervene-wait conflict. They argued cogently against "unwarranted" early intervention and pull together significant areas of information to suggest that remission rates are highest among children who are female, had a very early onset age, have some family history of remissions, actually show some decline in stuttering frequency in the year following onset, and seem to function normally in general speech and language development and in measures of nonverbal intelligence. Curlee and Yairi also point to a lack of data to support the values of early intervention. On the other hand, Lincoln and Onslow (1997) reported that early intervention (defined as ages 2 to 5 years) secured near elimination of stuttering and that these levels of achievement remained stable from 2 to 7 years posttherapy.

Of course, some questions raised by Curlee and Yairi about report data (particularly the original diagnosis accuracy) remain. Arguments for early intervention include rebuttals that reports of spontaneous remission are exaggerated, and that clinicians risk missing those in real need. Again, my personal orientation is that I would not have been contacted if the child either was not unusually disfluent or the parents unusually anxious or perfectionistic about speech. Either or all of the aspects can profit from evaluation and improvement. Adopting a wait-and-see approach creates the chance to miss real stuttering in its early, vulnerable stages.

Enrollment Decisions

Linked to early intervention is the decision point on whether or not to enroll based on symptoms, reports, test results, or other data. In some settings there are preset criteria and the SLP must determine if those criteria have been met. In other settings, the knowledge and philosophy of the clinician will make the determination. There are several factors that argue for early intervention or intervention at any time.

Test scores rarely make a decision for me. Decisions should not rest on a test score. Unfortunately, they sometimes do. When a professional opportunity to evaluate exists, the following items may influence a decision to intervene or not. I have gathered these items from my experience and a wide range of sources. For that reason, there will be some variations in figures, but I find no instances of actual disagreement or contradiction.

- Overall dysfluencies above 10%
- Three or more repetitions per unit of occurrence (Martin, Haroldson, and Woessner [1988] compared dysfluencies, including four levels of repetitions, disrhythmic phonations, tense pauses, interjections, and revisions or incomplete phrases. They found repetitions to be the best single identifier for separating stuttering and nonstuttering speakers.)
- Struggle (visible/audible) on 3% or more of utterances
- Observable struggle in one or more of the following areas (as the auditor's perceptions of stuttering increase, so also increases the probability that the stuttering label will be attached to the speech behaviors):
  - Speech mechanism (lips, tongue, larynx, etc.)
  - Face (facial expressions, grimaces, etc.)
  - Head-neck-shoulder involvement (rigidity, peculiar postures, jerks, shoulder elevations, etc.)
  - Body parts (fingers, hands, arms, legs, feet [tapping, snapping, jerking])
- Disrhythmic phonation
- Inappropriate changes in pitch, loudness, rate, and so on
- Appearance, dysfluency or not, of overinvolvement of head-neck-shoulder postures or movements during speech
- Part-word repetitions occurrences at or above about 2% of utterances
- Prolongations (determined to be atypical) on 3% or more of the words uttered
- Sound durations are longer than expected
- Stutterlike behaviors are about 3% more frequent compared with other children of similar age

- Genetic evidence of stuttering in the distant family (i.e., historical past [e.g., Grandfather Jones] or distant family [e.g., cousin Joe twice removed])
- Immediate family history of stuttering, especially if it did not remiss alone
- Delayed stuttering onset (see Yairi, Ambrose, Paden, & Throneburg, 1996)
- Delayed overall onset of speech and language
- Concomitant speech and language problems along with fluency problems (see Yairi et al., 1996, and Watkins & Yairi, 1997)
- Particular auditors or particular situations appear to be strong triggers for fluency problems
- The schwa vowel is used to replace the proper vowel in a syllable in repetitions
- There are observable associated behaviors such as direct word-specific avoidances (see earlier and in chapter 2) general antiexpectance avoidances (as above)
- Family concerns or demands are apparently punishingly high
- The child's concerns about speech or speech acceptance are too extreme
- The child labels herself or himself as a stutterer or uses self-derogating terms about her or his speech

Yairi et al. (1996) compared 32 stuttering children on several factors after dividing the children into three groups: early recovery (ER; remission after 18 months or less), late recovery (LR; more than 18 months passed before remission), and persistence (P; no recovery up to this time). They found that the P group started out with a lower dysfluency rate than did the other two groups, reported onsets that averaged about 5 to 8 months later than the ER and LR groups, and showed less symptom fluctuations over time. Interestingly, and perhaps related to the milder early stages, the P group averaged about 8.5 months' delay between perceived onset and efforts to secure help, whereas the ER and LR groups averaged only 2.5 months between the reported onset and securing help. In another study, Watkins and Yairi (1997) evaluated selected language measures on the three groups. Compared with fluent children norms, they found the groups all were within norm limits on their language measures. However, there was enough variability in results and in departures from norms (in individuals) in the P group to justify language assessment for all children suspected of fluency problems.

Zebrowski (1997) proposed an interesting organization for decision making and planning. She divides children into triage groups based on four time intervals identifying onset of fluency problems.

Stream I   0–6 months since onset
Stream II   6–12 months since onset
Stream III   1–2 years since onset
Stream IV   2–3 years since onset

Each group, or "stream," is assigned a point system based on various factors such as sex, associated behaviors, family history, and so on. Each item is scored 1 point. There are two therapy plans (A and B) for Stream 1; therapy plans C, D, and E relate to the other streams, depending on their scores. Plan D includes monthly clinic visits (or home visit by the SLP), and plan E appears to bring early (relative term) intervention on a direct child therapy basis. Although Zebrowski (1997) does not describe step-by-step procedures, she does provide excellent therapy structures and suggestions.

Schwartz and Conture (1988) provided another possible frame of reference in a more general sense. They tried to separate child stutterers by certain speech characteristics. Intervention decision was not considered, but their format could be used for planning intervention. They found that their stutterers (43), ranging from 3 to 9 years of age, seemed to divide into separate clusters:

- **Cluster 1**—higher within-word, sound/syllable repetitions, lower prolongations; also showed a comparatively low count on frequency and types of associated behaviors. Seventeen of the 43 stutterers were placed in this cluster.
- **Cluster 2**—higher counts on repetition; associated behaviors counts were lower than for the first cluster. Eight stutterers were placed in this cluster.
- **Cluster 3**—highest count on prolongations, with nonspeech behaviors and behavior variations that were close to both the previous clusters. Eleven stutterers were placed here.

- **Cluster 4**—high count on prolongation; higher count on associated behaviors and behavior variations than any other clusters. Four persons were placed here.
- **Cluster 5**—high count on prolongation, lower count on repetitions; highest of all the clusters on associated behaviors and numbers of different behaviors per stuttering. Three persons were placed in Cluster 5.

Chronicity and Stuttering

Many persons who stutter are not "cured" by therapy. Among those who are dismissed with "some residual dysfluency," there is a high relapse rate. The perseveration or chronic characteristic of stuttering is the greatest challenge and biggest millstone around our neck. For many years the topic was avoided, but it has been dealt with extensively in recent years. The bottom-line issue is the question: If results are so often incomplete, and relapse rates are so high, why don't SLPs look for it, plan for it, and prepare the client for it?

Cooper (1973, 1987) wrote concerning what he called the chronic perseverative stuttering syndrome (CPSS). He noted that too many mature stutterers have little hope that therapy intervention will eliminate their problems. It is of course often true in dysarthria, dysphagia, dysphasia, dyspraxia, certain voice disorders, and so on. Cooper advocated early counseling of stutterers about the possibilities and probabilities of CPSS (i.e., the client would have to live with residual dysfluencies, at best). His proposal caused a stir, and some recrimination, but he organized and stated clearly many things that needed to be said. Cooper brought out a significant issue and buttressed it with 10 observations on behaviors or occurrences that reinforce the probability of PS for any particular client. Taking his lead, I have developed an equivalent of the CPSS list and suggest the use of both because each addresses a number of different points. Prognosis shifts toward the negative as

1. Age increases.
2. Symptom age increases.
3. Occurrence age is later.

4. The number or percentage of current avoidance behaviors increases.
5. The number of avoidance behaviors per spasm occurrence increases.
6. The complexity and duration of avoidance behaviors increases.
7. The overall frequency of stuttering spasms increases.
8. The number of failed prior therapy experiences, and the strength of negative reactions to those failures accumulates.
9. There is the existence of past successful or semisuccessful therapies, which then culminated in relapse.
10. The person's level of anxiety and fear when she or he anticipates and experiences stuttering goes up.
11. The person's personification of stuttering as "it," and in control of person strengthens.
12. The person's tendency is to think, act, respond most of the time with "stuttering" being foremost in her or his mind is predominant.
13. The person has difficulty, or seems to, in hearing the disfluencies in the speech of nonstutterers and regards similar disfluencies in her or his own speech as being abnormal.
14. The person wants to place restrictions (session frequency or duration, transfer sites, not involving significant others, etc.).
15. The person's life environment is apathetic, barren, or hostile and nonsupportive toward therapy.

SUMMARY

In organizing a diagnosis and evaluation workup, it is important to stop and think. There will be some tendency to go for a prepackaged assessment inventory (there are a number of quality ones on the market and in various texts). This tendency is quite appropriate, up to a point. Beyond that point, the clinician needs to stop and think over a few considerations:

- Age and sex of the client
- The reported dysfluency severity and related problems
- Status and concerns of significant others
- Vocational significance, if any, of stuttering and therapy
- School significance, if any, of stuttering and therapy
- Any associated occurrences that might affect speech fluency

In other words, what is there about this particular upcoming diagnosis that makes it like or unlike other diagnoses? Although the clinician may not receive all the information needed before a session, it is nevertheless important to avoid mindsets that dictate that every child stutterer must have tests X, Y, and Z, and all mature stutterers must be tested by P, Q, and R forms. Conture (1996), among other things, urged the clinician to take the time to use several different tests of the same functions. He also recommended repeated observations over time. Commenting on 100 children seen for diagnosis, Conture felt that, after a thorough evaluation, about 45% of the children had a question mark on the "Needs therapy?" recommendation. This finding applies equally to adolescent and adult clients, and it expands to include the questions concerning the form and organization of therapy. By staying flexible in diagnostic and evaluation decisions, the clinician will be in a much better position to provide the level of service that the client deserves.

REFERENCES

Ambrose, N.G., & Yairi, E. (1994). The development of awareness of stuttering in preschool children. *Journal of Fluency Disorders, 19*, 229–246.

American Speech-Language-Hearing Association. (1998, Spring). Terminology pertaining to fluency and fluency disorders.

Andrews, G., & Cutter, J. (1974). Stuttering therapy: The relations between changes in symptom level and attitudes. *Journal of Speech and Hearing Disorders, 39*, 312–319.

Armson, J., Jenson, S., Gallant, D., Kalinowski, J., & Fee, E.J. (1997). The relationship between degree of audible struggle and judgments of childhood disfluencies as stuttered or non-stuttered. *American Journal of Speech-Language Pathology, 6*, 42–50.

Blood, G.W., & Blood, I.M. (1989). Laterality preferences in adult female and male stutterers. *Journal of Fluency Disorders, 14*, 1–10.

Bloodstein, O. (1993). *Stuttering: The search for a cause and cure.* Boston: Allyn & Bacon.

Bloodstein, O. (1995). *A handbook on stuttering.* San Diego, CA: Singular Publishing Group.

Boone, D.R., & McFarlane, S.C. (1988). *The voice and voice therapy* (4th ed.). Englewood Cliffs, NJ: Prentice Hall.

Conture, E.G. (1990). *Stuttering* (2nd ed.). Englewood Cliffs, NJ: Prentice Hall.

Conture, E.G. (1996). Treatment efficacy: Stuttering. *Journal of Speech and Hearing Research, 39*, 518–526.

Cooper, E.B. (1973). The development of a stuttering chronicity prediction checklist: A preliminary report. *Journal of Speech and Hearing Disorders, 38*, 215–223.

Cooper, E.B. (1982). A disfluency descriptor digest for clinical use. *Journal of Fluency Disorders, 2*, 355–358.

Cooper, E.B. (1987). The chronic perseverative stuttering syndrome: Incurable stuttering. *Journal of Fluency Disorders, 12*, 381–389.

Culatta, R., & Goldberg, S.A. (1995). *Stuttering therapy: An integrated approach to theory and practice.* Boston: Allyn & Bacon.

Curlee, R.F., & Siegel, G.M. (1997). *Nature and treatment of stuttering, new directions* (2nd ed.). Boston: Allyn & Bacon.

Curlee, R.F., & Yairi, E. (1997). Early intervention with early childhood stuttering: A critical examination of the data. *Journal of Speech-Language Pathology, 6*, 8–18.

Daly, D. (1993). Cluttering: Another fluency syndrome. In R. Curlee (Ed.), *Stuttering and related disorders of fluency.* New York: Thieme Medical Publications.

Daly, D.A., & Burnett, M.L. (1996). Cluttering assessment, treatment planning, and case study illustration. *Journal of Fluency Disorders, 3/4*, 239–248.

Darley, F.L., & Spriestersbach, D.C. (1978). *Diagnostic methods in speech pathology* (2nd ed.). New York: Harper & Row.

DeNil, L., & Brutten, G. (1991). Speech-associated attitudes of stuttering and nonstuttering children. *Journal of Speech and Hearing Research, 34*, 60–70.

Fletcher, S.G. (1972). Time-by-count measurements of diadochokinetic syllable rate. *Journal of Speech and Hearing Research, 15*, 763–770.

Ham, R.E. (1986). *Techniques of stuttering therapy.* Englewood Cliffs, NJ: Prentice Hall.

Ham, R.E. (1989). *Therapy of stuttering: Preschool through adolescence.* Englewood Cliffs, NJ: Prentice Hall.

Hixson, T.J., Hawley, J.L., & Wilson, K.J. (1982). An around-the-house device for the clinical determination of respiratory driving pressure: A note on making simple even simpler. *Journal of Speech and Hearing Disorders, 47*, 413–415.

Howell, P., & Au-Yeung, J. (1995). The association between stuttering, Brown's factors, and phonological categories in child stutterers ranging in age between 2 and 12 years. *Journal of Fluency Disorders, 20*, 331–344.

Howell, P., Sackin, S., & Rustin, L. (1995). Comparison of speech motor development in stuttering and fluent speakers between 7 and 12 years old. *Journal of Fluency Disorders, 20*, 243–256.

Ingham, R.J., Fox, P.T., & Ingham, J.C. (1994). Brain image investigation of the speech of stutterers and nonstutterers. *ASHA Magazine, 36*, 188.

Kalinowski, J.S., Lerman, J.W., & Watt, J. (1987). A preliminary examination of the perceptions of self and others in stutterers and nonstutterers. *Journal of Fluency Disorders, 12*, 317–332.

Kent, R.D. (1996). Hearing and believing: Some limits to the auditory-perceptual assessment of speech and voice disorders. *American Journal of Speech-Language Pathology, 5*, 7–21.

Lincoln, M.A., & Onslow, M. (1997). Long-term outcomes of early intervention for stuttering. *American Journal of Speech-Language Pathology, 6*, 51–63.

Martin, R.R., Haroldson, S.K., & Woessner, G.L. (1988). Perceptual scaling of stuttering severity. *Journal of Fluency Disorders, 13*, 27–47.

Martin, R., Parlour, S.F., & Haroldson, S. (1990). Stuttering and level of linguistic demand. *Journal of Fluency Disorders, 15*(2), 93–106.

Peters, T.J., & Guitar, B. (1991). *Stuttering, an integrated approach to its nature and treatment.* Baltimore: Williams & Wilkins.

Pool, K.D., Devons, M.D., Freeman, F.J., Watson, B.C., & Finitzo, T. (1991). Regional cerebral blood flow in developmental stutterers. *Archives of Neurology, 48*, 509–522.

Riley, G.D. (1972). A stuttering severity instrument for children and adults. *Journal of Speech and Hearing Disorders, 37*, 314–321.

Riley, G.D., & Riley, J. (1983). Evaluation as a basis for intervention. In D. Prins & R.J. Ingham (Eds.), *Treatment of stuttering in early childhood: Methods and issues.* San Diego, CA: College-Hill Press.

Riley, G.D., & Riley, J. (1989). Physician's screening procedure for children who may stutter. *Journal of Fluency Disorders, 14*, 57–67.

Schwartz, H., & Conture, E.G. (1988). Subgrouping young stutterers: Preliminary behavioral observations. *Journal of Speech and Hearing Research, 31*, 62–71.

Sherman, D. (1952). Clinical and experimental uses of the Iowa Scale of Severity of Stuttering. *Journal of Speech and Hearing Disorders, 17*, 316–320.

Shipley, K.G., & McAfee, J.G. (1998). *Assessment in speech-language pathology* (2nd ed.). San Diego, CA: Singular Publishing Group.

Silverman, F.H. (1980). The stuttering problem profile: A task that assists both client and clinician in defining therapy goals. *Journal of Speech and Hearing Disorders, 45*, 119–123.

Silverman, F.H. (1996). *Stuttering and other fluency disorders* (2nd ed.). Boston: Allyn & Bacon.

Silverman, S.W., & Ratner, N.B. (1997). Syntactic complexity, fluency and accuracy of sentence imitation in adolescents. *Journal of Speech and Hearing Research, 40*, 95–106.

Stocker, B. (1980). *The Stocker probe technique: For diagnosis and treatment of stuttering in young children.* Tulsa, OK: Modern Educational Corp.

Vanryckeghem, M., & Brutten, G.J. (1996). The relationship between communication attitude and fluency failure of stuttering and nonstuttering children. *Journal of Fluency Disorders, 21*, 109–118.

Wall, M.J., & Myers, F.L. (1995). *Clinical management of childhood stuttering.* Austin, TX: Pro-Ed.

Watkins, R.V., & Yairi, E. (1997). Language production of children whose stuttering persisted or recovered. *Journal of Speech-Language and Hearing Research, 40*, 385–399.

Watson, J.O., Gregory, H.H., & Kistler, D.J. (1987). Development and evaluation of an inventory to assess adult stutterers' communication attitudes. *Journal of Fluency Disorders, 12*, 429–450.

Wilkenfeld, J.R., & Curlee, R.F. (1997). The relative effects of questions and comments on children's stuttering. *American Journal of Speech-Language Pathology, 6,* 79–89.

Wingate, M.E. (1984). A rational management of stuttering. In M. Peins (Ed.), *Contemporary approaches to stuttering therapy.* Boston: Little, Brown & Co.

Woolf, G. (1967). The assessment of struggle, avoidance, and expectancy. *British Journal of Communication, 2,* 158–171.

Yairi, E., Ambrose, N.G., Paden, E.P., & Throneburg, R.N. (1996). Prediction factors of persistence and recovery: Pathways of childhood stuttering. *Journal of Communication Disorders, 29,* 51–77.

Zebrowski, P.M. (1997). Assisting young children who stutter and their families: Defining the role of the speech-language pathologist. *American Journal of Speech-Language Pathology, 6,* 19–27.

Zemlin, W.R. (1998). *Speech and hearing science, anatomy and physiology* (4th ed.). Englewood Cliffs, NJ: Prentice Hall.

CHAPTER 2

Initial Stages and Planning in Management

- Overview
- Procedural Options To Consider
- Associated Behaviors and Avoidances
- Summary

OVERVIEW

Titling a chapter as "Initial Stages" may be misleading for two reasons: (1) the possible implications that the procedures outlined here must be initial, or first, in the therapy plan, and (2) the possible implications that the clinician "should" use each or any of the processes delineated. Neither implication is intended. My personal point of view is that decisions concerning the use of items in this chapter should be made, or the processes actually started within, the first few therapy sessions. The decision well could be not to use one, another, or any. I do not use all of these items for all clients; for some clients, I have used none. However, I hope that each clinician pauses long enough to decide which, if any, might be significant. The chapter starts with factors to consider in planning therapy and then moves through a series of topics. As in chapter 1, and all subsequent chapters, I have selected and developed topics with which I have experience and that meet personal criteria I have developed over the years.

PROCEDURAL OPTIONS TO CONSIDER

The clinician can approach management of a new client with only one question in mind at first, What program can I use? That one word, "program," can be the knell for ethical behavior. Our code of ethics indicates that we will do the best for the client that we can. When a clinician starts with a "What program?" orientation, ethics may die and the welfare of the client may become insignificant. Unfortunately, the primary factor operating here may be *the welfare of the clinician.*

This is not a blanket condemnation of prepackaged programs but of their misuse. There are many good programs on the market. There also are some that are not so good. With all of them, there is a possibility that certain key elements in the therapy of stuttering, dysarthria, aphasia, dysphagia, and so on will be reduced to their lowest common denominator. I do not say "Don't use programs;" I suggest that thoughtful and careful planning go into the entire spectrum of management decisions. In the following divisions of this section, I want to call three areas to your attention:

1. Situational Constraints on Therapy Planning
2. Client Factors Affecting Therapy
3. Clinician Factors Affecting Planning

Situational Constraints on Therapy Planning

Factors beyond the clinician's control dictate the structure of many situations. These factors may be most evident in school settings, but they also function in private practice or general clinic settings. Group or individual therapy settings have strong influences on management selection. Group placement creates a real constraint on individual attention, is particularly useful with children, and can be valuable with adolescents and adults. Group therapy provides valuable opportunities for sharing, interaction, cross-monitoring, fluency analyses, desensitization, pseudostuttering, role play, and other shared activities. It limits individual attention, personal problems, individualized transfer programs, and problem solving on a personal level. Unfortunately, in some settings group work is mandated. It often happens in the schools, and language, articulation, fluency, and so forth are mainstreamed together to the despair of many clinicians and the frustration of many clients.

The frequency and duration of therapy sessions affect management options. What is the value of relaxation therapy for a hypertense stutterer (state/trait anxiety) if the clinician sees that client twice a week for 25 minutes per session? If the suggestions are, as mentioned previously, with a mix of problems in the group, then relaxation work for 5 minutes twice a week will not make it. A factor to be mentioned later—significant others—may rescue low frequency and/or short duration if somebody is available to bridge the gap between in-clinic and out-clinic communication. In planning, with individualized procedures or with programs, frequency and duration factors should be considered.

Equipment is a marginal consideration, because about 95% or more of dysfluency management procedures can be done without special equipment. Of course, *special* has a variable meaning. I am thinking of computers, delayed auditory feedback (DAF) units, metronomes, biofeedback drivers, airflow electronics, and so forth. I assume the availability of an audio cassette recorder. I hope for the availability of portable video cameras and playback units. Various P3 programs require special cards, objects, boards, score sheets, boxes and bags, board games, and other things that are fun and convenient but easy to lose, wear out, or use up. They also, except for that particular P3 program, are not very important in therapy.

Significant others (SOs) are very significant. Wendell Johnson believed that the significant others were the cause of most stuttering. Although that belief is no longer widely held, it is known that significant others can ignore, maintain, and even exacerbate stuttering. In other words, they can be important.

Prepackaged programs often are based on an expectation of outside support and assistance, and individualized programs work better with such support. The clinician needs to consider the availability, the interest, and the understanding of outside persons. Indeed, the lack of availability of significant others can argue against using certain procedures or programs.

Significant others are not only parents, but also teachers, spouses, friends, siblings, and other persons who may have an interest in the client. At times it will be worth a counseling session or two with the nonclients to asses their availability and motivation. This information can be considered in the selection of management approaches and the organization of those approaches selected.

Calendar of care might affect procedure decisions. University training programs routinely interrupt therapy every 8 to 14 weeks and start over again (after a 2- to 6-week break) with a new clinician. Parental vacations and school breaks operate similarly for children. Frequency and duration of sessions aside, the clinician's question should be, "How far can I hope to get on the road to dismissal in what specified period of time?" For adolescent and adult clients, without semester or quarterly vacation breaks, I try to target 18 months for in-clinic management and another 3 years for maintenance follow-up. In a university training program, that 18 months jumps to 3 years, and maintenance may be lost. The times I offer are very approximate and are never offered to the client as guarantees or specific goals. However, I think clients or parents deserve a time estimate.

Special situation factors can affect any management sequence, and that may not be known right away. However, some special factors will be obvious. A few are

- "I do not want my husband to know that Eddie is coming to therapy."
- "I am only coming here because my parents make me."
- "My commanding officer told me if I do not clear this up in 3 months I will not get my second looey [second lieutenant] bars."
- "Never ask me to do any practice or projects on my speech at work."
- "I have a botched-up cleft palate repair and if I change position of any of my articulators I honk like a goose!"

Other problems include finances, health, study schedules, court cases, and religious beliefs. Whether or not the requests are "real" is irrelevant, if they are real to the client. The clinician must consider each and make a decision. The clinician must be sure that it was a decision, and not the lack of a decision, that excluded a factor.

Client Factors Affecting Therapy

The medical model calls for the patient to do or take something so many times per day, in a set quantity, for a set duration, and so on. When instructions are interrupted, questioned, or disputed, frowns abound. Clinicians like to think they treat clients as unique individuals, but the rapid growth of P3 program practices makes these claims somewhat questionable at times. However, there are several client factors that should be considered in developing a management program. These factors are summarized briefly below.

Age

In general, fluency reinforcement options are stressed for up to 8 or 9 years of age (approximate), and significant others tend to be "significant" up through adolescence. Transfer may be automatic up to 5 or 6 years of age, and avoidances are uncommon. Self-monitoring and analysis usually do not function well in early years. Environmental counseling and manipulation may be very profitable early on.

Sex

Females generally tend to present milder spasm patterns, demonstrate subtler avoidances, and be more covert in stuttering. My personal experience suggests that females, at any age, lean more toward fluency reinforcement procedures and are less motivated by symptom modification.

Severity

In terms of spasm frequency, duration, struggle, and so forth, severity tends to affect attitudes toward therapy procedures. In general, I have found that the milder the dysfluency pattern, the greater the attraction of fluency reinforcement to the client and the lower the acceptance level for symptom modification. As in everything, it is not a universal truth, but it is fairly functional.

Motivation

My student clinician and I once dismissed a college-age client and suggested he not return for therapy. We felt his motivation was only to be able to say "I tried to do something about my stuttering, but they could not help me." For 6 months he had ducked, dodged, or outright refused every procedure, fluency, or symptom. His stuttering pattern was 99% avoidance and 1% spasms. Motivation can be internal from the client (I have to do this) or external from somebody else (you have to do this). Therapy programs that involve more client hard work and tolerance are wasted if motivation is low. Home assignments may become a waste of time. Early on, the clinician should check motivation levels and use these findings to guide selections.

Attitude

The attitude of the client is tied to motivation. The clinician hopes the client accepts responsibility for progress and improvement. What the clinician dislikes is a client who feels like a victim and does not accept responsibility. The weaker and the less responsible the attitude, the poorer the prognosis. Also, more clinician oversight and motivational work are required. It may be necessary to pay attention to bibliotherapy, thematic content, desensitization, and other basic areas.

Goals

Goals also relate to motivation. What the clinician needs to discern is what the client really wants out of therapy. Most children and adolescents want plain fluency, zero stuttering. In fact, they usually want to be more fluent than people who do not stutter at all. Adult fluency clients often will express goals of wanting to talk better and be in control. They also want fluency, but generally do not think it is likely.

In planning therapy, the stronger the 100% fluency goal is for the client, the more procedure choices lean toward fluency reinforcement. Of course, many fluency programs have a dismissal criterion of 0.5 or less stuttered words per minute (sw/m), or the equivalent. When mature clients are insistent on a fluency goal, I accept this desire and work toward it. Along the way, I mix bibliotherapy, self-analysis, and desensitization in therapy to the extent the client will accept them. I hope for goal attitude change.

As therapy progresses I look for residual dysfluency patterns that will motivate the client toward developing some problem-solving and maintenance control systems. In clients up to 8 or 9 years of age my target is a stable, fluent speech pattern. Another goal factor is the client's expressed time frame. Many adult clients will indicate they are willing to work for a few months; thus counseling and decision change need to be a part of the plan. Children usually do not put time constraints on therapy. Any amount of time is too much. Nevertheless, until adolescence, children usually will do what adults ask them to do.

Overt/Covert Stuttering Patterns

If the client is a very covert, quiet stutterer, prognosis is probably fairly poor for any therapy approach. If the client cannot be changed into a more overt, accepting stutterer, the clinician should employ fluency reinforcing procedures. Also, the clinician should incorporate bibliotherapy, desensitization, pseudostuttering (probably will be rejected), and monitoring of speech.

Avoidances

Avoidances create the approximate psychological situation found with the covert stutterer. The added problem here is the number and intensity of strongly habituated avoidance behaviors. A client I recently supervised, if asked his name, would say: "My name mm, hmm, hmm, hmmm, well, mmm, hmmm, yes, it's mmm. . . ." This response could go on for only 3 or 4 seconds, or up to 30 to 40 seconds. He rejected fluency-type Easy Onset work because he felt it drew attention to his speech. When challenged by recordings of 30 to 40 second postponements, he replied, "Well, that's just the way I talk!"

Avoidances can become part of the person. The clinician needs to decide whether certain avoidances have to be targeted early in therapy, whether some can be picked up later at opportune times in a program, or whether they are avoidances that will be dissolved or neutralized by progressive reductions in stuttering spasms. However, this decision needs to be a thoughtful one. It is unwise for the clinician to ignore avoidances and hope that Easy Onset will displace them.

Cognitive Factors

Cognitive factors need to be considered. Children and adults with inadequate intellectual capacity can, and do, stutter. Complexity of therapy concepts, attention spans, and multiple-step procedures may cause diffi-culties and need to be evaluated before selection. Children always will need simpler procedures than older persons, for example.

Graduate-degree speech-language pathologists (SLPs) often forget that many clients lack their educational and linguistic sophistication. Of course there is a reverse side to every caveat. One of my past clients was a European university professor, and his restatements and clarifications of my directions and definitions were wondrous (and embarrassing) to hear. Some clients will want to know everything; others just want to feel that the clinician knows everything.

Clinician Factors Affecting Planning

Therapy of stuttering is not popular with many clinicians. The frequent lack of satisfactory dismissal fluency and the high relapse rate are probable reasons. Another factor is the inadequacy of most training programs in fluency disorders. Still another would be that most SLP students graduate with management experience involving no more than (at most) two flu-ency clients for a total of 16 to 40 sessions.

What many clinicians fail to realize is that almost all stuttering therapy techniques are used routinely with other communication disorders. Dysarthria and aphasia need rate reduction, Easy Onset is used well with dyspraxia or hypertense vocal function, as is relaxation, and so on.

The clinician needs to assess his or her level of knowledge about stuttering, and progress from there. The American Speech-Language-Hearing Association (ASLHA) Special Interest Division #4 (Fluency and Fluency Disorders) has been working on definitions, guidelines for competency, and mentoring programs. Realization is yet in the future, and application farther. A clinician also needs to be aware of the differences between fluency reinforcement and symptom modification, historically and today. For earlier divisive statements, I direct the reader to my discussion (Ham, 1989, pp. 117–124). For more recent integrative developments I strongly recommend the 1991 text by Peters and Guitar, where the two approaches are discussed and combined. Finally, I recommend the information sources of the National Stuttering Foundation, and the support and advocacy organizations cited later in this chapter and in chapter 9.

First Meetings

I will not discuss client introductions and that mysterious process called establishing rapport. Exactly how the clinician proceeds with certain activities, and the depth or intensity of the activity, depends on the client factors discussed earlier. The time factor of first meetings also depends on the loquacity of the client. Just a few months ago I observed a student clinician go through three typed pages of questions in 17 minutes. She then began to panic when she realized she had covered her entire preparation and still had 43 minutes to go. Another client might have spent the entire hour on her first page.

I will not go too deeply into specific questions, but those presented in chapter 1 can be drawn on, as well as this discussion. The clinician should never hesitate to replicate questions from diagnostics. Clients may have thought of additional information, changed their mind, or wanted to ask some questions of their own. The reasking of questions applies whether a client is in for a 2nd, 5th, or 15th experience in therapy. Answers and situations can change, and so can the perceptions and understandings of the people involved. Areas in which questions can be formulated or information can be exchanged include, but are not limited to:

1. Statements of what the clinician wants to find out in this and the next few sessions, why this information is desired, and what the early goals of therapy are.
2. Early goals of therapy can include:
   - Asking numerous questions.
   - Securing information about the client.
   - Developing some start-up outside assignments.
   - Establishing the client's needs and goals.
   - Initiating a draft of the long-range therapy plan.
3. Statements to elicit the client's definition and description of his or her speech problem and the reasons for seeking therapy.
4. Identification of the terms the client uses to talk about her or his "problem" and their importance to the client.
   - What is the client's name for stuttering and how important is it to him or her?
   - Exactly what does the client do when she or he stutters?
   - Exactly what does the client do to prevent stuttering?
   - What people and situations cause the most difficulty?
5. Evolution of the client's stuttering over the years. The clinician may have to dig for information and model different patterns.
6. Identification of past therapy history. Obviously, past therapy failed, or the client relapsed, or she or he would not be here. Therefore, the client may be reluctant to discuss past history and feign forgetfulness. Probes and re-coverage are appropriate, and they may be inserted into sessions over periods of months to keep building the information bank. It is not at all unusual for a client to have "done everything" the clinician suggests. Clients also have a real tendency, when a new procedure is presented, to say "That's not the way I learned it before." This reaction should prompt exploration of the client's experience with the procedure. (*Note:* There is absolutely no barrier to using an approach previously used with a client. The situation, the clinician, the concepts, and even the client are not the same as before.)
7. Incorporation, on a regular, recurring basis, of "Tell me about you" questions. The clinician can never know too much likes and dislikes; family members, friends, and enemies; successes and failures; classes, teachers, bosses, and coworkers; jobs or job hopes; entertainment and hobbies; and so on.
8. Identification of current and perceived future burdens or problems created by stuttering.

9. Identification of client concerns about therapy (e.g., possibility of failure, the amount of work demanded, avoidance of embarrassing activities, and so forth).
10. Repetition, with expansions of the goals of early sessions, inviting questions and comments.
11. Assignment of tasks and bibliotherapy to make client feel that things are being done and therapy is under way.

Outside Assignments in Therapy

Orientation

Some clinicians avoid assignments because they doubt their value versus the time taken, do not like the extra work, and do not want to deal with clients who have to be pushed to perform at all, much less perform adequately. The clinician can make assignments fail, or be of little worth, in a number of ways.

- Do not give any.
- Give meaningless busy work.
- Give too many.
- Give assignments that are too easy.
- Provide no client choices.
- Fail to check on assignments.
- Fail to link assignments to clinical activity.

Why use assignments? The reasons are many and varied. Every time the clinician gives a client an assignment, he or she is transferring some management responsibility to the client. It takes learned behaviors from an in-clinic performance and establishes the idea of transferring that behavior to out-clinic life. Whether the client is 7 or 27 years of age, he or she will say "I just forget to use the ___ when you're not around to remind me." Outside assignments contribute, progressively, to a series of skills and habits that must be practiced.

- Self-monitoring—How/what did I do or not do?
- Self-evaluation and analysis—What were the characteristics and how well were they carried out?
- Self-consequation—What do I do about it?

Elements of Adequate Assignments

I learned the value of home assignments the hard way. My master's degree supervisor had clients come for therapy every day, 5 days a week. I assisted with one stutterer, originating three to five assignments every day of the week for the client to select two to three to perform. Grinding out 21 assignments a week for 15 weeks—315 different assignments—was hard. To ensure quality consistency, without warning, the supervisor would announce "role reversal" day and I would have to carry out the assignments he had drawn up, and the client acted as clinician. From that experience I offer seven suggestions about the characteristics of a good assignment.

1. Relevance. Assignments can review past work or expand current efforts, but they must relate to the current needs of the client and the therapy program.
2. Value. There has to be something in the assignment that is of current or future value to the client.
3. Reasonable. An assignment should be doable, in the client's terms. For some covert-type clients, one telephone call and one conversation is demanding; for some overt-type clients, 10 efforts at each activity might be reasonable.
4. Difficulty. Any assignment should be set at a difficulty level that already has been achieved in the clinic or under supervision. Failure can occur on any assignment, but it should not occur often. When it does happen, it calls for clinician self-evaluation. I am not referring to failure to try, but failure by the client in an honest effort.
5. Selection. Sometimes a particular situation or need of the client will dictate specific assignments. Otherwise, it usually helps to give the client a "do this" or "do that" choice. The assignment not selected can be saved for another time.
6. Reporting. The clinician should not create a lot of paperwork and assignment forms. Records should be kept, even if it only is a list of words stuttered on, situation labels entered, "good-fair-poor" ratings on eye contact efforts, and so on. Providing the client with simple report forms often is a help. Also, within a particular assignment, choices are useful, such as: "Prewrite your questions and then make

___3, ___5, or ___7 telephone calls each day for the next five days and. . . ."
7. Reward. An acceptable part of an assignment is a reward. It can be material (Buy yourself a ___ if you do well.) or psychological (Cancel your next assignment if you score above 85%.).

Application Methods for Assignments

At the end of a session, do not treat assignments casually. If an assignment is worth the client's time and effort, it is worth taking 5 or 10 minutes at the end of a session to go over it thoroughly and discuss it with the client. Content of the discussion includes

- The schedule (number of days, repeats, time spent, etc.)
- The task (explain and demonstrate if needed)
- Form and detail of any reporting
- Solicitation of questions from client
- Securing of commitment, or negotiation of revision

At the other end of the assignment continuum, the clinician must never forget to call for and review each assignment on its due date. The clinician must physically look at reports or summaries, ask for particulars, compliment or reward successful work (or genuine effort), and ask the client for her or his own evaluation as well as for suggestions of how the design could have been improved (gives basis for a future assignment or for the client to take over planning assignments gradually). If the client is young enough, a separate score sheet or visible record for assignment achievements can be used.

If feasible, the clinician should check on assignment performance with in-clinic repeats or with supervised out-clinic experiences. It keeps the clinician aware of client evaluation (and performance) standards and may reveal strong and weak areas of which the client is unaware. Occasionally, the clinician should perform assignments for the client so he or she can compare performances. A periodic review also helps the clinician keep an eye on a possible problem of "Let's don't, but say we did." It is not uncommon for clients who do not perform well to glorify their report, or who do not perform, to lie. Clients with a multitude of excuses can be a real problem as well. It is impossible to specify how to motivate specific individuals, but a regular monitoring and rechecking pattern will eliminate or reduce many problems. If a nonconforming client is over 9 or 10 years of age, the clinician should formally advise him or her that prognosis estimates have just dropped by about 50% due to failure to perform assignments.

Bibliotherapy

Orientation

Bibliotherapy originally referred to the use of printed material (biblio = book forms) but now includes audio and video materials. The method is used to provide background and historical information, and related material concerning stuttering and therapy. Its use saves in-clinic time, generates discussion topics for later sessions, and may steer the client in particular directions the clinician wants to develop. Subject matter may focus on theory, descriptions, specific topics, and therapy methods, or concern autobiographies and experiences of other stutterers.

Bibliotherapy is an adjunct to therapy that probably is too neglected today. Programs tend to organize around doing things rather than learning and talking about them. That is not bad, however, knowledge increases self-security, reduces the negative effects of the unknown, reduces victimization feelings, increases feelings of not being alone (I'm not the only person who stutters), and so on. Bibliotherapy is very useful with parents, with mature clients, and even with clinicians. I am not going to suggest how to use bibliotherapy material, but it has applications for group, individual, fluency or symptom orientations, first meetings and maintenance, outside assignments, and so on. One guideline is in order: If bibliotherapy assignments are made, the clinician cannot assume that good will come of them and forget about them. The clinician must check on progress, encourage questions, and ask questions to probe compliance and thought processes. The clinician must remember that reading ability levels of clients vary. I frequently use the Stuttering Foundation of America's *Self-Therapy for the Stutterer* and may ask the client to buy a copy (very inexpensive). On a reading level and motivation basis, some clients return 48 to 72 hours later and have finished the entire publication. Other clients are still less than halfway through the work by the end of 30 days.

Suggested Resources

Exhibit 2–1 is a resource list composed of texts and organizations that may be useful. Some of the sources are client oriented; some are clinician oriented; some are both.

Exhibit 2–1 Resource list

Arthur, R. (1964). *The mystery of the stuttering parrot.* New York: Random House. (A juvenile detective-adventure story.)

Berne, E. (1964). *Games people play.* New York: Ballantine Books. (A layperson's introduction to transactional analysis that covers a multitude of "games," including some that clinicians may play.)

Bloodstein, O. (1993). *Stuttering: The search for a cause and cure.* Boston: Allyn & Bacon. (A professional but easy-to-read history of people and developments in stuttering therapy circa 1930 to 1990.)

Conture, E.G. (1990). *Stuttering* (2nd ed.). Englewood Cliffs, NJ: Prentice Hall. (A text that contains useful explanations and models for use in therapy with young clients.)

Culatta, R., & Goldberg, S.A. (1995). *Stuttering therapy, an integrated approach to theory and practice.* Boston: Allyn & Bacon. (A text with some sophistication that has nearly 60 pages devoted to treatment programs.)

Curlee, R.F. (Ed.). (1993). *Stuttering and related disorders of fluency.* New York: Thieme Medical Publications. (A general text, by contributors; somewhat sophisticated, but contains some useful chapters, particularly Dill's chapter on school-age stutterers.)

Curlee, R.F., & Siegel, G.M. (1997). *Nature and treatment of stuttering, new directions* (2nd ed.). Boston: Allyn & Bacon. (A general text containing useful information areas for adult stutterers.)

Emerick, L.L. (1970). *Therapy for young stutterers.* Danville, IL: The Interstate Printers & Publishers. (A very brief, but useful, source for the age group.)

Ham, R.E. (1986). *Techniques of stuttering therapy.* Englewood Cliffs, NJ: Prentice Hall. (A wonderful text oriented to older stutterers and to symptom modification.)

Ham, R.E. (1989). *Therapy of stuttering: Preschool through adolescence.* Englewood Cliffs, NJ: Prentice Hall. (Text aimed at preschool and young clients.)

Kent, R.D. (1994). *Reference manual for communication sciences and disorders.* Austin, TX: Pro-Ed. (Not limited to stuttering, but very useful section on evaluation and management activities with stutterers.)

National Council on Stuttering, 558 Russell Road, DeKalb, IL 60115. (A support and advocacy group; useful early or late in therapy.)

National Stuttering Project, 5100 East LaPalma Drive, Suite 208, Anaheim Hills, CA 82807. (A support and advocacy group; useful early and late in therapy.)

continues

Exhibit 2–1 continued

Peters, T.J., & Guitar, B. (1991). *Stuttering, an integrated approach to its nature and treatment.* Baltimore: Williams & Wilkins. (Its integrated approach is its particular value.)

Selmar, I.W. (undated). *Help! My child is starting to stutter.* Danville, IL: The Interstate Printers & Publishers. (Very short, but useful, publication for parents.)

Shames, G.H., & Florance, C.L. (1980). *Stutter-free speech: A goal for therapy.* Columbus, OH: Charles E. Merrill. (A very interesting behavior modification approach to rate reduction therapy through delayed auditory feedback.)

Shipley, K.G., & McAfee, J.G. (1998). *Assessment in speech-language pathology.* San Diego, CA: Singular Publishing Group. (Useful for evaluation forms.)

Silverman, F.H. (1996). *Stuttering and other fluency disorders* (2nd ed.). Boston: Allyn & Bacon. (Text with very good chapters for disfluency/dysfluency counseling and good appendixes for evaluation and management forms.)

Speak Easy International, 293 Concord Drive, Paramus, NJ 07652. (Support and advocacy group, useful early or late in therapy.)

Starkweather, C.W. (1986). The development of fluency in normal children. In H. Gregory (Ed.), *Stuttering therapy: Prevention and intervention with children.* Memphis, TN: Stuttering Foundation of America. (Very useful in counseling parents and teachers.)

Stuttering Foundation of America, P.O. Box 11749, Memphis TN 38111. (The top advocacy organization and inexpensive resource for printed and video material about stuttering; write for resource list and costs.)

Wall, M.J., & Myers, F.L. (1995). *Clinical management of childhood stuttering.* Austin, TX: Pro-Ed. (Useful for the age group indicated.)

Pseudostuttering or Faking

One area of strife between symptom modification proponents and fluency reinforcement adherents is pseudostuttering, or faking. Those not involved in disciplinary philosophics have leaned away from faking because it is hard to do and embarrassing. I have discussed the philosophic conflicts extensively (Ham, 1986, 1989) and will not repeat them here. I will, however, advocate its use and support its value to both client and clinician, as delineated below.

Clinician. Pseudostuttering increases credibility with the client, provides the client with models, helps the client in early stages of spasm modification or analysis, and demonstrates the various changes possible in the client's personal stuttering pattern or how various disfluency modes of control can be used in fluency reinforcement or symptom modification.

Client. Pseudostuttering helps in desensitization, monitoring, and self-analysis. It enables the client to alter and simplify her or his own stuttering pattern; can be used in transfer and maintenance work; and helps in the development of self-efficacy (i.e., it is possible to be disfluent and not stutter).

Pseudostuttering divides into two categories—faking for the client and faking for the clinician. Both are addressed; however, the focus is on the clinician because the stutterer already is qualified as an expert in performing stuttering and mainly needs work on voluntary variations of it.

Pseudostuttering (Faking) for Clinicians

Definitions

Learning to stutter is a required element of my undergraduate and graduate fluency disorders classes. Every student, solo and with a partner, goes through a sequence to learn the various forms of pseudostuttering behaviors.

The basic stuttering spasm divides into two major categories, before subdividing and varying.

1. Clonic spasms (repetition)—alternating contractions and relaxations of opposing muscle groups. Spasms may be relatively slow or fast, relaxed or tense, rhythmic or disrhythmic.
2. Tonic spasms: (1) prolongations—where opposing muscle groups contract at the same time, to the extent that speech production components can move only at a slowed rate and prolonged duration and at a high tension level; and (2) stoppage—where opposing muscle groups are in a state of tetany (frozen, cannot move). There is no air release, no phonation, no articulator movement.

Stoppage has been called a "tense pause," which is a misleading label. A pause is a temporary interruption in effort; a stoppage can be either temporary or permanent (speaker gives up speech attempt). On the other hand, a tense pause may be a pause while an anxious speaker tries to think of the statement he or she so carefully memorized and now has forgotten. She or he is pausing to remember and is tense because of stage fright. All blocks or stoppages are tense pauses, but not all tense pauses constitute stuttering.

Repetitions, prolongations, and stoppages (blocks) constitute the forms of basic stuttering spasms. Over time and maturation, mergers occur where there are clonotonic (primarily repetition with partial prolongations and/or stoppages mixed in) or tonoclonic (primarily prolongation and/or stoppage with interrupting bursts of repetitions during release struggles) spasms, or both, in a client's speech.

In learning to stutter, clean, uncomplicated patterns are needed. The complexities are added later. Then some common associated behaviors (e.g., basic word-directed avoidances) are incorporated.

Acquisition Steps

It is best to work with a partner, preferably another SLP. However, spouses and friends also can be recruited. A mirror and an audio cassette recorder are required.

A word of advice is in order: Nonstutterers never achieve a comfort level with pseudostuttering. The value of being able to pseudostutter lies in the payoffs in therapy and counseling.

- *Step 1.* Below is a list of 45 words. Read the entire set aloud, in groups of three. In each triad fake a *repetition* on the first word, fake a *prolongation* on the second word, and fake a *stoppage* on the third word. Repetitions are to be easy and rhythmic, about three to five each time; prolongations and stoppages should last about 2 to 3 seconds each and should be tense but not too strong. Do not hit anything hard, and employ no struggle, no overflow, etc. Fake on the first syllable, but if a different syllable feels "right," hit that one. Look at each word and then, while faking, look at yourself in the mirror. Record this effort and play back.

is	fail	fasten	tease	fabulous
was	shoe	silly	ship	argument
near	ring	ever	dine	courageous

go	this	pester	turkey	cannibal
dumb	pet	dinner	rocket	fascination
bet	green	carbon	airplane	stability
aerial	sailor	happy	arguable	minister
comb	freshen	wonder	Halloween	capitalistic
gravy	greasy	candy	scary	political

The effort should sound rather artificial. Notice whether any personal preference has been displayed for one of the three disfluency types. Also, see if any syllables or phonemes seem to do better with a particular disfluency (e.g., initial vowels seem to work best with prolongations, and so on).

- *Step 2.* Repeat Step 1, with one change: on each triad's first word, use a *stoppage*; on each triad's second word, use a *repetition*; and on each triad's third word, use a *prolongation*. Record and analyze as before.
- *Step 3.* Repeat Step 1, with one change: on each triad's first word, use a *prolongation*; on each triad's second word, use a *stoppage*; and on each triad's third word, use a *repetition*. Record and analyze as before.

In the 135 productions of Steps 1 through 3, each word has been uttered three times, each time with a different major disfluency form. In the past, I have called for the three steps to be repeated with increases in effort and breaks in rhythmic patterns. However, my students suggested that the single-word practice, after the first round, was "not real" and that I should move on to sentences. I have done so, but further practice with the isolate words in the first three steps may be performed if desired.

- *Step 4.* Below are nine sentences, also divided into triads, each sentence with an underlined word. Read each triad of sentences aloud, looking in the mirror and recording self. In each triad, the underlined word in the first sentence gets a *repetition*, the underlined word in the second sentence gets a *stoppage* fake, the underlined word in the third sentence gets a *prolongation* fake. Repeat this on the second triad, and then on the third triad. As before, keep the tension and duration levels fairly low. Record and play back for evaluation. Do fakes sound more real in sentences than they did in single words?
  1 <u>Most</u> people have trouble trying to fold up road maps.
  2 He went slowly down the <u>bank</u> of the river toward the bushes.

3 Insert tab A into slot B while bending <u>along</u> the dotted line.

1 The trouble with <u>hobbits</u> is that they are so small when you meet them.

2 The <u>dog</u> backed off slowly, growling at me.

3 Watch out for <u>cabs</u> on rainy days, because they will splash you.

1 The <u>Russian</u> peasant has very little concept of space travel.

2 <u>Try</u> to do the very best job you can.

3 How do I get there from here if I don't <u>know</u> where I am now?

- *Step 5.* Repeat Step 4, but rotate the three disfluency modes and alter the severity aspects as follows:

  – Repetitions—5 to 10 per unit, faster and irregular, some audible forcing

  – Stoppages—3 to 8 seconds each, in the mirror show visible signs of effort and forcing

  – Prolongation—last 3 to 8 seconds each; visible facial and neck tension, audible sounds of vocal effort

  Record, play back, and evaluate. What happens to the disfluencies as efforts intensify?

- *Step 6.* Repeat Step 4, but rotate the disfluency modes again and increase severity as follows:

  – Repetitions—10 to 15 each, hard, loud, irregular repeats. Several times let it merge into an in-out prolongation or stoppage.

  – Prolongations—8 to 12 seconds each, loud, visible, and audible tension. Several times, try to "escape" via a repetition, but fail. Several times, try so hard that you freeze into a stoppage and then back to a prolongation.

  – Stoppages—8 to 12 seconds each, squeeze eyes shut, then open, distort face, etc. Break into repetition or prolongation and then return to stoppage.

  Look at self while faking. Record and evaluate playback.

- *Step 7.* Use the mirror (if no partner) and tape recorder. Read aloud the five sentences below. Each sentence has three words underlined. In this first run-through, in each sentence: fake a moderate-to-severe repetition with the first underlined word; fake a moderate-to-severe stoppage with the second underlined word; and fake a moderate-to-severe prolongation with the third underlined word. On playback (and with partner's feedback) ask: How real are you starting to sound? Which disfluencies seem more real? How tiring is it? (*Note:* If any fake sounds mild, repeat that particular sentence with all three fakes.)

> Washington is noted for its sunny climate and gentle warmth. A sense of honor requires first an awareness of others' needs. Florida students wear snow parkas when the first frost occurs. Dive bombers were extremely vulnerable to any kind of defense. Stutterers have a tendency to avoid speaking opportunities.

• *Step 8.* Repeat Step 7, including recording and play back, but use any fake patterns. All 15 fakes can be repetitions, stoppages, or prolongations, or use a mix. All severity levels should be moderate to severe. Same penalty factors as in Step 7 for mild fakes. Also, in each sentence try to include up to five avoidance behaviors for the whole sentence. Create any mix you want. Select from the options below:
  • postponement
  • substitution
  • starter
  • release
  • revision
  • retrial
  • circumlocution

Mix different forms of the same avoidance, for example:

> Postponement—[silence]; uh; well now; uh well; hmm, hmm; etc.

If you need further information, review avoidances in chapter 1 or later in this chapter.

• *Step 9.* Use the paragraph provided below, and record the effort. First, read the paragraph aloud to establish a baseline standard. As soon as you finish, read it again for faking practice. The paragraph has 152 words, and your target is to be an "average stutterer," stuttering on about 10% of the words. You will want to fake on at least 15 words (you pick them), with no mild spasms, and all but two or three spasms involving one or more avoidances. As soon as you have finished this second reading, perform a third reading. Try to fake stutters on the same words, but absolute imitation is not required. Do not try to stutter in the same way on the same words. Rewind the tape and play back all three efforts. Compare them and evaluate performance. If satisfied, progress to Step 10. Otherwise problem solve and work it out before you continue.

> The question of uncertainty haunts every stutterer. Experience has taught him the words on which he is most likely to stutter, and the situations that cause him the greatest difficulty. However, he always falls short of perfect predictability and, therefore, must anticipate stuttering at any time, regardless of the word or the situation. For many stutterers, this causes anxiety development that spreads to most speaking functions and leaves them prey to all the fears that feed on anxiety. The usual result of anxiety and fear is an exaggeration of the stuttering spasm itself. This comes about in two ways—first, the actual struggle or core behavior of the spasm itself becomes intensified and extended over time and, second, the stutterer develops an increasing supply of avoidant speech production behaviors. The outcome of his efforts to control or avoid stuttering spasms is generally that the stutterer increases his dysfluency and intensifies his anxieties.

- *Step 10.* Set up the mirror and recorder. Ten topics are listed below. Talk aloud to yourself in the mirror (or to a partner, or both) for at least 1 minute on each topic. Fake a moderate-to-severe spasm, with avoidances, somewhere between 5 and 10 times in 1 minute (i.e., every 6 to 12 seconds, or about once in every 10 to 15 words). In 10 minutes of talking, 1 minute at a time, you will generate somewhere between 60 to 120 fakes. After the first topic, stop and play back your effort and see if anything needs fixing. Repeat this after the second minute. Then finish the final eight topics.

  1. My best vacation
  2. My worst class
  3. My first date
  4. My best friend
  5. The last movie I saw
  6. What animal is the best pet? Why?
  7. Defend your political preference

8. Do you work to live, or vice versa? Explain
9. My most embarrassing experience
10. My most rewarding experience

- *Step 11.* Use your partner, or enlist friends. Record. Talk to at least one person you know fairly well, face to face, for at least 5 minutes, explaining what you are doing and why. Explain types of disfluency, avoidances, and so forth. Fake at least three spasms per minute, moderate to severe. Ask auditor what she or he observed about your eye contact, their reactions, etc. Evaluate recording.

Other exercises could include talking to another person on the telephone and following the preceding exercise exactly. Or, stop 10 strangers (e.g., store clerks, restaurant workers, etc.) and ask questions or give orders. Fake (moderate-to-severe spasms with avoidances) at least twice with each person. Afterward, evaluate responses, feelings, levels of severity, realism, and so on.

Pseudostuttering for Clients

Rationale

Why should a stutterer learn how to stutter when he or she already stutters and has come to therapy to stop stuttering? There are at least nine reasons.

1. To aid the client in monitoring, self-analysis, and development
2. To decrease sensitivity and increase tolerance for disfluency
3. To compensate for in-clinic adaptation (very common) so that the client has "stuttering spasms" to use in practicing fluency controls or symptom modification techniques
4. To increase feelings of self-efficacy
5. To help get started on various steps of therapy
6. To teach the stutterer firsthand that a spasm consists of different levels of complexity and effort and that these can be progressively reduced
7. To help the stutterer control spasms
8. To practice (or negatively practice) targets specifically selected for reduction or elimination
9. To use in maintenance practice after dismissal

Acquisition Steps

There is no set way for the client to learn to fake stuttering, except perhaps to make sure that he or she receives careful preparation in monitoring, self-analysis, and desensitization either before, or as a part of, faking. Being able to stutter may not be the problem; being willing to stutter may very well be. Faking can be one of the first steps of therapy, or the clinician can wait until the client is well on the way in applications of fluency controls or symptom modification techniques. Some of the approaches require developments that typically occur later in therapy, but client variations will dictate actual form and pressure levels. The easiest approaches are:

- Use all or any part of the 11 steps sequenced for clinicians.
- Have an experienced clinician model different stuttering patterns for the client to imitate.
- Have the client observe other stutterers (tape, group work) and practice imitating their different patterns.

Having the client imitate his or her own pattern is widely used, and I have separated it from the above for one reason. For a client, any faked spasm is likely to turn real, but much more so in efforts at self-imitation. At all times, the client must understand that it is all right. In fact, that tendency can be pushed deliberately for clients who adapt too quickly and provide little or no stuttering for fluency measurement or symptom controls. This phenomenon can be used later in therapy to look for "trigger" points in abnormal articulatory preparatory sets (see chapter 8). Five additional values of having the client imitate self include:

1. Gain awareness of avoidance behavior and work on elimination.
2. Develop the idea that the client can control stuttering by learning to stutter differently.
3. Exaggerate or otherwise alter the intensity, struggle, duration, or other characteristics of typical spasms.
4. Provide rehearsal for symptom modification techniques such as cancellation, pull outs, or preparatory sets.
5. Provide rehearsal for fluency controls models such as Easy Onset, Light Contact, and so on.

Sample Client Assignments

Ten sample client assignments are as follows:

1. Use a list of 50 words; read aloud and record. On each word, use one of your own avoidance behaviors. If there is more than one, rotate them. If a word turns into a real spasm, let it. However, note to see if any particular avoidance seems more likely to trigger a spasm than others.

2. Take a paragraph of about 300 words and underline the 20 words you might stutter on if you were reading to an audience. As you read aloud, try a variation of your usual spasm on each underlined word. If it turns real, take note, and go on. Repeat this exercise with eight or nine more paragraphs over several days. Now look back and see if you can find any common factors on the words where stuttering turned real.

3. Use a word list or a paragraph. On any real stuttering, immediately repeat the word with a slowed, exaggerated version of the spasm you just had.

4. Read a list of 50 words aloud while the clinician or a friend marks any words on which you stuttered on a copy of the list. Exchange sheets. Read and fake on all newly marked words (only). If any fakes become real, accumulate all such words and run them again. Try three more times.

5. Take a list of 10 words on which you have actually stuttered in the recent past (in-clinic or out-clinic experiences). Read each word aloud, faking a different pattern than your usual. If it turns real, finish the word, pause and breathe, relax, and try the same thing again with an easy Bounce (see chapter 6).

6. Have clinician read single words aloud (can be put on tape for home assignments), faking various types of spasm. Have clinician pause about 5 seconds between words. During pause, imitate the modeled spasm.

7. Select one of your most common avoidance behaviors and deliberately insert it (as a fake), stuttering or not, ___20, ___40, ___60 times a day. Record how many times the fake avoidance triggered a real spasm.

8. Set a target, during free speech with the clinician, that you will fake a certain number of spasms as the two of you talk. After each fake,

have the clinician imitate it and guess if it was a real or a fake spasm.

9. Identify several situations you experience fairly regularly that are not particularly stressful. For a period of 4 days, try to fake five stuttering spasms in one such situation each day.
10. Teach a significant other how to fake. Model extensively and evaluate their efforts. Make the lesson last for at least 30 minutes.

Other uses of pseudostuttering will depend on the particular management program that is used. A clinician who cannot fake is asking the client to do something that she or he cannot do—change the way he or she speaks. A clinician who cannot fake is a person who has failed to acquire a useful therapy device, has failed to deal with their own fears and anxiety, and has shown minimal tolerance for dysfluency, but expects the client to achieve in all of these areas.

ASSOCIATED BEHAVIORS AND AVOIDANCES

Overview

Working on associated behaviors is useful and productive early in therapy, but must be done thoughtfully to avoid premature, discouraging failure. Some habits will be very hard to eradicate. In chapter 1, these behaviors were extensively described and defined for evaluation purposes. Exhibit 2–2 delineates associated behaviors and avoidances. The list can go on and on. Some stutterers have 90% or more of their symptomatology covered by physical struggle categories, in terms of time taken and effort expended. Other clients' time and effort are focused on one or both behavioral avoidance categories. In clinical evaluation and the first few management sessions, the clinician needs to establish the exact nature of the syndrome. That information will affect the management plans.

Rationale for Avoidance Reduction

In the early stages of therapy the clinician generally does not try to reduce or eliminate the physical struggle aspects of associated behaviors. These struggles are so intimately a part of the stuttering spasm itself that

Exhibit 2–2 Associated behaviors

Physical struggle
- Spasm struggle (the actual stuttering spasms)
- Proximal struggle (in and physically close to the speech mechanism)
- Distal struggle (overflow to other parts of the body)

Behavioral struggle—Avoidances
- Word-specific avoidances
  - Postponement
  - Retrial
  - Substitution
  - Mutism
  - Release (struggle?)
  - Starter
  - Revision
  - Circumlocution
  - Eye contact
- Communication-general avoidances
  - Mutism/withdrawal
  - Louder/softer volume
  - Stereotyped inflection
  - Belligerence
  - Broad humor, joker
  - Eye contact loss
  - Increased/decreased speech rate
  - Monotone inflection
  - Reduced/varied prosodic stress
  - Subservience
  - Physical movement distractions
  - Dialect, accent variations

early direct work usually leads to failure and frustration. This caution does not apply if the clinician uses a fluency reinforcement approach, because replacement of stuttering with fluency is the primary goal of such therapy. However, in fluency reinforcement or in symptom modification, early work on other associated behaviors can be valuable. In fluency reinforcement programs, there typically is a grinding period of time when the client is practicing, for example, 30 to 40 or 50 to 60 words per minute (wpm) rates, or metronome rates set at 40 to 60 beats per minute (bpm), or DAF settings around 250-ms delay, or Easy Onset at the "leaky tire" sounding stage, or breath chewing at the "hot potato speech" stage. At those times, clients are sure of one thing—they sound terrible and never want to talk like that. While working through such frustrating levels to more speech-natural levels, avoidance reduction activities can be intermingled. The client can feel, "I am working on my stuttering," and usually will see some tangible progress. Also, in fluency reinforcement, when it reaches the usual termination criterion of 0.5 or less sw/m, there will still be residual stuttering. Where there is stuttering, there will be avoidances (Ham's law). As a result, avoidance reduction will reinforce the maintenance of fluency and hopefully contribute to relapse resistance. On the symptom modification side, avoidance reduction or elimination is important at every stage of therapy, from first day to dismissal. Indeed, for programs such as those developed by Sheehan (1970), avoidance reduction is the primary focus of therapy.

Thus, attention to physical struggle behaviors occurs in therapy aimed at controlling or eliminating stuttering moments. Word-specific avoidances are a good target early on for nearly all types of programs, and they can be dealt with throughout therapy. The communication-specific avoidances will vary in terms of their concern in therapy. Some will disappear, without extra attention, as speech and sense of speech control improve. Other aspects are part of the client's personality and her or his adjustment to life. If these aspects are to change significantly, they can be addressed best by professionals trained in counseling and psychotherapy.

Selection of Avoidance Behaviors

The general rule of thumb in selection of avoidance behaviors is to go first for the psychological effect on the client, rather than for the most significant effect on the dysfluencies. Sometimes they coincide. Early in therapy, clients need to have some visible or audible signs that therapy is worth it all. Changes in speech behavior typically are the signs desired most, and avoidances (some at least) are the easiest to change. From diagnostic reports and observations the clinician must categorize the various associated behaviors and describe them. Over the weeks and months of therapy, additions to the list can be made. The clinician's selection from the list may be easy, or they may be confusing. Some factors to consider are as follows:

- *Client awareness.* The more aware the client is of a particular behavior, the easier it should be to control or eliminate it.
- *Obviousness of behavior.* Awareness or not, the more overt, gross, or extended a behavior is, the easier it is to bring to awareness. Quiet little "mmm, mmm" behaviors may be hard to control, while "uh HEH uh HEH!" two to five times in a very loud voice should be easy to eliminate.
- *Client preference.* The behaviors that bother the clients, or significant others, the most are candidates for elimination. This factor links to awareness, but carries feelings and attitudes as well.

- *Frequency of occurrence.* Some avoidances occur only under special circumstances, at very high levels of anxiety, on particular words, and so forth. Common behaviors offer more opportunities and incentives.
- *Longevity.* The life history of a particular behavior is important. The "older" an avoidance is, the harder it will be to eradicate. Unfortunately, clients rarely have very good recall as to when a behavior was adopted.
- *Proximity.* The distance between the behavior and the actual spasm is very influential. Proximity has two dimensions:
  1. Space—the nearer, physically, an avoidance movement is to the speech mechanism, the more difficult it will be to gain control (e.g., a lip-licking postponement is harder to get hold of than a head-scratching behavior).
  2. Time—the nearer in time to a spasm a behavior is, the more difficult control will be. Postponements are more difficult than substitutions, but easier than starters. In turn, starters are easier than release efforts.
- *Singularity.* The more unusual or nontypical a behavior is, the easier control will be. This factor often equates to obviousness. A postponement of "Well uh . . ." is much less obvious than one of "Aw, heck. . . ."
- *Isolation.* A postponement of "uh . . . uh . . . uh" without further insertions is easier to handle than "Well now, uh, you see, uh, uh, it's, well, I think. . . ."
- *Effectiveness.* Nothing succeeds like success, and avoidances are no exception. If a client feels the avoidance is really effective (i.e., really helps reduce stuttering), then enthusiasm for elimination may be minimal. This feeling will be increased if, during early control efforts, the stuttering spasms increase in frequency or intensity.

Attack on Avoidances

As I have stated before, the attack on avoidances may never stop in therapy. The reasons are many, including the number and complexity of avoidances some clients display, the lack of client cooperation, the need to postpone addressing some behaviors until later in therapy, and Jost's law (my paraphrase)—old habits tend to return and displace the new behaviors that originally replaced them. The clinician should assume that attention to associated behaviors will never stop.

Monitoring

In order to be aware of avoidances, identify types, categorize them, and evaluate effects, the client must work at watching and listening. Many avoidances are so automatic that nothing can be done until they are successfully monitored. Some avoidances, like other habits, can be reduced or eliminated just by monitoring (i.e., as long as someone is watching [e.g., nail biting] no biting occurs). Two basic steps are:

- *Step 1: Establish a baseline.* The clinician must define the client's associated behaviors and then focus on the word-specific avoidances. This effort will lead the client to become aware of all the avoidance behaviors that she or he performs. The client should not be advised of what they are, but be allowed to find them out personally. If the client seems to lack such ability or knowledge, the clinician may read aloud or talk to the client while faking the various avoidances the client typically uses. After 1 minute or so, the clinician should stop and ask, "What avoidances did I use on what words?" After doing this about 10 times, it is time to record the client (audio or video), play it back, and inquire, "Now, what do you do when you speak?"
- *Step 2: Combine resources.* The clinician should use mirror work, audiotape, and videotape while the client reads and talks aloud. After replaying recordings and referring back to earlier definitions, the clinician may ask, "Do you see or hear any starters . . . was that a long pause or a real postponement . . .?" and so on.

The latter step usually needs to be sampled several times. From this preliminary effort the clinician will want to move up to activities such as in-clinic telephone calls, in-clinic visits from strangers, and supervised out-clinic projects. The discussion of monitoring in chapter 3 will provide examples of activities. Also, the client should be performing regular home assignments as fast as he or she shows competence at monitoring and evaluation. If the client decreases (or eliminates) any behaviors, that is fine but it is not the goal yet.

Self-Analysis

Self-analysis is a vital part of avoidance attacks (and especially crucial in fluency therapies). In monitoring eforts, the client worked on tasks to stimulate listening and awareness behaviors. Now the client needs to find out a number of things about each avoidance. The specifics of exactly what is done, how it is done, and when it is done need to be identified. Other elements discussed earlier—obviousness, frequency of use, space and time factors, singularity, isolation, and effectiveness—also need to be defined. The last element is particularly important early on. In the process of self-analysis, some clients may spontaneously elect to reduce or eliminate some behaviors. Chapter 3 contains material relevant to this discussion.

Ranking of Behaviors

Ranking covers another element discussed earlier, client preference. It basically is the action of letting the client set personal priorities, and the clinician interacting with the client to make sure the client considers relevant factors such as behavior longevity, complexity, and so on. A ranking of behaviors helps the client have some idea of where to start, increases the early effort to have the client take responsibility for therapy, and can be referred to over time as therapy progresses.

Trial Runs

Trial runs on behavioral change are a good idea, especially when they are presented to the client as just that, trial runs. The clinician does not want a client early in therapy to try and control a behavior and fail completely. On the other hand, a very successful trial run can be a signal to go full out on the attack against a certain behavior or set of behaviors. In general then, it is better psychology to suggest exploratory efforts at first, rather than all-out attacks. Two examples follow:

1. For the next ___ days, try to collect, each day, five instances where you tried to eliminate the following behaviors (examples follow):
   - The starter, "uh"
   - The postponement, "Well uh . . ."
   - Failure to hold eye contact during a stuttering spasm

If you stutter, go ahead. Best to try only one control per spasm. Report on results, and which behavior was easiest to control.

2. For the next 10 days, try to stop using your postponement avoidance (identify). Each day persevere until you reach the goal set below, then let it go for the rest of the day:

Day 1	1	postponement	Day 2	2	postponements
Day 3	4	postponements	Day 4	8	postponements
Day 5	10	postponements	Day 6	15	postponements
Day 7	20	postponements	Day 8	25	postponements
Day 9	30	postponements	Day 10	40	postponements

If you do not have enough opportunities to control avoidances, then readjust the goals. If you have the opportunities, but find the goal level too much to handle, reset the goals. Handle the schedule as you wish (i.e., start and keep at it until goal is reached; do one third in the morning; one third in the afternoon; one third in the evening; etc.).

Decision Levels

The decision point or level is reached when the trial run information is considered and the clinician and client decide on one of the following:

- Go full-steam ahead after one specific avoidance behavior, or make the avoidance one of several targets.
- Go full-steam ahead on several different avoidances at once, or make the several avoidances one of several targets.
- Delay any avoidance work until the client can relax more, has had some desensitization, and has greater self-confidence.
- Delay any avoidance work until the effect (on avoidances) of other therapy activities is observable.

Avoidance Reduction Summary

As I wrote earlier, if functional avoidances remain in the speech of the client, relapse is almost guaranteed. Avoidances will not "take care of themselves" if they are word specific. Any time stuttering, even infrequent stuttering, occurs on a word, the old avoidances will tend to appear and reinforce the stuttering struggle. On the other hand, avoidances that are communication specific often do respond to general treatment. Greater self-confidence, work on speech naturalness, and so forth may reduce or eliminate many generalized behaviors, even if some stuttering spasms still occur.

SUMMARY

This chapter was placed to follow immediately the chapter on diagnosis and assessment. It contains areas (with those in chapter 3) that I think need to be considered before major therapy activities begin. All too often in teaching and supervision I see new therapy plans that start off with variations of, "The client will begin work on Easy Onset . . . on rate reduction . . . on cancellation. . . ." I smile and begin with a series of suggestions that the student clinician might want to consider before jumping feet first into curing stuttering. These suggestions comprise the bulk of chapters 2 and 3.

REFERENCES

Ham, R.E. (1986). *Techniques of stuttering therapy*. Englewood Cliffs, NJ: Prentice Hall.

Ham, R.E. (1989). *Therapy of stuttering: Preschool through adolescence*. Englewood Cliffs, NJ: Prentice Hall.

Peters, T.J., & Guitar, B. (1991). *Stuttering, an integrated approach to its nature and treatment*. Baltimore: Williams & Wilkins.

Sheehan, J.G. (1970). *Stuttering: Research and therapy*. New York: Harper & Row.

Stuttering Foundation of America. *Self-therapy for the stutterer*. Memphis, TN: Author.

CHAPTER 3

Methods of Monitoring, Evaluation, and Self-Evaluation for the Stutterer

- Rationale for Clinicians
- Rationale for Clients
- Dysfluency Monitoring
- Attitude Evaluation
- Listener Evaluation
- Loci of Stuttering
- Consistency
- Fears and Fear Hierarchy
- Speech Naturalness
- Summary

RATIONALE FOR CLINICIANS

To function adequately in the areas of therapy acquisition, application, transfer, and maintenance, the clinician must be able to evaluate the client's behavior in terms of its *appropriateness, completeness,* and *adequacy.* To be less than capable in these areas of evaluation is to risk (for the client) partial learning, poor self-efficacy, or outright failure. Evaluation of final point behaviors cannot occur if there was no initial evaluation, or if it was incomplete. Likewise, evaluation cannot occur without having the capacity to *monitor,* or to be aware of, variations in behavior. However, monitoring must be consistent and constant.

RATIONALE FOR CLIENTS

It is all well and good for the clinician to monitor and analyze, but what about the client? The client may balk and ask why she or he is "wasting time" on self-monitoring and self-evaluation when it is the clinician's job to work with the stuttering problem. If the client clings rigidly to this point of view, then therapy probably is a waste of everybody's time. Otherwise, the client needs to understand that monitoring and analysis value can extend to, but not be limited to

- Additions to, or corrections of, diagnostic information
- Selecting the major mode(s) and minor techniques to be used later
- Accurate awareness of problem behaviors, rather than overreaction, misinterpretation, or fearful ignorance
- Knowledge of self, behaviors, and feelings
- Abolition of the "all stutterers are alike" stereotype
- Awareness of the frequent fluency problems found in "normal" speakers

A valuable step in therapy management is to have the client confront her or his stuttering as soon as possible to set the tone for future work. One of the best, and most profitable, ways to do so is to focus directly on monitoring and evaluating the actual dysfluencies presented by the client.

DYSFLUENCY MONITORING

Preliminary Questions

In monitoring, clinicians initially want to find out what clients truly know about their speech, as opposed to what they think they know. Questioning the client may be a starting point in that arena. The clinician must try not to answer any of the questions accidently but rather push the client to dig and find answers. If the client denies knowledge and requests information, the clinician must resist the impulse to be an "authority" and suggest that those answers will be uncovered along the way. Starting points for questions include the following queries:

- Physically, what do you do with your tongue, mouth, throat, chest, hands, and body when you stutter?
- What happens to your eye contact when you stutter?
- What is your eye contact like when you are not stuttering?
- Does your head jerk, bob, turn, or otherwise move when you stutter?
- How do you shape your mouth during a block?

- Do you do anything with your hands, arms, feet, or legs when you stutter?
- In general, what do you do to try and prevent stuttering from happening?
- If you are hit with a block, do you fight it or try to escape from it?
- How do other people look when you stutter?
- What are your personal feelings when you think you are going to stutter?
- How do you feel, physically, when a stuttering spasm is over?
- How do most people act when you stutter?
- What behaviors by listeners do you like least?
- What behaviors by listeners do you like most?
- Do you stutter more, less, or the same as you did 1 year ago? Three years ago? Five years ago?
- Do you physically stutter more severely, less severely, or about the same as you did 1 year ago? Three years ago? Five years ago?

These questions touch on areas such as attitude, auditors, and so forth, but just scratch the surface. Based on information already known about the client, the clinician will want to edit this list and add to it. In general, the clinician should listen to and note answers without comments, except to be encouraging and to add spin-off questions as warranted by the client's answers.

Dysfluency Specifics

In this series of questions, which is keyed to the actual moment of stuttering, the clinician must be ready to model, demonstrate different forms, and help the client. This process can be a significant step in desensitization for the client. Also, it usually is a valuable activity in building the credibility and expertise of the clinician (in the eyes of the client) to be able to fake all those different models.

The list that follows can be amended based on knowledge already possessed about the client:

- Do you produce repetitions when you stutter? [Model several patterns.]
- Do you prolong when you stutter? [Model.]

- Do you mix prolongations and repetitions? [Model.]
- Do you produce stoppages when you stutter? [Model silent and voiced.]
- Do you mix stoppages with the other forms? [Model several varieties.]
- If you mix, what mixes seem to predominate?
- If you mix, what percentage of spasms seems to mix?
- On repetitions, does the vowel involved keeps its form (oo, eee, ooo, etc.) or does it seem to become "uh, uh, uh"?
- On repetitions, are the repeats slow/fast, easy/hard, rhythmic/irregular, and so forth?
- Usually, how many times do you repeat on one effort?
- Are repetitions usually phrases, words, part words, syllables, or sounds? If there is a mix, can you divide by percentages?
- What sounds are you most likely to repeat on?
- Do repetition movements seem to be mostly in the tongue? Jaw? Lips? Throat? All of these?
- If your stutterings are divided into short, medium, and long, about how many seconds does each type usually last? Guess if unsure.
  - Short about _____ seconds or less
  - Medium about _____ seconds
  - Long about _____ seconds
- In seconds, about how long did your longest spasm ever last?
- If you prolong in a spasm, do you tend to prolong on the syllable, like "saaa" or on the first sound, like "ssss"?
- Is the spasm form (repetition, prolongation, stoppage) consistent or does it vary from spasm to spasm?
- On stoppage blocks, do you usually get stuck after starting to say the sound you stick on, or do you get stuck before you can get anything out?
- When/if hit by a repetition, what seems to get you unstuck?
- When/if hit by a prolongation, what seems to get you moving?
- When/if hit by a stoppage, what seems to get you unstopped?

It is best to avoid an interminable cross-examination here. The client will tire of it and may become irritable. The list may be accomplished over a series of meetings, mixed in with other early program activities. The clinician may share "what other stutterers have done" to keep interest up, refer to bibliotherapy, work on a little relaxation, and so on. As suggested before, the clinician must resist the impulse to tell the client everything noticed about her or his speech. It is important to let the client figure it out without the clinician's help.

Listening Analysis Tasks

These activities help the client assess his or her ability to notice and remember moments of stuttering. The analysis occurs on three levels: word, sentence, and spontaneous speech.

Word Level

The clinician gives the client a list of words (see below) and asks her or him to read aloud each column, in descending order, until all 32 words have been produced. The client is not to hurry. The clinician records the exercise on tape and marks the words producing a stutter on a copy of the word list.

car	bet	board	past
act	eave	oats	up
devote	number	because	kitchen
under	error	apple	asking
davenport	security	maintaining	likelihood
conspiracy	additional	television	strangulated
dictatorial	impresario	erratically	irritatedly
confidentiality	materializing	insensitivity	superintendency

The clinician should know how to pronounce all the words, but should not help the client. If asked for help, the clinician should encourage the client to do his or her best without modeling. As soon as the client is finished, the clinician makes the following requests:

- "There were 32 words in that list. Tell me how many you stuttered on." No comment is made on the answer.
- "Now, look at the list of words and mark each word you stuttered on."

If the client did not stutter on any words, the clinician moves on. If there were some marked words, the client reads only those aloud in a second round, while the clinician records the effort.

The clinician plays back the tape, without stopping, and directs the client to listen. The clinician unobtrusively watches the client to see if she or he shows overt reactions. After running the complete recording, the clinician completes the following sequence:

- Asks the client, "Did you stutter as often here as if you were reading aloud by yourself, at home? To a friend? To a large group of people?"
- Repeats the above question but changes "as often," to "as severely."
- Asks the client, "Would anything else have been different in these various situations, for example, rate, loudness, inflection, or other variations?"

The tape is rewound and played back, stopping after every stuttering spasm. If, for example, the client stuttered more than 12 to 15 times, the clinician chooses 10 to 12 spasms and asks the client, "What did you do physically, etc., when you stuttered there?" The clinician probes and questions, even replays the tape if it will help. If the client is still not too cued in, it is all right to help with the answers.

If the client complains of not being alerted ahead of time to monitor and analyze, the clinician should tell the client that it was done deliberately to check his or her basic monitoring level and to create a first reminder that constant monitoring is needed. When satisfied that all value has been obtained from the word list (several different lists can be used if the client seems to need it), the clinician moves to the sentence level of evaluation.

It is a good idea to have the client practice self-analysis at home. With a different word list, the client could record and play back the tape, listening for and analyzing spasms. On return to the clinic, the client can play the home tape, and an evaluation of any differences from the clinic efforts can be performed, indicating where improvement may be needed. Another home assignment could be to have the client perform a daily analysis of 10, 20, 30, or 50 spasms, keeping notes on index cards.

Sentence Level

After complimenting the client on word-level performance, the clinician's attention moves to phrases and sentences. The client is asked to read 10 sentences aloud and, after each sentence, answers the following questions:

- Did you stutter on any word? If so, name them.
- What part of the word was stuttered on?

- What was the form of each stutter (repetition, prolongation, etc.)?
- Rate the severity of each stuttering spasm

The following sentences may be used:

- Few people know how to sail a ship.
- Carol liked to play with the Shetland Sheepdogs.
- Big bears can usually beat careful cats.
- Linda's favorite author was Camus, that sad and lonely man.
- I don't know if I can keep up with the rest of the class on calculus.
- Patsy was a mean, smart, persistent, and very intelligent dog.
- The chorus conductor had the upsetting habit of breaking his batons when he was frustrated.
- Ann had that enviable capacity of being able to start a conversation with a doorknob at a party.
- Don stared at the dentist's chair and wondered how it got on his desk.
- One of the problems with trying to monitor stuttering is that you get so tied up with trying to get through a word that you forget to keep score or remember the details.

In no particular fashion, the sentences become longer and more complex. The clinician may want to stop the client at a particular linguistic complexity level and work there. All efforts should be recorded and analysis follows the line of questioning presented previously. However, there are some additional questions made possible by sentence constructs:

- If you stuttered, where in the sentence did it tend to occur?
  - Right at the beginning?
  - Right at the beginning of a phrase within the sentence?
  - On longer or shorter words?
  - On proper names?
  - On stressed syllables?
  - On stressed words?
  - On important words?
- Did one stutter seem to lead quickly to another, or did it give you some "time off?"

- On the longer sentences, did you breathe as often as you needed to?
- If stutterings occurred, did they tend to occur right after a breath?
- Did you tend to slow down or to speed up as you came up to a stuttering? Which did you do right after the stuttering?
- How often did you know a few words in advance that you probably were going to stutter on a particular word?

The clinician is free to add other questions and make up more sentences as needed. This exercise can be used for more than one session unless the stutterer no longer stutters in the clinic due to adaptation. The exercise also can be performed as a home assignment.

Spontaneous Speech

Spontaneous speech nearly always needs to move in graduated steps. The initial level is described first.

While being recorded, the client answers closed-end questions using some of the question words to formulate the answer (reduced communication responsibility). Samples are provided below, but the clinician will need to make up 30 or 40 more questions.

> What is your name?
> My name is Bill Charlton.
> How old are you?
> I am 23 years old.
> How long do you remember stuttering?
> I remember stuttering for 17 years.

The foregoing should be used as an example of how to cue answers to questions, and keep things brief. When the remaining questions are presented, the clinician tells the client to stop if a stuttering occurs when responding. The clinician should be attentive to whether the client stops right after the spasm, or not until the answer is completed. If the client misses a stuttering spasm, he or she is stopped after the end of the reply, and asked if a stuttering occurred. If the reply is "no" or "not sure," the tape is played back.

Some clients will take several sessions to function well at this sentence level, especially if spasms are quite mild. A few clients will knock off the first 10 sentences so thoroughly that this level can be relegated to home assignments.

The next level of spontaneous speech analysis uses a more open-ended question form. As always, the procedure is recorded. The client is instructed to stop as soon after a stuttering spasm occurs as possible. Then, he or she is to perform as thorough an analysis as possible. When the client is finished, the clinician adds his or her analysis. If possible, the analysis should be more thorough than the client's without overwhelming him or her. Then the clinician indicates that these analytical comparisons will occur each time.

Possible cue questions for the client include the following:

- What are the directions to follow to get from here to where you live?
- What is a typical Saturday at your house from getting up to going to bed?
- What would you say if a person asked you, "Well, what do you do when you stutter?"
- Should we allow people to vote before they pay taxes?
- Do you think our legal system meets our needs today?
- What sort of person do you think is qualified to be president of the United States?
- What is your opinion concerning the state of education today?
- Does a male or female make the most reliable friend you could have? Why?

Responses to such questions may be quite long. Rather than wait for a post hoc analysis, the client may be instructed to stop immediately following a spasm.

The clinician should be aware that some published sources contain prewritten questions. Some are quite thought provoking and well suited to therapy.

Stop Capacity

Using the same pattern as before (questions eliciting spontaneous speech), the clinician will want to move closer to the actual moment of stuttering and combine spasm awareness and a capacity to stop or interrupt ongoing speech. The stop capacity is important for several reasons:

- Desensitizes the client; he or she cannot run away from stuttering spasms.
- Represents the first real experiences at controlling stuttering; the client's attitude changes and he or she experiences self-efficacy.
- Increases awareness and monitoring skills.
- Develops information lodes for future use.
- Is a necessary element of most symptom-oriented therapies.
- Is a prerequisite to the later use of cancellations (see chapter 8).

This procedure uses the same types of sentence (closed and open) material, and question/answer formats as used in the prior sections. Paragraph readings and monologue topics also can be used. The client's directions are presented below.

> If you stutter on a word, go ahead and finish the word. Do not stop then. Finish the word. Then, you stop. Pause for 2 or 3 seconds. During the pause, tap on the table with the pencil so the recorder will pick up your signal. The tapping will be something to listen for when we rewind and evaluate. Ready?

After recording about 5 minutes of words, sentences, or discourse, the tape is rewound. Before playing it back, the client is asked to estimate how many times he or she stuttered, if he or she remembers any of the words stuttered on, what kinds of spasms were performed, and so on. In particular, the client should be asked if he or she missed any stuttering spasms; that is, did the client

- Catch a spasm, but fail to stop immediately after?
- Completely fail to be aware of a spasm?

The exercise targets specific aspects more intensely. The characteristics are as follows:

- Awareness—Is awareness excellent, good, or partial? If the answer is "partial," is it because the missed or delayed-response ones are 1 second or less in duration? Client speech rate is too fast? Client is presently a poor stopper? What is the percentage of spasms caught versus spasms produced? 30%? 50%? 90%?

- Stop capacity—Can the client stop right after a stuttered word is completed? Any errors in this area should be corrected. Also, if mild spasms are so brief that following words come too quickly for a precise stop, a percentage of stop targets based on length, severity, type, and so forth will need to be set.
- Analysis—How is the client's analysis capability progressing? The client should be consistently (but not always) asked questions such as
  – What was the form of the spasm?
  – How long did it last?
  – Where was it located at first (larynx, tongue, jaw)?
  – Did struggle spread to face, head, neck, other areas?
  – What happened to eye contact?

For variation, the clinician can have the client talk at length, and then stop her or him randomly after some of the spasms and test her or his analysis skills (with the preceding questions or those from earlier lists).

Specific performance areas can be targeted based on the individual client. For instance, if the client has shown a tendency toward noticeable overflow behaviors, or has a habit of closing his or her eyes or breaking eye contact during spasms, these behaviors can be targeted. Eye contact will be expanded further in a subsequent section of this chapter, but a few suggestions can be offered here.

- Instruct the client that when he or she starts to stutter when reading, that is a signal for the client to look [at the clinician, at himself or herself in the mirror] until the word is finished and then to look back at the page and continue reading. Target 5 minutes where every spasm generates good eye contact. Add 1 minute for every missed eye contact.
- Have the client read aloud a paragraph with 10 words underlined. On each underlined word, the client is to fake any kind of a spasm and create good eye contact with himself or herself. The penalty is the same as before.
- Have the client talk with the clinician for a total of 5 minutes. Instruct the client that the split second a stuttering spasm begins represents a signal to establish and hold eye contact. Each eye contact failure will require the client to repeat the same word with a fake spasm and good eye contact.

The clinician can work out other penalties for failure to maintain eye contact, to stop, or to perform other monitoring tasks. Illustrative examples include the following:

- Add another word, another sentence, or another 15 seconds of talking time.
- Repeat the entire sentence, read or spontaneous, with "perfect" eye contact, regardless of whether or not stuttering reoccurs.

Throughout the monitoring, self-analysis procedures, the clinician will want to work with the client on transfer of monitoring and analysis capabilities. That extension will not be covered here, except to provide a general structure. In most cases, on an out-clinic basis, it is important to use a cassette recorder and a mirror so the client can talk to himself or herself in the mirror and listen to the tape playback. Often people are not consistently available (and willing or able) to perform the auditor role, much less the evaluator function. The clinician can work with the client on transfer of monitoring skills as part of regular management sessions. Again, this activity is covered later and needs only a few specifics here.

- Prewrite telephone calls, make them, and record the client (only). Then analyze and discuss; play back for further evaluation and discussion.
- Make unscripted telephone calls, following the same procedure as above.

Avoidance Behaviors

Once monitoring and analysis are fairly well established at the simple levels described previously, the clinician may wish to monitor and evaluate avoidance behaviors. The clinician may need to "teach" at this point in order for the client to understand what avoidances are, why they should be eliminated, and so on. Definitions must be clear, and each avoidance must be demonstrated by pseudostuttering. The following material is designed to help the clinician with these tasks.

Definition: An avoidance is spasm specific. It is any behavior (audible, movement, pause, gesture) designed to avoid, reduce, or escape stuttering on a specific word.

Common avoidances are:

- Postponement—any behavior designed to delay a speech attempt. Model silent pause, an "uh, er, well, you see," and a shrug.
- Starter—any behavior whose production coincides with and gives support to an attempt to utter the feared word. Model, such as "uh Richard."
- Retrial—when an identifiable attempt to say a word is terminated (not just repeated), there is a pause (long or brief), and a completely new attempt. Model such as "My name is, uh, my name is. . . ."
- Release—any movement, gesture, or audible behavior inserted during the production of a spasm to try and break the spasm cycle. Model a gesture, a sudden pitch shift, and so forth.
- Circumlocution—use of a phrase or multiple words to replace one feared word. Model "I like the spread, the stuff from cows. . . ."
- Substitution—use of a synonym or other replacement word instead of the word originally targeted. Model "Do you have sss . . . any bread?"
- Release—any interjected sound, word, gesture, or movement to try and escape from a specific stuttering spasm in process. Model "My name is Riiiii (sudden gesture) chard." (It can be argued that this is not an avoidance behavior because the spasm already has started, but the speaker is trying to escape and avoid the rest of the spasm.)

The client should be asked whether he or she uses any of these behaviors. The clinician should model the behaviors and discuss any to which the client admits (how often, what situations, when adopted, how effective, etc.). In particular, a goal should be to help the client recognize those behaviors used unconsciously. In-clinic work on a variety of language hierarchies and situations should be followed with solo home practice, out-clinic supervised efforts, and transfer assignments.

Avoidances can be hard to detect because they are so often automatic and difficult for the client to see. Initially, it is easier to target the grosser, physical avoidances that can be felt and can be observed in a mirror. On the other hand, substitutions and circumlocutions may sound very normal and hard to detect, and they also have the added value of being quite effective in avoiding stuttering. In addition to spasm-specific avoidances, there are avoidance behaviors that are keyed to stuttering in general, but not to a specific word/spasm production. They are antiexpectancy behaviors.

Antiexpectancy Behaviors

Avoidance actions in the form of antiexpectancy behaviors are important, but they can be very difficult to handle. The avoidance behaviors cited earlier are word specific, aimed at avoiding stuttering on a specific word. On the other hand, antiexpectancy behaviors are aimed at reducing or preventing the occurrence of any stuttering at any time. These behaviors are endlessly variable. A few are cited below:

- Changes in overall speech rate, loudness, prosody, pitch, and so forth
- Unique accents, pronunciations, dialects
- Generalized gestures, rhythmic or jerky patterns of movements
- Mutism, refusal to speak
- Compensations (written message, prerecorded tape communications, whispers to a "symbiote")

Usually the clinician delays this area of self-analysis until there has been some progress in control of word-specific avoidances. This delay occurs because some clients need experience in easier analytic tasks and desensitization to the experiences of listening to self. Also, and very important, this level of self-analysis cuts very close to the bone of the essence of the individual client. Changing any of the behavior types cited previously may be very difficult because of their widespread character and effects. In addition, change may occur spontaneously as therapy progresses and the client reduces stuttering, increases self-confidence, learns methods of symptom control, or develops skills and confidence in fluency reinforcement. However, it is useful early on to recognize antiexpectancy behaviors and monitor any changes over time. The clinician probably will need to lead the client in monitoring for antiexpectancy behaviors through the following approaches:

- Didactic instruction—teaching the client about antiexpectancy behaviors some stutterers have used and explaining and modeling them.
- Group discussions—having clients discuss antiexpectancy behaviors in group sessions and analyzing one another relative to their occurence.

- In-clinic client assignments—having the client listen to the radio, watch television, and be alert for different kinds of overall speech patterns that could be used in stuttering defense.
- Out-clinic assignments—having the client hunt for different types of patterns or behaviors in home, school, work, and social settings.
- Listening sessions—play audiotapes or videotapes of stutterers to look for antiexpectancy patterns in their fluent speech.

As noted, antiexpectancy behaviors often are "food for thought" rather than a call to action early in therapy. In fact, some stutterers should be protected from too much knowledge early in management sessions because they can develop renewed feelings of inadequacy and cowardice. However, this information can be very useful in later transfer stages when a major target is "speech naturalness" and maintenance of therapy gains.

Eye Contact

Few aspects of interpersonal behavior are more important than eye contact. Our language is replete with "eye" expressions: "eye to eye," "keep an eye on that," "the mind's eye," "tell me that and don't blink," "look me in the eye and say that," and so on. Judgment of a person's friendliness, sociability, honesty, accuracy, veracity, courage, and other aspects can depend on eye contact. A person with poor eye contact can be regarded as shifty, sneaky, unreliable, cowardly, nervous, or submissive. On the other hand, too much eye contact can make a person seem harassing, overbearing, aggressive, domineering, and so on. Eye contact is important.

Among our diverse cultures, there may be times when strong eye contact is counter to the client and his or her cultural grouping. The clinician, if not sure, should query the client as to what is proper eye contact in that person's social milieu.

Specific Eye Contact

Stutterers often tend to have poor eye contact. Some develop poor eye contact as part of their overall speech pattern, more or less as one aspect of their antiexpectancy behaviors. Those having poor eye contact will vary. Some will have it on almost everything they say. Some will display it starting a word, or several words, prior to the stuttering and for several words following a completed block. Some will break eye contact only during actual stuttering moments. A few will have excellent eye contact. There are many variations. Therefore, as part of both symptom and fluency programs, avoidance reduction, desensitization work, or assertiveness training, eye contact may be quite important. Thus it must be evaluated in monitoring and self-analysis.

Eye contact activity might include an exercise in which the clinician sits in front of a tripod video camera, with the camera shooting over his or her shoulder. The camera is focused on the client. After recording for a period of time, the clinician and client review the tape together and evaluate

- How many times did the client's eyes shift away from clinician contact?
- How many times did the client's head shift away from center?
- On stutterings, did the client's eyes close or blink multiple times?
- On stutterings, did the client's gaze shift?
- On stutterings, did the client's eyes glaze or lose focus?

In another exercise, the clinician can instruct the client to signal and stop conversation any time the clinician breaks eye contact during a stuttering spasm by the client. The clinician should make sure to break eye contact deliberately several times. Likewise, the client can watch himself or herself in a mirror while talking with the clinician. The client must stop any time eye contact is broken while stuttering. After the spasm, the client must analyze and describe what happened during the exercise.

General Eye Contact

The preceding exercises can be combined with desensitization work, spasm analysis, and other management activities. Another monitoring check can be made without prior notification to the client. In this activity, the clinician makes an effort to dress distinctively or use makeup (female clinicians), hold a ring hand near their face, and so on, for several minutes of conversation with the client. Then the client is asked to swing around 180° (facing away from the clinician) and stay that way while the following questions (apply clinician gender where appropriate) are asked:

- What color is my lipstick?

- Am I wearing eye shadow? If so, what color?
- Am I wearing a necklace? If so, describe.
- Am I wearing earrings? If so, describe.
- Am I wearing rings? If so, describe.
- What does my shirt/sweater/blouse/coat look like?
- What do my glasses look like?
- What writing instrument am I using?
- What does my watch look like?

The observation of others can be assigned as an out-clinic activity where the client is told to go to a mall (or elsewhere) and observe 10, 20, or 30 males and an equal number of females. The client must keep score (provide the card illustrated in Exhibit 3–1) on particular observations. The items to be checked can be varied according to season, locale, or other factors.

Another exercise involves taking the client out and having him or her observe strangers while the clinician asks (fluently) for directions or some other information. After each contact, the client reports on the eye contact witnessed. The clinician must be sure to have good eye contact, but not too much.

The preceding exercise can be repeated, but this time the clincian should fake a few stuttering spasms with each stranger. After each contact, the client must report about overall eye contact by the stranger. The clinician

Exhibit 3–1 Observation scorecard

Observation	Male	Female
Wears glasses		
Wears some type of tennis shoe		
Wears earrings		
Wears shorts		
Has white/gray/silver hair		

should check the client's view of the stranger's eye contact during the fakes. Again, the clinician must remember to have good eye contact.

Another variation involves having the stutterer replicate the clinician's performance and, after each experience, have the client compare his or her observations with the clinician's observations of eye contact concerning

- Client's overall eye contact
- Stranger's overall eye contact
- Client's eye contact during stutters
- Stranger's eye contact during stutters

Further eye contact monitoring work can be done with family, peers, classmates, coworkers, friends, and so forth. In all instances, the goals and actions will be approximately the same as those described previously.

ATTITUDE EVALUATION

Attitude is an area of self-monitoring that often is ignored because the clinician either does not think of it, or because she or he is uncertain about dealing with it. At the early stages of self-monitoring and analysis it is better to keep concepts simple and focus on basic speech and stuttering attitudes. In those two domains, inquiry can be separated broadly into questionnaires and test approaches and self-inventory. In the following text, examples of both approaches will be offered. Frequently, the content areas of questionnaires, forms, and tests range outside "attitude" and into avoidance behaviors, auditor awareness, and other aspects.

One of the older attitude measures—almost 60 years old—is the Iowa Scale of Attitude toward Stuttering (Ammons & Johnson, 1944). It is a dated test, socially and functionally. However, it can be used to some advantage. Forty-five statements are made concerning stuttering. The reader agrees, or disagrees, with each statement on a 5-point scale. The resulting scores can be translated into a good-to-poor attitude toward stuttering. The halo effect applies to any question or statement where the "politically correct," socially acceptable, ego preserving answer is obvious. On this scale, it is very obvious, and the client will need specific instruction and motivation to overcome this problem. Despite its age and simplistic attitude, the Iowa Scale is still a useful starting point for the client to start thinking about attitudes and how they can affect behavior.

For this 45-item form (administration time is usually about 20 minutes), it is suggested that it (and similar forms) be used early on as a home assignment to begin, among other things, to habituate the client to outside work and self-direction. The client should respond to the first four or five items in the clinic (discussing halo effect).

A more recent attitude probe is the so-called Erickson S-scale, or S-24 scale. This very simple measure has 24 statements to which the stutterer responds with "true" or "false" (Erickson, 1969). Again, the halo effect is strong. Occasionally, some clients will cognitively agonize over the "true-ness of true . . . and the falseness of false" and hesitate to designate. The client should be instructed as follows:

> None of these statements are true or false 100% of the time. Go with your first reaction that comes in as "generally true" or "generally false." If a statement happens to fall outside any experience you have had, make a best guess answer.

In general, higher Erickson scores reflect poor attitudes. As scores go up, negative aspects increase. Anything above about 15 for males, and 10 for females, is into the typical stutterer range. I had 75 college seniors take the S-24 during class, and several scored above 15 on the measure. Clearly, poor speech attitudes are not limited to stutterers.

Another old-but-good questionnaire form is the Stutterer's Self-Ratings of Reactions to Speech Situations (Darley & Spriestersbach, 1978). It contains 40 situation statements concerning communication activities that often occur, such as conducting telephone calls, meeting people, asking questions in a group, and so on. All 40 situation statements are read by the client, and rated (1 to 5) on each of the categories below (each statement is rated four separate times):

- The degree to which each situation is regarded as *enjoyable*.
- The strength of the client's tendency to *avoid* each situation.
- The amount or severity of *stuttering* likely to occur in each situation.
- The *frequency of occurrence* of each situation for this client.

The 1 through 5 ratings can be added separately for each category, and the sum divided by the number of items responded to. The four resulting averages can be compared with norms provided by Shumack in 1955.

It is feasible for the clinician to prepare a reaction list tailored to fit a particular client, such as a younger person in a school setting encountering the following situations:

- Volunteering to answer a question in class
- Answering when volunteered by the teacher
- Reading aloud in class
- Talking with teachers before or after class
- Delivering oral messages to school personnel
- Presenting original speeches with few notes
- Presenting memorized material aloud
- Engaging in small talk with students of the same sex
- Engaging in small talk with students of the opposite sex
- Calling a classmate for a date

A similar specialized list could be developed for a work setting. Self-evaluations also could be formulated around specific category activities, as shown below.

> *Rate each telephone situation below on a 1 to 5 scale where 1 is "like much" and 5 is "dislike much."*
>
> | | |
> |---|---|
> | When I am talking on the telephone with my father | 1 2 3 4 5 |
> | When I am talking on the telephone with my mother | 1 2 3 4 5 |
> | When I am talking on the telephone with my sister | 1 2 3 4 5 |
> | When I am talking on the telephone with Grandmother Jones | 1 2 3 4 5 |
> | When I am talking on the telephone with a telephone salesman | 1 2 3 4 5 |
> | When I am talking on the telephone with a store clerk | 1 2 3 4 5 |
> | When I am talking on the telephone with a potential social date | 1 2 3 4 5 |

A comparatively recent development among attitude questionnaires is the Inventory of Communication Attitudes (Watson, Gregory, & Kistler, 1987). This inventory covers 39 situations that can be grouped into 13 triads of similar situation types. The client must go through the 39 situations five times, each time rating the 39 items on a 7-point scale. The five scales are structured so that a "1" first indicates an enjoyment of the speech situation identified, and a "7" suggests an intense dislike for that situation. On the second run-through, probing the level of the client's fluency, a "1" equals excellent, while a "7" equals very poor. On the third and fourth repetitions, the same situations are checked in terms of the client's perception of, or belief in, what other people enjoy or hate and their levels of fluency and disfluency. The last repeat is for the client, as in other scales, to rate the frequency with which she or he meets each of the 39 situations.

Thus the clinician can compare across situations, compare the stutterer with his or her perceptions of other speakers, relate frequency of occurrence to reality (checking probable situation avoidance), and relate situation frequency to client enjoyment and to client speech status (stuttering severity).

LISTENER EVALUATION

Monitoring and evaluation of listeners can be of significant value early in the management program. First, it is necessary to admit that some people are poor listeners. Stutterers can (and do) experience teasing, imitation, laughter, overt rejection, and other lacerating reactions. It is particularly true among children and adult bonding groups ("the boys" or "the girls"). However, many or most auditors fall into an attitude range from surprise and overdone sympathy (Oh, you poor thing!) to a neutral or accepting tolerance. Many stutterers, however, project their own feelings of embarrassment and irritation on their auditors and construe rejection whether or not it occurs. Combine such a tendency with a stutterer's minimal or nil eye contact, and one witnesses a self-perpetuating and self-reinforcing cycle of negative experiences.

There is another dimension to auditor awareness. It occurs when the stutterer engages in the EB-MIF (Everybody But Me Is Fluent) game. The client can be so focused on her or his own dysfluencies that others' disfluencies occur without notice, or are minimized to naught. In monitoring and self-evaluation the stutterer needs to know that other people have disfluencies and that the client has both *dis*fluencies and *dys*fluencies. It should be added here that training and assignments dealing with the stutterer's communication environment usually contribute significantly to client desensitization. Because presumed auditor reactions can be a very negative influence in the anticipation/apprehension/hypertension cycle of many stutterers, breaking that cycle can be important. Guided observation and evaluation can be of assistance.

Auditor evaluation and monitoring can involve separate, short periods of in-clinic teaching by the clinician to explain measures, rationale, and procedures. In general, those aspects will not be covered here because the age and sophistication of the client will affect the length and content of such instruction. Several activities follow that can be used with the client after discussion of individual differences among speakers.

- The clinician videotapes 2 minutes of a major network news reader, and 2 minutes of a guest on a late-night talk show, selecting opposite ends of the continuum of verbal smoothness. The client views both segments and answers the following questions:
  - Which person was the better speaker? Why?
  - Which speaker was most like the average speaker?
  - Who was louder, faster, higher in pitch, better in pronunciation, and so forth?

  Any differences between speakers are discussed and expansions of definitions of different disfluencies are offered. Any similarities between the speech of the client and either individual on the tape are emphasized.
- The client is given a solo out-clinic assignment to scan television and find
  - The speaker who tripped or stumbled over words the most
  - The speaker who uses the most hand gestures
  - The speaker who was loudest, fastest, slowest, softest in speech
  - The speaker who seemed to be most disfluent

The in-clinic and out-clinic assignments can be rewritten and used several times, until the clinician feels the client is generally "tuned in" to the broad area of being aware of other speakers. More specific attention can be focused using the exercises that follow.

- The clinician plays an in-clinic tape, audio or video, of a person who is supposedly fluent, but shows frequent word breaks, repetitions, incomplete statements, or other disfluent practices. The client is asked to look for these fluency breaks and identify them.

- Clients who are students (fourth grade through graduate school) are instructed to listen to classmates in various verbal activities during classes and identify specific behaviors such as:
  - Uh, er, hmmm, you know, ya see, well
  - Incomplete phrases
  - Broken words
  - Repetitions (phrase, word, syllable)
  - Unique behaviors
- The client is assigned an out-clinic task such as listening to five different conversations, pairs or groups, for about 5 minutes each. Then the client must fill out the card in Exhibit 3–2 on the appropriate lines. The client is told not to actually count, just form an impression. For each category rated, the client uses a 1 to 5 scale where 1 equals "little or none" and 5 equals "frequent."

LOCI OF STUTTERING

As clients pass the initial levels of ability to be aware of stuttering generally, and then learn to count spasms, rate them for severity, categorize spasms by type, detect avoidances, and so forth, another monitoring area for analysis emerges. This monitoring area is determining the loci of

Exhibit 3–2 Behaviors displayed by fluent speakers

Situation	Repetitions	Fillers	Broken Sentences	Overlong Pauses	Interjections	Other
1						
2						
3						
4						
5						

stuttering for the specific client. This topic is also discussed under headings in diagnosis, preparatory sets, and other management activities.

General Loci

Loci monitoring can be found in a number of management venues. They include

- Initially in diagnostics
- Early when self-analysis is a major therapy target
- In symptom modification to target probable specific moments of stuttering
- In fluency reinforcement to anticipate need to switch to fluency induction behaviors
- Problem solving for specific difficulties

Loci analysis can occur early in therapy, or it can be applied intermittently. On the basis of many different research studies, a number of suggested loci have been proposed over the years. Those locations or factors that are associated with higher probabilities of stuttering include

- Feared (Jonah) words unique to a specific client (e.g., aluminum, Dr. Fucci, May I)
- Feared (Jonah) words typical for many stutterers (e.g., own name, address, telephone number)
- First three words (in decreasing order) starting a new utterance after a pause
- Stressed word in an utterance
- Stressed syllable in a word
- Consonants more than vowels
- Plosives/stops more than fricatives/continuants
- Longer utterances
- Information value of word
- Longer words (over five phonemes)
- Unfamiliar words
- Proximity of previously stuttered word

- Stressful topics or situations
- Emotional situations (any type)
- Stress-causing people

Special loci factors can be added for particular individuals. Many of the in-clinic and out-clinic (supervised and unsupervised) activities described on previous pages can be used to work on identifying loci factors. If it is possible to retain early in-clinic audiotape and videotape recordings, they can be used for practice. Otherwise, suggested sequences for phoneme characteristics and word-length factor are presented.

Phoneme Characteristics

The words arranged in phoneme triads (vertical) below are read aloud:

goat	three	even	door	army
fun	cat	shall	where	puddle
air	oar	bet	over	fizzle

Each triad contains an initial plosive, initial continuant consonant, and initial vowel. The clinician should make up 20 to 30 more triads of varying word lengths and have the client go through them three times. On each run-through, the clinician marks any stuttering with a 1, 2, or 3, depending on the reading.

The client then repeats the triads just used, only he or she repeats them as the clinician reads each word aloud. The clinician should not read too quickly, or set a rhythm. Stuttering is marked as before.

After both exercises, the client and clinician examine the markings to see if there are any phoneme loci, word-length factors, and so forth. If there are any such indicators, they are discussed with the client and home assignments are arranged so the client can monitor his or her speech in real situations—just enough to verify, contradict, or expand on the initial indicators.

Word-Length Factor

Following the same procedure for phoneme characteristics, the client runs through the material below twice. Some sample word lengths are offered below, but the clinician will need to formulate additional ones.

season	tunic	glider	former	babble
seasoning	opportune	glycerin	formerly	bobolink
unseasonable	opportunity	glioblastoma	formidable	brachiating

The client is not assisted in the pronounciation of any words. When marking any stuttered word, the clinician circles the number of the trial if the client has a pronunciation problem. The clinician should be able to pronounce all the words in order to judge the client's pronunciations.

After discussing the topic in the clinic, the client may be asked to work at home and develop a list of words most likely to be stuttered on. The clinician can help the client get started, and ask him or her to enlist help from any familiars who are around often enough to know her or his patterns. When the list is returned, the clinician goes over it with the client, looking for commonalities, and discusses findings. The list is retained for future use.

The clinician also can provide a series of sentences and have the stutterer read them aloud. On each reading, the clinician checks for loci factors on any stuttering, especially after breath breaks or other pauses. Again, a few samples are offered below, but the clinician will need to make up 20 to 30 more.

- How are you today?
- I am feeling fine, but John Wolf says I look a little pale.
- Do you think you have a fever, or is there some bug going around that we are all likely to catch?
- I feel fine when I first get up, but I get more and more fatigued as the day goes on and my energy level seems to go lower and lower.
- My doctor told me that what I should do is go to bed earlier, drink lots of liquid, and don't worry so much.

All of the foregoing activities are offered as examples of beginning efforts. They are structured mainly for in-clinic use, and the clinician definitely would want to expand loci monitoring to out-clinic activities. One activity frequently of concern to the stutterer is the telephone. The clinician will want to check monitoring and analysis on telephone calls, starting with closely supervised and pre-scripted calls. Whenever possible, the client's side of a telephone call should be recorded for later replay and analysis. The procedure for monitoring and analyzing telephone calls includes the following steps:

- Begin with 10 to 20 prewritten telephone calls that are short and familiar, involving topics such as movie start times, goods carried by a grocery store, or hours that a restaurant serves breakfast.
- Move to longer pre-scripted calls that will have several utterances prewritten, but the speech in between the prewritten parts is up to the client.
- Assign unscripted calls to people the client knows. Some of these should be solo home assignments, with the client recording only his or her side of the conversation.
- Have the client make unscripted calls from the clinic involving content that is not familiar. Possible tasks include calling the library to find out how to reserve a new book [supply a title], responding to several employment advertisements in the newspaper, or soliciting details on how to become a member of an association.
- Hand out a series of home assignments of increasing difficulty. Have the client record only his or her side of the conversation and bring the tapes to the clinic for analysis and discussion.

General Concerns

Previous paragraphs have focused on specific aspects of stuttering loci. There are also concerns of a more general, less specific nature. Some of those addressed are as follows:

- Have the client secure a helper (wife, mother, sibling, friend) and, with the helper, repeat the word and sentence/paragraph reading activities. Does the amount of stuttering go up or down with the new auditor? Do spasms occur on the same words as before? Do spasms occur on fewer or more words? On the same or different words? If different, do the same loci "rules" apply as in the clinic? Record.
- Repeat the auditor procedure with telephone calls and answer the same questions. For some clients, friendly auditors may not be available due to time constraints or lifestyle. In some instances, the "near and dear" are not that "dear" and/or the client will resist performing before them for personal embarrassment reasons. Such attitudes probably need review, but such review is probably outside the purview of the clinician.

• Check the desensitization assignments in chapter 4, and use them to hunt for loci factors.

CONSISTENCY

Consistency of stuttering behaviors also is covered in chapter 1 and in several other sections. It is included here because it is a factor that is approachable in most monitoring and self-evaluation exercises. Consistency monitoring is accessible when working on loci of stuttering, so iteration (of consistency work) is almost required. In stuttering, *consistency* is the degree to which a stuttering on one particular word is followed by a new stuttering *on the same word* when that word occurs in another location. A word stuttered on consistently is, in effect, a Jonah word. Stutterers vary in consistency. Activities to evaluate consistency are those used to determine loci and related measures, so there is no need to develop new or special activities. Reuse the same activities.

Two other considerations deserve attention here. First, consistency does not have to be limited to specific words. It can relate to other loci factors, such as the initial word following a pause for respiration. Second, consistency may emerge only after therapy management chips away at total dysfluency counts and reduces them to more of a "core group" of stutterings where consistency patterns become more obvious. Lower consistency factors early in therapy may appear to change to higher consistency, over time, when actually it is the reduction in nervous anxiety and tension spasms allowing that core to become more apparent.

FEARS AND FEAR HIERARCHY

Situation fears certainly figure prominently in client management. There was a time when some early fluency reinforcement clinicians stated flatly that situation fears no longer deserved attention because "elimination of stuttering" by fluency expansion would eliminate any reasons or causes for situation fears. Unfortunately, this rule did not function as planned—nobody told the clients—and "residual disfluencies" bore a suspicious resemblance to stuttering. We went back to considering situation fears.

The whole concept of fear hierarchy use in therapy is covered separately elsewhere, but it deserves attention here. The clinician can direct his or her attention to forms (discussed earlier) such as the Stutterer's Self-Ratings of Reactions to Speech Situations (Shumack, 1955), or to the Erickson S-24 scale (Erickson, 1969). This time around, the clinician concentrates on the situations, not the attitudes or reactions. The situations can be used as a starter list for the client to rate for stress production. Another way is to build a from-scratch list of situations. First, with the client, the clinician develops a gross list of situation categories, such as:

- Telephone
- Home
- Employment
- School
- Friends
- Strangers
- Special
- Other

From that beginning, clinician and client confer to expand the gross categories into subcategories, such as:

Telephone

To immediate family	Salespersons, fundraisers, etc.
From immediate family	Opinion pollsters
Brief business calls	Being asked to volunteer
Complex business calls	Asking others to volunteer, buy, etc.
From named persons	To named persons
Professional calls to	Professional calls from
To request a date	To be asked for a date
To beg a favor	To be asked for a favor
To "sell" an idea	Special aspects

The "special aspects" category is meant to indicate specifics of broader categories, such as:

- Any telephone conversation I have with Grandfather Smith
- Annual telephone ticket sales for the theater guild
- Weekly call to my parole officer
- A call to my ex-father while Mom listens in

Additional telephone categories can be broken down similarly; there will be overlaps between and among categories. The overlaps are not important because the final arrangement of situations will almost certainly scramble the categories.

Next, the clinician and the client arrange the situations in a hierarchy of stress or dislike. For some it will be easier to start macro and then go micro by first grouping the situations by low, medium, and high stress levels. The client is asked to look at each situation and consider: How much stress and anxiety does that situation cause me most of the time? As each decision is made, the clinician puts an L, M, or H by the item, until every item belongs to one of the three groups. The client should operate on the premise that this ranking is for "most of the time" and to ignore unusual occurrences or levels. Rankings now may group as shown below.

> **Low:** Immediate family, opinion polls, Aunt Dorothy, any of my friends
> **Medium:** Most strangers, being asked to volunteer, Uncle Ernest
> **High:** Asking others to volunteer, Grandmother Jones anytime, asking for a date

There is no set number, but it is not unusual to have 50 or 60 situations— sometimes the list goes over 100, especially later in therapy. The next step is to instruct the client as follows:

> Now, take all the *low* stress situations and arrange them in rank order of stress, from lowest to highest in that low category. When that is done, number each one, starting with "1" for the lowest, and going up consecutively. Absolute precision is not important. Whether a "low" is 2 or 12 is significant, but whether it is 5, 6, or 7 really isn't. When you have numbered all the lows, move to the *medium* stress group and number them, starting with the number following the highest item from the low group. Repeat the process a third time with the *high* group.

A consecutively numbered set of situations now exists. The client looks over the list and changes the rankings of any situations desired. The revised set will provide the basis for a fear or stress hierarchy structure. Future additions can be made by putting any late add-on situations into the judged number and adding an alpha indicator (e.g., 23a, 47c, 52a, etc.). The primary purpose of the hierarchy development at this early level is to orient the client to evaluating stress objectively, facing up to the fact that there are fears to be dealt with, and helping the clinician make early assignments.

SPEECH NATURALNESS

At first glance, speech naturalness seems very much out of place in the early stages of therapy management. One of the significant drawbacks (after the relapse problem) in early fluency reinforcement programs was that the fluency achieved often sounded worse than the dysfluency displaced. Clients might drone, tick, and whisper/gasp their way through speech that even then might still have dysfluencies at "0.5 or less stuttered words per minute." Aside from this distorted and dysfluent fluency, clients often found fluency reinforcement to be onerous, tiring, irritating, and too demanding to be used consistently after the maintenance phase of therapy, if that long. Subsequently, along with relapse concerns, many clinicians paid more attention to what supposedly fluent speech sounded like after therapy. Studies demonstrated that listeners, experienced or naive, often could differentiate normally fluent speech from nonstuttered fluent speech. In some cases, mild stuttering was preferred by listeners, compared to fluent speech. At least 25 years ago, Curlee and Perkins (1969, 1973) emphasized the need to reintroduce prosody and naturalness back into delayed auditory feedback (DAF) rate control fluency work with stutterers. Wingate (1966) stressed the significance of prosody in therapy and transfer stages of stuttering. In 1953, as his graduate student clinician, I found that Van Riper routinely used post-program time to rebuild and expand speech naturalness of stutterers who had such needs after primary therapy was completed. Onslow and Packman (1997) wrote extensively concerning management approaches aimed at shifting away from extreme alterations of speech parameters early in fluency therapy. They favored approaches that were closer to normal speech rates and built sequentially on extended length of utterance (ELU) or graduated increments in the length and complexity of utterances (GILCU) development. Their orientation will be considered elsewhere. At this point, there is no question that many management techniques, including those in symptom modification, can have deleterious effects on the naturalness of speech. However, as implied in the opening sentence of this section, management techniques are not the only possible source of speech naturalness problems.

Many stutterers adopt certain antiexpectancy behaviors to reduce the overall probability of stuttering occurrence. These behaviors may involve the basic speech parameters of loudness, rate, and pitch. In addition, inflection, stress, accent, pronunciation, and other factors may be altered. Over time, these alterations become strongly habituated, unconscious behaviors that occur whether the speaker is actually stuttering or not. Many therapy programs that may effectively reduce or eliminate stuttering may not remove, or even affect, these reactive behaviors. Moreover, any management procedure that requires close attention from the client over extended periods of time will tend to generate effects on the overall speech pattern. Whenever close attention is paid to any behavior, related behaviors tend to be altered to some degree. Last, many stutterers will be convinced that, in addition to stuttering, their supposedly fluent speech is substandard when compared with the hypothetical norm. Sometimes they are right, but often they are not. Therefore, most clients need some monitoring and evaluation input on the naturalness of their speech early on. They certainly will want the information much later in therapy, as indicated below.

Speech naturalness has gained a great deal of attention in recent years. The emphasis is deserved. Surprisingly, few people (to my awareness) have done objective work in speech naturalness until fairly recently. In 1984, Martin, Haroldson, and Triden published a 9-point scale of speech naturalness, reporting adequate reliability for the scale, adequate consistency, and agreement among naive listeners. A rating of "1" reflects a judgment of "highly natural" about a speech sample; a rating of "9" denotes a judgment of "highly unnatural" about a speech sample. I have applied this scale in management and found it useful. I have used it at the end of therapy in transfer and maintenance work, and I have used it early in therapy as one exercise in self-analysis. I have developed my own concept of speech naturalness, finding a 5-point scale more applicable. In addition, I use the referents for the client to evaluate production aspects on the basis of "like" and "unlike" rather than "natural" and "unnatural." Clients seems to have responded to this judgment aspect well, deciding if

- My speech sounds *like* that of other people I know.
- My speech sounds *unlike* that of other people I know.

The five points of rating are:

    1 =   sounds completely unlike the speech of people I know

2 = sounds rather unlike the speech of people I know
3 = some of it is like, and some of it is unlike, the speech of people I know
4 = most of the time it sounds like the speech of people I know
5 = my speech sounds just like the speech of people I know

In discussions with the client, the clinician emphasizes that she or he is making comparisons to a peer group and not to some imaginary icon of good speech. Any physical format can be used, but I typically have the client monitor 1 to 3 minutes of spontaneous speech and then rate the sample using the form in Exhibit 3–3. In these uses, employing audiotape or videotape, I have the client review the activity and first rate the overall speaking effort.

Exhibit 3–3 Speech naturalness evaluation

Parameter	Evaluation 1 2 3 4 5
Rate of speech	
Loudness, including variation	
Pitch, including variation	
Quality, resonance	
Stress on syllables, words	
Inflection in general	
Pauses, frequency and duration	
*Dis*fluencies*	
Eye contact, general and specific	

**Dis*fluencies: the ordinary disfluencies that help speech sound natural, not artificial.

Possible limited use of naturalness evaluations at this point might include:

- *Step 1.* Discuss the naturalness concept with client and then have him or her rate several people he or she knows very well (rate from memory). Then have the client rate himself or herself. As a home assignment, have the client listen to the live speech of the people rated at the clinic and decide if any of the ratings should be changed.
- *Step 2.* In the clinic, have the client listen to audiotapes and watch videotapes of his or her own speech (several minutes each) and rate himself or herself again. Compare the results to those achieved in Step 1. Discuss.
- *Step 3.* Have the client listen to or watch a sample of the clinician's speech and rate it. Remind the client that the criterion is like or unlike, not good or bad.
- *Step 4.* In the clinic, have six or so segments on videotape of people talking (look for variety), and have the client rate them based on the like or unlike criterion.

This level is about as far as naturalness needs to be taken at the early stages of therapy. It helps sharpen the self-monitoring, monitoring, and evaluation skills of the client. It also helps the client compare himself or herself to others on more dimensions than just stuttering.

SUMMARY

The practice of some packaged programs is to restrict responses to a pre-set pattern of stimuli or formulas ("do it this way") with little call for analysis and evaluation. In the long run, this approach will serve the client poorly. Imitation without thought can carry only so far into sophisticated levels of behaviors. Monitoring and evaluation cannot be overstressed, but they can be overused. One can spend too much time on any activity, to a point of negative returns. The cut-off points are not constant across clients, and the clinician will need to answer the question "What does this client need?" *not* "How much is enough?

REFERENCES

Ammons, R., & Johnson, W. (1944). Studies in the psychology of stuttering: 18. The construction and application of a test of attitudes toward stuttering. *Journal of Speech Disorders, 9*, 39–49.

Curlee, R.F., & Perkins, W.H. (1969). Conversational rate-control therapy for stuttering. *Journal of Speech and Hearing Disorders, 34*, 245–250.

Curlee, R.F., & Perkins, W.H. (1973). Effectiveness of a DAF conditioning program for adolescent and adult stutterers. *Behavioral Research Therapy, 1*, 395–401.

Darley, F.L., & Spriestersbach, D.C. (1978). *Diagnostic methods in speech pathology* (2nd. ed.). New York: Harper & Row.

Erickson, R.L. (1969). Assessing communication attitudes among stutterers. *Journal of Speech and Hearing Research, 12*, 711–724.

Martin, R.H., Haroldson, S.K., & Triden, K.A. (1984). Stuttering and speech naturalness. *Journal of Speech and Hearing Disorders, 49*, 53–58.

Onslow, M., & Packman, A. (1997). Designing and implementing a strategy to control stuttered speech in adults. In R.F. Curlee & G.M. Siegel (Eds.), *Nature and treatment of stuttering, new directions* (2nd. ed., pp. 365–375). Boston: Allyn & Bacon.

Shumack, I.C. (1955). A speech situation rating sheet for stutterers. In W. Johnson (Ed.), *Stuttering in children and adults: Thirty years of research at the University of Iowa.* (pp. 341–347). Minneapolis: University of Minnesota Press.

Watson, J.O., Gregory, H.H., & Kistler, D.J. (1987). Development and evaluation of an inventory to assess adult stutterers' communication attitudes. *Journal of Fluency Disorders, 12*, 429–450.

Wingate, M.E. (1966). Prosody in stuttering adaptation. *Journal of Speech and Hearing Research, 9*, 550–556.

CHAPTER 4

Dealing with Anticipation, Apprehension, and Hypertension

- Overview
- Communication Fear Hierarchy
- Relaxation
- Desensitization
- Reciprocal Inhibition
- Attitude Changes
- Summary

OVERVIEW

Practically every stutterer, even the very young one, has developed an anticipation that speech attempts can be very difficult and frustrating. Apprehension usually follows anticipation (when the anticipation is negative)—or becomes part of it—as the person develops feelings of fear and anxiety associated with the anticipation of stuttering. For some speakers the emotion is an icy lump somewhere south of the diaphragm. It is a feeling that, at the very least, makes speaking an unenjoyable experience.

For some stutterers, the anticipation and anxiety reach disabling levels, and the negative feelings overwhelm communication. On a simple neurological basis, emotional states cannot exist without an excess of muscle tension. The hypertense state is a whole-body experience, but inevitably it tends to focus on the body areas that are crucial to the feared performance—in this case, speech. Therefore, tension in respiratory, phonatory, resonance, and articulatory muscles is liable to be greatest just at the time when smooth coordination and rapid adjustment are needed for fluent speech. Therapy typically targets the problem that causes tension and anxiety. It also targets the actual tension and anxiety states, working on their control or elimination while therapy of dysfluencies goes on.

COMMUNICATION FEAR HIERARCHY

The fear hierarchy in communication, and in therapy, has been mentioned in prior chapters and will be addressed in subsequent chapters. The hierarchy idea has been a mainstay in therapies for generations. Initially, many fluency reinforcement clinicians suggested that fear hierarchies (among other things) were no longer needed in therapy. Their rationale was that fluency therapy removes stuttering and, if stuttering is removed, then there is nothing to fear or to be tense about. The validity of that concept was undermined over 20 years ago, and fear hierarchy development and use are viable in all sorts of therapies.

Development of the Fear Hierarchy

In analysis procedures the client may have developed a fear hierarchy, or an approximation of one. If this task has not been accomplished, the clinician must ensure its completion. This requirement applies to both fluency enhancement and symptom modification. It may not apply below client ages of 8 or 9 years, but procedures for young children will be discussed. Therapy cannot have a reasonably favorable prognosis if the clinician (and the client) lacks an awareness of out-clinic practice and transfer venues and the stress potentials associated with various venues. Even if relaxation therapy, desensitization, or other activities are not part of the therapy plan, fear hierarchy identification is an important part of management. At the very least it will be useful in describing the client's communication environment and the degree of his or her involvement, or lack thereof.

Preliminary Structure of the Fear Hierarchy

First, the situations met by the stutterer need to be identified. In this initial step the clinician will want to identify and divide communication into rough categories and have the client estimate his or her contacts in these situations on a weekly basis, as demonstrated in Exhibit 4–1. The "Other" category can be used to add any initial communication contacts typical for that individual. It might be unique to a job or some other factor. Of course, any nonapplicable categories (school for an adult, business for a school child) are omitted.

Exhibit 4–1 Weekly communication situations

General Situation	Met Each Week	Avoided Each Week
Telephone calls	_____	_____
Classroom questions/answers	_____	_____
Social conversations, one on one	_____	_____
Social conversations, small group	_____	_____
Family conversations, one on one	_____	_____
Family conversations, group	_____	_____
Clerks, waitresses, drivers, etc.	_____	_____
Response to strangers' questions	_____	_____
Business conversation, superiors	_____	_____
Business conversations, peers	_____	_____
Business conversations, customers	_____	_____
Other	_____	_____

Refining the Preliminary Structure

At this point, some material for discussion has been amassed. The client can compare his or her contacts and (particularly) avoidances with non-stutterers he or she knows. The client also can be asked to track the amount of time spent on speech, compared with others. The Talking Time Log (Exhibit 4–2) can be used to delve into this aspect. However, it can be left to later transfer and maintenance activities, or not used if the client turns out to be a reasonably verbal stutterer-communicator.

The clinician also may continue from the ending point of the initial listing and open discussions of each rough category that he or she has entered a count report on (the clinician should be ready to add more generic situations the stutterer forgot to mention initially). For example, the clinician could start with the "Telephone" category. Then the client would identify what situations occur (e.g., calls from family, calls from friends, meaningless calls from strangers [fundraisers, wrong numbers, etc.], calls from business persons—job site, calls from business persons—customers; calls to each of the categories above) or other categories of calls that might occur just because of the uniqueness of the client. When the generic "Telephone" category has been refined, the clinician moves to the next category and breaks it down into subcategories. After completing all categories, the clinician goes back over each generic category and asks for "numbers" (received/accepted and avoided) for each subcategory. The subcategory totals often will disagree with the original generic category totals, and this inconsistency will need to be straightened out and justified.

Exhibit 4–2 Talking time log

Situations	*Face to Face*	*Telephone*
Number of times for brief contacts today with friends or family, less than 1 minute each	_____	_____
Number of times for family conversations today, over 1 minute each	_____	_____
Number of times for conversations with friends, over 1 minute each	_____	_____
Number of stranger contacts of less than 1 minute	_____	_____
Number of contacts with strangers, more than 1 minute	_____	_____

It is quite possible that the expanded generic list might have 10 or 15 categories, with 5 or 6 subcategories each, for a total of 60 to 70 communication situations. Together, the client and the clinician review the list to see if there are any situations, unique or ordinary, that were omitted.

Sorting and Weighting the Refined Structure

Next, the client goes through the total list of situations and selects two situations:

1. The situation causing the least anxiety and the least stuttering
2. The situation causing the most anxiety and the most stuttering

The client may vacillate and say that any one situation, when repeated, can vary in its difficulty, depending on a number of factors. The clinician should acknowledge this fact but apply the "in general" criterion and force the selection. When the selections have been made, the client is instructed as follows:

> Look over the remaining situations and find one situation that you feel falls almost in the middle, halfway between the two extremes you picked earlier.

The same variability problem cited above will operate here as well, but the client should be led to make a median choice. Then the client is asked to number the low-end choice as 1, the high-end selection as 100, and the in-between selection as 50. Next, the client is asked to take all the remaining situations and divide them into two groups, those above a 50 ranking and those below a 50 ranking. After that grouping, the final list will be organized as follows:

1—selected situation	10	20	30	40
50—selected situation	60	70	80	90
100—selected situation				

The client is to look at each unassigned situation and give it a numerical grouping as 10, 20 . . . 80, 90. The end result is a rough-cut fear hierarchy, measuring stress from 0 to 100, in units of 10. This list is similar to Wolpe's (1973) Subjective Units of Disturbance Scale (SUDS), which that psychotherapist developed as part of a program of systematic desensitization and reciprocal inhibition.

The clinician now possesses a summary of speech situations encountered by the client; an estimate of the situation frequency of occurrence on a weekly basis; an estimate of the frequency with which situations are avoided; and a tentative ranking of situations in terms of the anxiety, tension, and stuttering levels of each situation. This hierarchy is valuable (and applicable) for planning out-clinic sessions with the clinician, for devising solo outside assignments for the client, for transferring any and every management procedure or behavioral change, and in planning for maintenance programs. The list will need to be revised over time as the client gains experience and goes through attitude changes.

Variations in Hierarchy Methods

Fear hierarchies can be structured in various ways. Any of the situation-frequency-reaction checklists described elsewhere in this book could be given to the client for editing of situations and assigning of a numerical value to each situation. The clinician also could have the client list all the probable situations and then rate each situation on a 1 to 10 scale, as shown below.

Situation	*Value*
Telephone call from mother (easiest)	1 2 3 4 5 6 7 8 9 10 (hardest)
Telephone call from stranger	1 2 3 4 5 6 7 8 9 10
Introduce self to strangers	1 2 3 4 5 6 7 8 9 10

Another procedure is to use any method desired to accumulate identified situations associated with the client. Each situation is written on a file card or slip of paper. When the list is fairly complete, the clinician "deals" all the cards or slips of paper out onto a table and has the client rearrange the sequence of situations, ranging from low anxiety to high anxiety until all situations have been set in a hierarchical sequence. If desired, items can be numbered at this point. An advantage to this method is that items can be inserted later, items can be withdrawn, and rankings can be rearranged as a result of therapy experiences and discussions.

With children, estimation of frequency, expectations of refined judgment, and so on may be too demanding. The basic list of situations can be drawn up, with the clinician providing many of the suggestions. The clinician can secure situation suggestions from experience or by asking the child's parents, teachers, or other contact persons. The resulting situations are best written down, one at a time, on slips of paper. The clinician then addresses the child in the words that follow:

> All right. We're going to make two piles of situations. Okay? Here on the left is easy and that means you have very little speech trouble then. Here on the right will be hard; that means that you may have more speech trouble then. Okay? Here's the first one, talking to your sister. Is that easy or hard? Good. Now, here's talking to Uncle Ernest. Is that usually easy or hard?

The clinician then can take the "easy" stack and try to elicit some subdivisions and variations there. The "hard" pile is left until later in therapy, because therapy very likely will be fluency based, with emphasis on easy interactions with significant others. There also may be home therapy or practice with favored (easy) persons, and minimization (at least for awhile) of any possible conflicts with negative or hard situations. Environmental counseling also can be built around the generalized categories and individuals that are identified as easy or hard at first.

Final Comments on Fear Hierarchy

The sheer act of formulating a fear hierarchy helps many clients from the aspects of desensitization and introspection. Treating things that tend to cause anxiety, tension, and fear in a calm, cognitive, make-a-list manner usually increases a client's positive feelings. Making a list of fears rarely cancels them, but it usually helps reduce them somewhat. At the very least it helps the client feel that he or she has a definable problem rather than an anxious mystery. The other values of a fear hierarchy in various aspects of therapy have been discussed earlier, and I will just iterate that it is a valuable tool. It is particularly useful when used in conjunction with relaxation techniques, either alone or in a program leading to systematic desensitization.

RELAXATION

In one of my early experiences as a dysfluency clinician a client told me "If I could relax, I wouldn't stutter . . . and I wouldn't be tense if I didn't stutter!" In fluency disorders of all types, tension plays a major role. Patients with recent Broca's aphasia quickly develop tension and anxiety to accompany their dysfluencies, so that neurogenics develop a behavioral overlay. Muscular tension, to a degree, is normal and mandatory in all activities, including speech. Excessive tension—hypertension—is antagonistic to all normal functions, including speech. The rate, rhythm, timing, language formulation and selection, and motor coordination of speech are disrupted by excess tension.

Strong emotion, positive or negative, is associated with muscular tension states. Whether wonderfully happy, extremely angry, or very anxious, high tension levels will accompany the emotion. The linkage between the central nervous system (CNS) limbic system and the rest of the nervous system (especially the basal ganglia) is well known. It links anxiety and tension. As will be noted later, it is nearly impossible to be relaxed and to be anxious simultaneously because of the interrelationship just cited.

Relaxation has been used in fluency disorders management for generations. Bloodstein (1995) noted that relaxation has been around for a long time. However, he also noted that few stutterers are able to transfer to out-clinic use the relaxation learned during in-clinic teaching and practice. As a result, few speech-language pathologists (SLPs) use pure relaxation therapy. Some clinicians combine relaxation with systematic desensitization and reciprocal inhibition. Most SLPs use relaxation for six more specific and limited purposes:

1. Initial reduction of in-clinic dysfluencies in order to facilitate communication with the therapist (Generally, I am opposed to this rationale and application.)

2. Early experience of fluency, or significantly reduced stuttering, in order to motivate the client, create early credibility of the clinician, and so on (I have concerns about the validity and wisdom of this rationale.)

3. As part of an instruction program to help the client differentiate between tension and hypertension, learn monitoring skills, and so on

4. Relaxation needs related to specific task acquisition, such as initial practice and learning of Easy Onset, dissociation of neck and shoulder girdle muscles from vocal production area, and so forth

5. Problem-solving activities where a fluency or symptom control approach hits a rough spot, such as performance on plosives, particular phonemes, or sensitive "Jonah words"

6. As the initial step of a program leading to reciprocal inhibition

The decision on whether or not to use relaxation may also depend on secondary, but significant, factors that include, but are not limited to, the following:

- Client willingness and motivation for therapy
- Clinician self-confidence in management, and ability to project it
- Unique characteristics of the clinician as a person (e.g., her or his tension level, state/trait anxiety, obvious vocal tension, "genuineness" quality, and so on)
- Client willingness to "surrender" tension defenses and trust the clinician
- Client's prior positive experiences with relaxation

In addition, other factors include aspects such as time of day of appointments, frequency and duration of appointments, environmental noise, physical characteristics of therapy room, room temperature, furniture comfort, room light, and so on.

In the following sections of this chapter I will suggest several informal relaxation activities, and I will finish the relaxation unit with an example of formal or extended relaxation activity. The latter will be stressed less than I have done in past publications, mainly because of the limited transfer values of extended relaxation therapy. Instead, I will give more stress to informal and partial relaxation activities used for purposes 3, 4, 5, and 6 mentioned earlier. Also, in the last decade or so I have found students and new clinicians are more at ease with "doing relaxation." This ease may stem from the growing practice of yoga, transcendental meditation, mantras, out-of-body searches, inner core searches, and just plain tension reduction procedures.

Informal Relaxation

I assigned an Easy Onset (EO) learning project to 70 fourth-year SLP majors and instructed them to "Relax your pseudoclient partner in whatever way seems best" and waited to see what they did. About 90% of the students used a close approximation of the following:

• Dimly lit or darkened room with one lit candle or a nightlight bulb
• Taped background music, usually nature sounds or quiet classical or mood music
• Instructions to the client about even, deep respiratory cycles
• Instructions to the client to "clear your mind," picture a relaxing scene, or mentally repeat a mantralike phrase
• Directions to try and feel tension, try and release tension, and try to "sink into" relaxation

The 70 students divided more or less evenly between having the client lie supine (on his or her back) and having the client seated in a soft, comfortable chair. The use of vocally induced relaxation seemed to be minimal after the initial instructions and reinforcement of those instructions cited in the last three items above. Most of the student reports indicated that satisfactory relaxation (for acquiring and practicing EO) was instated after about 10 minutes, but it needed to be reestablished for each session on EO.

Informal relaxation also can be achieved through, or as a part of, breathing exercises. This approach may be particularly useful with children who might not concentrate on a multi-instruction relaxation exercise, but would follow instructions such as:

I want you to breathe in very slowly, like this. [Model inspiration.] Hold your breath until I tell you to let the air go, and then breathe out slowly like this. [Model expiration.] I'll do it again.

[Model inspiration, pause, expiration.] Now, you try it. Breathe in and hold—hold—hold, breathe out, slow—slow, breathe in, hold, breathe out.

Overstake (1979) felt that his "block breathing" facilitated relaxation. In this approach, the four stages of a respiratory cycle (in, hold, out, hold) are cued or timed in equal time intervals to the client's cardiac pulse rate. Another common approach to relaxation is to ask the client to list the things that help him or her relax and then use that information appropriately. Occasionally it is impossible, or at least inappropriate, to use the client's information. Still another method is to schedule a high-tension activity and then follow it with a "now relax"–type activity. For instance, the client reads a paragraph aloud as fast as possible, and then is given the following instruction:

Stop, take a deep breath, and let it out slowly; take another deep breath and read the same paragraph aloud in a slow, easy, relaxed way.

A discussion of the physical sensation and reading differences in terms of tension, loudness, reading rate, pitch, articulation errors, or any other relevant signals follows.

Relaxation and Young Children

Relaxation is usually easy to do with children, but often it is hard to maintain in a clinical setting. Transfer, as relaxation, is very poor, but the effects of relaxation on speech often will transfer spontaneously with minimal out-clinic practice. Modeling to young clients is very important.

Listen to me and watch me. Try and do just what I do. I'm feeling really slow and easy, real tired. . . . I can sag down like this . . . my head's too heavy to hold up . . . my arms just hang down . . . when I talk it's slow and draggy like this . . . I sort of whisper when I talk. . . .

The old symbols of Raggedy Andy, Lazybones Scarecrow, Sagalong Sleepyhead, and other suggestive characters can be used. As noted earlier, children tend to be good at mimicry and usually adopt imitative relaxation easily. However, they will "unadopt" it just as quickly, so relaxation is used best when teaching a particular mode of speech (usually fluency reinforcement modes) rather than trying to teach the cognitive concepts and uses of relaxation.

Intensive Relaxation

The title of this section has an oxymoron quality to it. Intensive relaxation exercises are still used but (I think) not as often as in the past. I developed an outline for intensive relaxation (Ham, 1986, pp. 127–129) that I have revised and am presenting here. The preliminary aspects of light level, atmosphere, and other environmental concerns are presumed to be under control and satisfactory.

- *Step 1: Explain relaxation concepts to client.* Demonstrate physical tension and relaxation. Describe the general procedure and determine if any aspects cause concern or embarrassment. Query the client to make sure she or he understands what is to be done. For female clients, suggest wearing slacks or shorts rather than dresses (or longer, full skirts rather than short-and-tight skirts). Advise all clients to avoid very tight clothing. Find out if physical anomalies require special surfaces, padding, support cushions, and so on. Determine if the client requires any special posture adjustment to avoid discomfort during relaxation efforts.
- *Step 2: Have the client lie down, supine, on the mat; close his or her eyes and "try it on."* Is the client comfortable (e.g., clothing loose enough, uncomfortable jewelry removed, agreeable light level, adequate back support, and so on)? Have the client adopt the posture to be used (generally, legs together, arms parallel with and touching body, head centered and facing up, eyes closed) and see if any changes need to be made.

If necessary, for understanding or personal ease, the clinician should model the posture and behavior desired. In fact, on the activities in subsequent steps, the clinician should either go through the entire exercise for the client to observe, or should have the client do it first for familiarization and then observe as the clinician does a follow-up model.

- *Step 3: Initiate preliminary relaxation procedure.* Have the client position herself or himself as described previously. Then, go through the preliminary relaxation procedure decided on. It can involve the use of special lights, background music, suggestion, and instruction, such as:

> I want you to close your eyes and just listen to the music and concentrate on breathing slowly and evenly. Breathe in, pause, and then breathe out. Breathe in . . . Breathe out. In . . . Out . . . In . . . Out. Just clear your mind; let it drift while you relax. Feel yourself settle into the mat as your body relaxes. In . . . Out, Breathe in . . . Out.

In the first session it is a good idea to stop after several minutes and check with the client. Many are settling right into relaxation, some are still tense and distracted and need further instruction and adjustment, and a few get the giggles and have to be calmed down. Once or twice (only) I have found clients who felt threatened and nervous by this approach, and I changed the menu to lights on, seated posture, and a more physical therapy approach to relaxation.

- *Step 4: Establish a command sequence with the client for each action.* Develop the sequence at each step in the process. An example follows.

> When I say "up," I want you to lift your right leg about 6 inches off the floor and hold it there until I say "relax." Then just let it drop. . . . Okay, "Up . . . Hold it . . . Hold it . . . relax."

In most cases, the client should hold any posture for about 5 seconds, or a little more.

In most of the commands, I use the wait time to direct the client's attention to the weight, or the tension, and, afterward, to feel the difference relaxation makes. Once the client clearly understands the command sequence and the duration of most hold commands, I run through the entire sequence. The sequence will vary with each client. I might skip some items with older clients because of physical discomfort. I might add a couple extra shoulder-girdle commands for a client who has shown a lot of upper chest and neck tension in stuttering spasms.

- *Step 5A: Feet and Legs*
Run through the entire sequence.

> Raise the right leg 6 inches above the floor, hold, relax, and let drop. Raise the left leg 6 inches above the floor, hold, relax, and

let drop. Repeat the right leg raise and also dorsiflex (point) the foot. Repeat the left leg raise and also dorsiflex (point) the foot.

Have the client relax all over and reinforce the suggestion with words about relaxing moments, images, and the like. Continue with the seriers of commands that follow.

Raise right leg and flex it at the knee (pulling it up toward the chest), feeling the pull on the back of the thigh, and ventroflex (toward the knee) the foot; hold it, hold it; straighten leg and foot slowly while gently dropping the leg back to the mat. Repeat this action with your left leg.

- *Step 5B: Stomach and Hips*

  Take a deep breath and hold it; now clench your fists and contract your stomach muscles real hard; hold it; relax and breathe out. Repeat.

I usually skip other hip, stomach, and lower back exercises. Then I have the client relax and breathe deeply and easily several times. Then I check the general relaxation of the client's lower body, while uttering a relaxation suggestion monologue. Exercises are repeated as necessary.

Place one of your hands on your abdomen. Press down with your hand and push up with your stomach; push hard and hold it, hold it; relax; put your hand down.

- *Step 5C: Hands and Arms*

  The client is left with both arms paralleling the body. Continue with the following commands:

  Clench fists, make arms rigid with tension; hold; feel the tension, hold; relax. Do it again. Flex both arms, leaving upper arm on mat, turn hands toward each other and press them together; push your hands against each other; harder, harder; feel the tension; hold it, hold it; relax and return; let your arms back; feel the relaxation; breathe deeply; hold it; let it go slowly; relax.

- *Step 5D: Thorax, Shoulders, and Neck*

  As we get up around the thorax, shoulder girdle, neck, and face, there will be more exercise items per area than there were for the lower body. Often, after sufficient initial run-throughs, I will drop the lower body exercises and concentrate on the upper body and the speech mechanism.

> Keep your arms at rest. When I tell you, shrug your right shoulder up from the mat and toward your right ear; hold it; feel the tension in shoulder and neck; hold it; relax; breathe; relax. Notice how your chest feels more relaxed. Breathe, relax.

Have the client repeat this exercise with the left shoulder. Then have the client do the exercise with both shoulders at the same time. Move to the next sequence.

> Keep your arms at rest; turn your head strongly toward your right shoulder; turn until you feel the pull on your neck and shoulder muscles; turn, turn; hold it; relax.

Have the client repeat this exercise, turning the head to left. Continue with the relaxation procedure.

> Press your head back against the mat, arching your neck up as you press harder against the mat; hold it; press hard; hold it; relax.

> Remain lying flat but tilt your head up and forward; press your chin against your chest and hold it, hold it; feel the tension on your neck and shoulder; hold it; relax and let head relax back.

> Lie back and relax; breathe in and out deeply and slowly several times. Enjoy the sense of sinking down into the mat.

- *Step 5E: Facial Areas*

Check to see if any body areas need renewed relaxation. If not, proceed with the following commands:

> When I say "forehead" I want you to wrinkle your forehead as hard as you can and hold it tight until I say "relax." When I say "eyes," I want you to squint your eyes shut as hard as you can and hold it tight until I say "relax." When I say "nose," wrinkle your nose up as tight as you can and hold it tight until I say "relax." When I say "jaw," clench your teeth together as hard as you can and hold it tight until I say "relax." When I say "tongue," press your tongue up against the roof of your mouth and hold it tight until I say "relax." When I say "lips," grin as widely and hard as you can, and hold it until I say "relax." Now, when I say

"tight," I want you to tense everything—your whole body, your face, shoulders, legs, arms, everything—until I tell you "relax."

If the client is concerned and questions whether to tense a specific part of his or her body, just reply that the object is to become as tense as possible, and not to worry about parts. Tell the client you will monitor to see if any body area seems neglected. When this is accomplished, give the following instructions:

Relax. Just relax. Keep your eyes closed. Breathe in deeply and hold it, exhale. Just keep a steady breathing pattern while you listen to the music. Keep your mind clear, don't hurry, relax, slow your breathing down, relax and feel it.

Usually the client is brought out of relaxation slowly. Tell the client to open his or her eyes and wake up a bit. Inquire how the client feels, how things went, and so forth. If it can be done, bring lights up slowly as you talk, or turn on a distant light in the room first. When the client sits up or gets up, be near and be watchful for any temporary dizziness or acclimation problems. Take note of the client's speech, and record it if desired. Clinicians often use the early return stage, just described, to practice relaxed speech patterns, Easy Onset, Light Contacts, and so on.

DESENSITIZATION

Sensitivity is the capacity to detect and respond to threshold-level stimuli. Part of maturation is learning when to be sensitive to small signals, and when to place signals (large or small) into a personal perspective. Stutterers, with reference to communication, tend to lack or warp that perspective. To be hypersensitive is to respond to stimuli that otherwise would be ignored, and to exaggerate the sensitivity to ordinary or minimal stimuli. A stutterer's communication hypersensitivity is linked directly to his or her fear hierarchy, and this document should provide a picture that simultaneously identifies sensitivity (anxiety) factors and assigns a sensitivity sensory value to each factor. A discussion of how to lower sensitivity and allow the client to respond with less exaggeration and distortion follows.

Desensitization in Management

Desensitization is one of the fundamental elements of classical symptom modification therapy, and it probably has State of University of Iowa links to early analytic theories of stuttering. At any rate, Johnson (Bloodstein, 1995), Bryngelson (1966), Van Riper (Eisenson, 1958), and many others emphasized desensitization. Fluency reinforcement therapy initially rejected desensitization (Ham, 1989), but produced many clients who could not retain fluency in situations where they felt pressure and anxiety. As a result, in the last decade or so, integration of management procedures has created a resurgence of desensitization applications.

Areas Affected by Hypersensitivity

Using the fear hierarchy, the clinician and client can compile a list of sensitivity areas to examine. An example is shown below.

Telephone	Coworkers	Strangers	Superiors
Groups	Social	Specific words	Specific persons
Gender	Family	Topics	Feelings

Next, the clinician uses the fear hierarchy to rank those situations. The clinician selects one or more categories to start with, based on two selection factors:

1. The situations selected are low(er) on the fear hierarchy.
2. At least some situations in each category can be performed in the clinic, and/or performed out of the clinic with the clinician present.

On a hypothetical case, I will draw up a desensitization activity list, one that would apply to many real clients.

- Make any type of telephone call.
- Receive any type of telephone call.
- Respond to questions or requests of strangers.
- Talk about own stuttering, therapy, and so on.
- Read material to learn about stuttering.
- Talk with other stutterers.

This list can be supplemented with activites unique to the client.

Telephone calls almost always can be made from in-clinic locations and used to transfer clinic experience to out-clinic solo telephone activity. Similarly, the clinician can make arrangements to have friends (clinician's or client's) call into the clinic to speak with the client. Contact with strangers usually can occur first with receptionists, custodians, or colleagues in the clinician's building.

Having the client talk about his or her stuttering is almost unavoidable in the clinic, and the clinician should note if the client shows any tendency to avoid discussing personal aspects of stuttering. The latter attitude may be marked by statements such as "uh, let's not talk about it; let's do something about it!" Changes of topic or a sudden series of questions are other common responses. Once the client is able to talk freely to the clinician about his or her personal stuttering, assignments outside the clinic can be devised. Four examples follow:

1. Keep a diary about your daily experiences with stuttering.
2. Tell three friends about your history of stuttering and past therapy.
3. Tell one (different) person each week about your therapy work and progress.
4. Interview an older family member about your stuttering past.

Bibliotherapy, gathering information, can be very useful, and it is discussed in chapter 2. Talking with other stutterers may be impossible, unavoidable in a group setting, or possible with some extra effort. A client can be assigned to talk with another stutterer, intermittently share therapy sessions, or just scheduled to observe another client's therapy. The clinician must ensure that permission is obtained from all clients involved. As just mentioned, use of existing and available stutterer support groups can be valuable (see chapter 9).

There are, perhaps, three keys to securing desensitization. First, the stutterer must be brought to the point where he or she is willing to perform the activities needed to desensitize. This process may go smoothly and quickly, or it may take quite a bit of time and careful planning because of client weakness and sensitivity. Next, the clinician must gauge the demand levels, and therefore the stress levels, of situations. Third, the clinician must secure a smooth transfer to solo client performance at a frequency level that should serve to stabilize the desensitization.

The client should be made aware of desensitization values and the targets selected. The client must be willing to face anxiety and perform, which means the clinician must set levels and goals that the client can tolerate in order to move progressively through the hierarchy. It is best if the client and clinician reach an agreement concerning stress levels and specific targets. Typically, the clinician carries desensitization far enough at any one stage of therapy to assist or enable other therapy activities, be they symptom or fluency oriented. Few clients will remain in therapy if desensitization is the only goal activity, week after week. The goal for the clinician is to get into desensitization, reach a level or target, ease off while bringing in another therapy dimension, and, at a proper time, return to further desensitization.

In-clinic performance targets, if wisely chosen, should approximate the following goals:

> Do not refuse, retreat from, or cut off a situation 100%
> Be able to construct an overall good postsituation report 95%
> Supply a "fairly accurate" report on one or more of the
>   following 80%
> • How many stuttering spasms occurred
> • Eye contact, general and specific (during spasms)
> • Breakdown of mild, moderate, severe spasm count
> Can describe other person's reactions, speech, etc. 75%

For out-clinic experience and practice, I would initially drop the percentage requirements by half, and slowly raise them as self-efficacy feelings and performance improve. Also, as control or fluency methods increase desensitization needs, criterion percentage targets can be raised. Sample out-clinic assignments are suggested below.

- Make 5, 10, 15, or 20 [select one] telephone calls per day to strangers and, after each call, total your spasms, count your avoidances, or evaluate your feelings [select one]. Bring in a report.
- Make 1, 3, 5, or 7 [select one] 10-minute telephone call(s) to people you know. Total your spasms, count your avoidances, or evaluate your feelings [select one]. Bring in a report.
- Arrange for 1, 2, or 3 [select one] friend(s) to call you each day and talk for at least 10 minutes each. Total your spasms, count your avoidances, or evaluate your feelings [select one]. Bring in a report.

- Call 5, 10, 15, or 20 [select one] strangers over the next 5 days; say you are conducting a telephone study of stuttering and have five questions to ask [make up questions in advance]. Keep calling until you reach the target number of people. Total your spasms, count your avoidances, or evaluate your feelings [select one]. Bring in a report.

These assignments are examples only; it is not a complete list, does not necessarily contain the best items for all clients, and explores only one area of communication. Obviously, while working on desensitization, these same activities can be used to stress self-monitoring, practice pseudostuttering, study listener attitudes, and so on.

The results of desensitization activity will vary. The competence of the clinician, session frequency, client stability, group or individual sessions, and other factors will interact. Leaving those factors aside, I would make five empirical observations:

1. Desensitization usually is a minor need for very young children, is very important and attainable for elementary school–age children, and is very important and not too attainable for many adolescent fluency problems.
2. Desensitization is more important, and harder to achieve, for female stutterers than it is for male stutterers.
3. Desensitization problems tend to be inversely correlated to stuttering severity; that is, the milder the stutterer the more difficult it will be to secure desensitization.
4. Pure fluency reinforcement therapy is completely compatible with desensitization work. Unfortunately, even now, desensitization does not occur when it would be most useful.
5. Desensitization (or lack of sensitivity) is positively correlated with transfer success, early on, and with final maintenance stability after the conclusion of therapy.

RECIPROCAL INHIBITION

Desensitization discussion leads to a concept or procedure that has been called "systematic desensitization," also known as "reciprocal inhibition." Wolpe (1973) linked relaxation and desensitization to the simulation or recreation of anxiety and tension. As noted elsewhere, relaxation and tension/anxiety are incompatible states. In its classical form, relaxation therapy of the intensive type is applied until whole-body relaxation is instated (35 to 40 or more sessions). When client control of relaxation is thoroughly in place, the SUDS concept (see earlier this chapter, under "Communication Fear Hierarchy") is applied to develop very detailed information about client fears. With the client in "maximum relax," the clinician verbally creates situations while monitoring the client's tension level, starting over and over again if tension rises too much. Transfer is complex and is broken into ministeps.

Brutten and Shoemaker (1967) applied Wolpe's ideas with stutterers. Over the years I have become less inclined to use reciprocal inhibition in the Wolpe style. It is extremely time consuming; frequently meets client resistance (on several points) among all but the most severe stutterers; has (as far as I am aware) a poor transfer capacity for stutterers; and requires an SLP who is simultaneously learned, skilled, and experienced in aspects of neurology, counseling psychology, and stuttering. It is difficult to find significant experience in the third aspect, much less the other two.

ATTITUDE CHANGES

The importance of attitudes is seen from instruments such as Cooper's (1973) Chronicity Prediction Checklist. Emphasizing attitude importance does not signify that there is a typical stuttering personality. Shames and Florance (1982) explored this question, as have other authors, and rejected the idea. I feel that most stutterers are about as well adjusted as most non-stutterers—a thought that can be somewhat worrisome. However, without going through a literature review, I would suggest that stutterers' attitudes toward communication tend toward the undesirable or unhealthy. These attitudes can be so intense as to be socially and communicatively disabling, or they may be mild enough to lose effect in therapy with ordinary progress and evolution of fluency or control systems.

Assessment of Attitudes

Evaluation of attitudes was discussed in chapter 1, in reference to diagnostic assessment. It also has been mentioned in this and other chapters to varying degrees. Without extended discussion, instruments to aid in assessing attitudes are presented in Exhibit 4–3.

One also could develop a communication attitude scale for personal use. Applications for planning therapy activities are obvious, and such personal lists can be readministered periodically to check on progress (i.e., changes in attitudes). A partial example is presented in Exhibit 4–4.

Exhibit 4–3 Instruments to assess attitudes

- *Children's Attitudes about Talking, Revised (CAT-R)*. DeNil, L., & Brutten, G. (1991). Speech-associated attitudes of stuttering and nonstuttering children. *Journal of Speech and Hearing Research, 34*, 60–66.
- *Inventory of Communication Attitudes*. Watson, J. (1987). Profiles of stutterers' and nonstutterers' affective, cognitive, and behavioral communication attitudes. *Journal of Fluency Disorders, 12*, 389–405. It is somewhat unwieldy to use, but informative.
- *Iowa Scale of Attitude toward Stuttering*. Ammons R., & Johnson, W. (1944). Studies in the psychology of stuttering: 18, the construction and application of a test of attitude toward stuttering. *Journal of Speech Disorders, 9*, 39–49. A well-constructed measure, but some items are archaic in reference and some have an air of inadequate political correctness. I have hoped for years that some person would revise and update it.
- *Perceptions of Self Semantic Differential Task*. Kalinowski, L.S., Lerman, J.W., & Watt, J. (1987). A preliminary examination of the perception of self and others in stutterers and nonstutterers. *Journal of Fluency Disorders, 12*, 317–321.
- *S-Scale*. Erickson, R.L. (1969). Assessing communication attitudes among stutterers. *Journal of Speech and Hearing Research, 12*, 711–724.
- *Speech Situation Checklists*. There are many forms of these around. A number of tools listed in this attitude section involve rating speech situations. They are, as noted elsewhere, useful for fear hierarchy construction, desensitization, transfer work, and so on. They also will provide input on attitude variations and problems.
- *Stutterers' Self-Ratings of Reactions to Speech Situations*. Darley, F.L., & Spriestersbach, D.C. (1978). *Diagnostic methods in speech pathology* (2nd ed.). New York: Harper & Row.
- *Stuttering Problem Profile*. Silverman, F.A. (1980). The Stutterer Problem Profile: A task that assists both client and clinician in defining therapy goals. *Journal of Speech and Hearing Disorders, 45*, 119–123.

Exhibit 4–4 Communication attitudes scale

Rate your agreement with each statement below. 1 = Strong disagreement, 2 = Disagreement, 0 = Uncertain, 4 = Agreement, 5 = Strong agreement.	
I talk as much as others do.	1 2 0 4 5
I don't mind talking on the telephone.	1 2 0 4 5
I have no "feared" words as far as stuttering is concerned.	1 2 0 4 5
I rarely substitute words to avoid stuttering.	1 2 0 4 5
I usually feel self-confident about my speech.	1 2 0 4 5
I am fluent more often than I am dysfluent.	1 2 0 4 5
In general, my luck is pretty good.	1 2 0 4 5
In speaking, I usually have pretty good eye contact.	1 2 0 4 5
My friends don't mind the fact that I stutter.	1 2 0 4 5
Usually I am fairly relaxed when I speak.	1 2 0 4 5
Most of the time, I think I am in control of my speech.	1 2 0 4 5
I am quite willing to talk about my stuttering to my family.	1 2 0 4 5
I am quite willing to talk about my stuttering to my friends.	1 2 0 4 5
I am quite willing to talk about my stuttering in the clinic.	1 2 0 4 5
I am quite willing to talk about my stuttering to strangers.	1 2 0 4 5
I am quite willing to talk about my stuttering to groups.	1 2 0 4 5
I would like to attend a stutterer support group meeting.	1 2 0 4 5
I am in charge of my life.	1 2 0 4 5
I really don't care what others think of me.	1 2 0 4 5
I wouldn't mind if I just stuttered "a little."	1 2 0 4 5

One could use different word choices and develop an attitudes list for younger stutterers (about 7 to 12 years), such as shown in Exhibit 4–5.

In the absence of formal tests, or the informal checks just suggested, the clinician can just listen for client statements that indicate attitudes. Such statements include, but are not limited to:

- I'm a victim. When my stuttering takes over, I try and fight, but "it" wins.
- Past therapy hasn't helped; I'm a real slow learner. I don't like slowing down . . . relaxation, gimmicky stuff.
- SLPs don't really understand what stuttering is like; nobody really understands me.
- Most of your techniques really are just tricks; what you call fluency gestures sound like avoidances to me.

- People listen to me and laugh; girls/guys don't want to go out with me because I stutter.

Observable behaviors tend to follow the lines suggested above. Situation avoidances, poor performance on outside solo assignments, lying about or "editing" assignment reports, rationalizations for nonattempts, incomplete efforts, or failures are a few behaviors that suggest poor attitudes.

In assessing attitudes and their significance, the clinician can attempt to categorize the client into one or more of the following four categories:

1. The client's attitudes seem rather typical, and the hoped-for success and progress in therapy should patch or mend any weak spots.
2. The client's attitudes, overall, are within acceptable limits, but specific areas (e.g., feelings of self-efficacy, concerns about quality of their nonstuttered speech, etc.) may need specific attention at the right time(s).
3. The client's attitudes, generally and specifically, are sufficiently undesirable to make them an early major and ongoing goal in management planning.
4. The client's attitude problems are major and may reflect underlying emotional problems. Referral for further evaluation and possible counseling should be considered.

Significance of Attitudes

Attitudes determine, or at least shape, a number of management aspects. Tolerance for dysfluency is a major attitude factor. Early professionals

Exhibit 4–5 Attitude list of young stutterers

	Rating			
Item	Almost Always	Often	Sometimes	Almost Never
I feel upset when I stutter.				
People don't like me when I stutter.				
I don't like to talk about my speech.				
Teachers give me a hard time.				
I get teased a lot about my speech.				

stressed the importance of the client being able (and willing) to say, "yes, I am a stutterer!" and stutter openly and willingly. Bryngelson (1966) stressed the tolerance and toughness factors in symptom therapy. Fluency reinforcement, in part, has come to recognize the value of a "tough attitude." After all, when fluency is typically defined as up to 0.5 stuttered words per minute (sw/m), tolerance attitudes had better be part of the therapy plan.

Responsibility or self-dependency is another part of attitude concerns. The stutterer needs to recognize that most of what he or she calls stuttering actually is what he or she is doing in an effort to avoid stuttering. The speaker, not the symptom, is the responsible agent.

Self-efficacy is the firm foundation or collapse factor in recovery and maintenance. The clinician must make sure that she or he does not project an attitude of "Do just what I tell you . . . how I tell you . . . when I tell" so that the client fails to develop a feeling that he or she can plan, perform, evaluate, and control his or her own behaviors. These three factors—tolerance, responsibility, and self-efficacy—are the products of the attitudes a client has plus the attitudes the clinician teaches or fosters.

Attitude Aspects

No one can possibly cover all the potential attitude variations of different clients. In an earlier section I described some personalized attitude characteristics. Below are some categories that are more generalized.

Perfectionism—any stuttering event, no matter how slight, is failure; not sounding like a television anchorperson is failure. These feelings relate to the next category.

Either/Or—an aspect of perfectionism that makes no allowance for "better" or "improved." A 10-second stuttering spasm and a fractional-time dysfluency are "stuttering" and therefore are failures.

Yes, But—a category I borrowed from Berne's *Games People Play* (1964). It is a passive-aggressive behavior where the client agrees with the clinician's purpose or analysis, but immediately negates it with a but: "I'm willing to try cancellations, *but* my mother doesn't want me to use them."

Prove It—the client protects himself or herself by challenging the clinician to prove that a feeling, attitude, point of view, or other thing is true, real, applicable, or so forth. Often, such proof is impossible to offer.

Been There, Done That—an attitude that is the bane of clinicians. Many stutterers receive their first therapy early in life and may have known a dozen clinicians before today's session. Obviously, past therapy has failed, or they have relapsed. Half-baked, incomplete therapy programs, or good programs and half-baked clinicians, provide source and justification for this attitude. Of course, for some stutterers it is just a defense mechanism. My response is to have clients relate their experience and then have them do it again my way.

Shifting Attitudes

Some attitudes cannot be shifted. Logic, persuasion, past experience, trial success, and other factors just may not change the attitudes of some persons. Where attitudes have been cemented by years of embarrassment, rejection, speech failures, and other negative reinforcements, amelioration, not elimination, may be the most for which we can hope. Amelioration is almost always possible; elimination is sometimes possible. Approaches to facilitate attitude change include

- Incorporating initial discussion, establishing rapport, sharing of treatment plans, and securing client commitment in the earliest stages of therapy
- Employing self-monitoring, self-analysis procedures
- Having the stutterer analyze the speech behaviors of "fluent" speakers
- Using self-study of attitudes and feelings through assessment instruments such as the S-Scale (Erickson, 1969) and other instruments
- Using carefully selected and graduated outside solo assignments to foster transfer and feelings of self-efficacy
- Using carefully planned in-clinic activity to foster the development of self-evaluation and consequation as part of every learning sequence
- Placing attention on bibliotherapy, both informational and inspirational
- Facilitating positive responses and attitudes, in the clinic, by the client

Shames and Egolf (1976) discussed thematic response (TR) therapy. Client statements about their speech, themselves, and stuttering are rated as either TR+ or TR–. Illustrative examples are provided below.

TR+	TR–
I came here because I decided it was time to do something. When I stutter, why I just tough it out and keep talking. I've got to quit avoiding things.	I've given up. I can't handle it. You wrestle with it! Stuttering has ruined my life. Just don't ask me to go out and talk to a lot of people.

The clinician, by voice inflection, facial expression, and verbal response, makes the client aware of what is TR+ and what is TR–. Ground rules are not laid out for the client. Clinician responses are restrained and understated as follows:

- MmmmHmmm [inflection indicating + or –]
- Oh? [plus facial expression and inflection]
- I like to hear you saying that
- Sounds sort of no-win
- Do you think that works?

Challenge points can be used when the clinician and client have a good rapport. The clinician suggests that a certain attitude (or a behavior expressing it) needs work. If the client agrees, then it is made a specific therapy target and plans are made. The clinician also can work to develop basic skills in problem solving with the client, approaching personal problems with a balanced view. Easy examples can be worked through together, and then more complex attitude problems can be broken down into steps and targeted.

Transfer work probably is the biggest support of attitude shifts in therapy, if it is done thoughtfully and continuously. What is learned in the therapy room is often in conflict with what is done (and what was believed in for years) outside the clinic. Therefore, work on transfers is imperative. There are SLPs who feel their job is done when in-clinic "instatement" occurs. I am at a loss for words when I hear this opinion.

SUMMARY

This chapter presented a collage of topics. Fear hierarchy, relaxation, desensitization, reciprocal inhibition, and attitude certainly are linked. Keeping them in balanced perspective is, however, difficult. Manipulating them all in therapy is harder, much harder then mixing mechanical symptom or fluency techniques. The elements in this chapter tend to require more finesse or sophistication (and self-confidence) on the part of the clinician. This fact may explain why those elements may be emphasized too little, or even omitted, from some management plans.

REFERENCES

Berne, E. (1964). *Games people play*. New York: Ballantine.

Bloodstein, O. (1995). *A handbook on stuttering*. San Diego, CA: Singular Publishing Group.

Brutten, E.J., & Shoemaker, D.J. (1967). *The modification of stuttering*. Englewood Cliffs, NJ: Prentice Hall.

Bryngelson, B. (1966). *Clinical group therapy for problem people: A practical treatise for stutterers and normal speakers*. Minneapolis, MN: T.S. Denison.

Cooper, E.B. (1973). The development of a stuttering chronicity prediction checklist: A preliminary report. *Journal of Speech and Hearing Disorders, 38*, 215–223.

Eisenson, J. (1958). *Stuttering, a symposium*. New York: Harper & Row.

Erickson, R.L. (1969). Assessing communication attitudes among stutterers. *Journal of Speech and Hearing Research, 12*, 711–724.

Ham, R.E. (1986). *Techniques of stuttering therapy*. Englewood Cliffs, NJ: Prentice Hall.

Ham, R.E. (1989). *Therapy of stuttering: Preschool through adolescence*. Englewood Cliffs, NJ: Prentice Hall.

Overstake, C.P. (1979). *Stuttering: A new look at an old problem based on neurophysiological aspects*. Springfield, IL: Charles C Thomas.

Shames, G.H., & Egolf, B.B. (1976). *Operant conditioning and the management of stuttering*. Englewood Cliffs, NJ: Prentice Hall.

Shames, G., & Florance, C. (1982). Disorders of fluency. In G.H. Shames & E.H. Wiig (Eds.), *Human communication disorders, an introduction*. Columbus, OH: Charles E. Merrill.

Wolpe, J. (1973). *The practice of behavior therapy*. New York: Pergamon Press.

CHAPTER 5

Control Methods for Fluency Reinforcement and for Symptom Control—I

- Overview
- Light Consonant Contact
- Easy Onset
- Whisper Speech
- Continuous Phonation and Blending
- Summary

OVERVIEW

This chapter discusses some closely related procedures: Light Contact, Easy Onset (EO), ventriloquism, and so forth. Two other techniques—continuous phonation and blending—are also presented; they are unrelated to the foregoing but are, themselves, linked together. In terms of relationship, the last two procedures are linked more to control methods discussed in other chapters but they can be, and are, used separately or with methods other than rate control.

This linkage confusion is compounded for many speech-language pathologists (SLPs) by their own past learning experiences with and exposure to package therapy programs. All too often student clinicians are taught to use one or more package programs and, as a result, assume that certain procedures are inextricably linked. In this chapter, and the next several, techniques will be presented as unitary phenomena, not as part of a package. References will be made to possible combinations, but most presentations will emphasize the unitary factor.

For instance, Curlee and Siegel (1997) tend to combine Light Consonant Contact (LCC) with airflow and suggest that it be offered in an extended length of utterance (ELU) context. They also suggest using it through a delayed auditory feedback (DAF) sequence, noting that voluntarily pro-longing (prolongation) the initial syllable of a word requires the use of a reduced or light articulatory contact (LCC). This combination is arguable. One can teach DAF (or other prolongation) techniques by combining a strong, slow-dragging articulator movement, while using blending and continuous phonation in order to maximize the tactile speech cues, thereby minimizing the auditory cues that stutterers usually monitor. One can note the combination of several techniques in the same package.

LIGHT CONSONANT CONTACT

LCC is a very old technique; nobody knows how old. Certainly, tech-niques to reduce or alter the stress and duration of articulator contacts have been around for centuries. Froeschels (1950) described an LCC method (ventriloquistic speech) about 50 years ago and, despite claims to the contrary, he was not the originator (Silverman, 1996). Every speaker develops habituated sets of articulator preformation and contact patterns, patterns that include the shaping modulations in the vocal tract, the energy or effort with which sounds are formed, and the durations of the various segments of the pattern. Stutterers tend to exaggerate or distort all parts of a production pattern—shaping, force, and duration. With use, the distorted preparatory set can actually become a trigger for stuttering spasms, as generalized anxiety and tension responses come to focus on specific areas of the speech production mechanism. It results in an habituated pattern of tense, prolonged, interrupted, distorted production. LCC, like most tech-niques, is aimed at changing this self-perpetuating cycle by reducing the motor speech tension and altering the preparatory set preformations. In LCC, the preformation is more important than the tension reduction.

LCC was the first control technique in stuttering I observed. The instructor invited a stutterer to visit and, as he spoke, the class became aware of a "hot potato" quality to his speech. He used the LCC method on almost 100% of his utterances, and we thought it was quite noticeable.

LCC and EO

There tends to be some confusion and overlap between LCC and EO, as there is between continuous phonation and blending. There is also overlap between fluency reinforcement and symptom modification. Actually, all techniques are tributary variations of the mainstream of motor speech pattern alteration. LCC does not necessarily involve EO. The prolonged breath components and relaxation of EO are not found in pure LCC, but often do occur together. In its pure form, LCC is restricted to reducing the force and duration of articulatory contacts, with any other effects being secondary. I will use "CP" to indicate continuous phonation, and assume blending will be covered by CP.

Silverman (1996) questions whether methods such as LCC can be used effectively where moments of stuttering are brief in duration. He cites Zebrowski (1991), who reported that stuttering children averaged 750 ms or less duration for both prolongations and repetitions. If true, then this finding applies to any technique used to regain control (see "Pullouts" in chapter 8) when stuttering occurs. Of course, it would not apply to preparatory sets, cancellations, or to generalized or limited fluency reinforcement applications. Also, Riley and Riley (1984), in their program for children, include LCC as part of their therapy program.

Teaching LCC

Ventriloquism

The simplest way to teach LCC is to have the client utter a short phrase aloud, and then repeat that phrase with his or her mouth open as wide as possible. Instructions to the client are of the nature, "You can move things, but nothing can touch." An example follows.

> *First utterance*: Hello, my name is Wendell Johnson.
> *LCC utterance*: eh oh I a ih ih uh ah uh

Emil Froeschels (1950) proposed this ventriloquistic approach, and many SLPs have used it (with stutterers and flaccid tongue problems). When clients first start this sequence, the initial response is to laugh, be embarrassed, and want to stop. Do not let them. The next problem is the temptation for both client and clinician to jump immediately to a slight degree of LCC because it sounds so much better. Resist the temptation. The client should keep working until he or she develops a sense of vowel formation and tract shaping as the articulators create minimal modulations.

Productions should be relaxed, not loud, and the vowel output should assume something of a melodic quality as syllable stress is reduced. Once the client can move smoothly from vowel unit to vowel unit, the clinician can use various types of practice material (word lists, sentences, paragraphs, discourse) until the client reaches a level or degree of LCC that balances intelligibility favorably against firmness of contacts. It usually is necessary to direct the client to increase relaxation of the articulators as he or she reduces the amount of articulator separation. When the desired level of LCC is reached, the clinician will need to decide whether its best use(s) is:

- As a fluency induction mode in all general speech output
- As a fluency induction device in specific speech loci and/or in specific communication situations
- As a preparatory set, pullout, or cancellation method (any one or all of them, as needed) on specific words when stuttering occurs or is anticipated
- To be combined with one or more added control modes

LCC is one of those techniques that should be recalled by the client for practice on a scheduled basis. Without repetition, it may slip from control and disappear.

Mechanical Separation for LCC

In 1951, I was required to buy a therapy device for a methods class. The device, which was to be used with sluggish or paralyzed tongues and for teaching LCC, was called a "bone prop" because it originally was made of bone and was used to prop the mouth open. By 1951, it was made of plastic and shaped and textured like a piece of bone. A bone prop (as I saw them) was about $\frac{3}{16}$-inch wide at each end, and perhaps $\frac{1}{8}$-inch wide across the middle. The surface at each end had a slot cut in it, like the slot in a common screw head. A small hole in the middle of the prop took a disposable string, so that one could hold onto the prop when it was in the client's mouth and prevent any accidental swallow or inhalation. Lengths of bone props were varied, and some SLPs kept a set of graduated lengths.

In use, the bone prop string usually was placed necklace-style around the client's neck. He or she then placed the prop more or less at midline of the mouth, with the maxillary (upper) central incisors set in the top groove and the mandibular (lower) central incisors set in the bottom slot. Placement slightly impeded interdental thrust, but not seriously. Usually, the client started with the shortest length prop and worked upward through various lengths, and then reversed the pattern until a length was found that combined acceptable production with tolerable comfort. Practice, articulatory or fluency, then helped set the contact force and pattern desired for transfer to nonprop speech. For sanitary control, it is better if each client buys his or her own bone prop (or equivalent). After each use, the item should be dipped in alcohol, dried with a clean tissue, and stored in an appropriate container or plastic bag.

Rather than bone props, which do slightly hinder lingual projection, dental blocks can be used. An inert block-shaped substance with a stick-like handle is inserted between the back molar teeth on one side of the mouth. The handle projects forward, along the inner cheek and out the mouth. Dental blocks come in graduated sizes and can be reusable (with sterilization) or disposable.

In an economic world of minimal support budgets, oral expanders can also be manufactured. I have used a sterile razor knife to score and split wooden tongue depressors into desired widths, placing them on the edge between molars, as described for dental blocks. They are discarded after each session. An SLP I know collected plastic swizzle sticks of various thicknesses and sterilized them between uses. A public school SLP bought packages of several sizes of Popsicle sticks and wooden stirrers for coffee and tea for use as discardable separators. Ingenuity, with due regard for safety and antisepsis, can provide an array of dental separators for LCC use.

Acquisition Steps

The steps described can be performed with a bone prop, with sizes of dental blocks, or with some of the creative items listed. The steps also can be used for LCC without mechanical aids (as described subsequently).

Preparatory Actions

First, the clinician prepares practice material in the form of a preliminary set of words for acclimation practice and two sets of 20 (or more) practice sentences. These practice items should be separated into "easy" and "hard" production groups. Easy predominates with fricative and other continuant productions and "hard" has more stops, plosives, and polysyllabics. Clinicians can develop their own lists, or use the items provided in the following steps. The word list is intended for initial, awareness practice, stimulation of monitoring awareness, and setting degrees of oral separation.

Hay	Fin	Sew	View	Go	Doe
Who	Fan	Sea	Vet	Gay	Dare
He	Foe	Sue	Van	Gas	She
How	Fat	Sir	Coy	Deal	Lie
Hoe	Fell	Son	Can	Do	Ray

Ten samples of easy and hard sentences follow.

Easy	*Hard*
How are you?	Give it to me.
I see some flies.	Butter the bread thickly.
Feel free to sing.	Most people don't do that.
Have some more mush.	Jump when you hear the gun.
Phil, where are you sir?	Don't ever do that again!
Have you seen Evelyn?	Nobody does that in October.
Where have all the fish gone?	Give me time to pack it up.
Send me some furry ones.	Calculate your best approach.
Feel the wave rush through.	Buckle your boots and jump up.
Haymows are fun to fall on.	Grab the brass ring and dance.
[Add 10 more of your own.]	[Add 10 more of your own.]

The hard and easy separation may not be needed, but some clients are initially more comfortable with it. The sentences above, plus personal additions, should provide adequate clinical practice material.

Suggested Practice Steps

The client and clinician discuss LCC mechanics and the rationale for LCC. The clinician models extensively what the client is to do and has him or her try LCC on a few, random words until assured that the client understands what is to be done. Once an understanding is achieved, the following steps are performed:

- *Step 1.* Use word list, and record on tape. Have client utter a word normally, then repeat it with a maximum oral opening. Have client slowly repeat the word four more times, reducing the oral opening each time. Repeat several times, labeling degrees of oral opening as "Regular, 1, 2, 3, 4, Maximum." Do this several times. Stop, rewind tape, play back. Discuss quality, intelligibility of different levels, and identify where the degree of separation and positive intelligibility seem best.

- *Step 2.* Use sentence lists (easy and hard). Record on tape. Have client read all 40 sentences aloud, in production pairs. That is, have client read a sentence aloud normally and then repeat the same sentence aloud with maximum oral opening. Judge readings on the bases of vowel accuracy, prosody normalcy, and minimal amount of observable production tension. After each four or five normal/maximum pairs, stop tape, play back, analyze, and discuss. If necessary, remodel, and try again. When client is satisfactory on 30 to 32 (80%) of the 40 sentences, move to the next step, or follow own criteria. Ask the client not to try LCC outside the clinic.
- *Step 3.* Use sentence lists (easy and hard). Record. Repeat the procedure in Step 2 but start at Level 4. Judge as before, and set an 80% criterion level.
- *Step 4.* Use sentence lists (easy and hard). Record. Repeat the procedures used in Steps 2 and 3, but start at Level 3. Evaluate as before, but judge production more closely, watching for slippage toward too much oral closure. During pause periods for evaluation, have the client do evaluations first. Then compare the two evaluations.
- *Step 5.* Use sentence lists (easy and hard). Record. Repeat the procedures used in the previous tapes, but start at Level 2. Evaluate as before, increasing the judging emphasis on "normal sounding" speech. At this point, speech should be understandable at the level of mild "hot potato" speech. Increase the client's evaluation responsibilities. Periodically, have the client utter a sentence at Level 2, and then say again at Level 3 or 4 (approximately). At this level, give the client solo home assignments, recording parts of them for evaluation in the clinic.
- *Step 6.* Use sentence lists (easy and hard). Record. Repeat the procedures used in Step 5, but start at Level 1. Repeat contrasting Level 1 with normal production and with Levels 2, 3, and 4. Have client do all evaluations now. Continue home assignments. Find out if client has been trying LCC on his or her own, and the results.

It will not be unusual if the client has tried to use LCC on his or her own. In fact it will be more surprising if he or she has not. If it has occurred, the clinician should take time to find out the details, consistency of efforts, results, attitudes, and so forth. The clinician should problem solve, motivate, scold, and reward as needed. At some early point in the home assignments, the client should be asked to start building a written list of words actually stuttered on outside the clinic. The client is to underline the syllable(s) on which the stuttering occurred. Sample instructions follow.

> Every day for the next 5 days you are to write down 10 words you stuttered on, marking the syllable you had trouble with. Bring the accumulated 50 words to our next session. I will add to the list by making a note of the specific words you stutter on in our clinic sessions.

The specific numbers may need to go up or down, depending on the frequency and severity of the stutterer's spasms. The clinician saves the word lists for use in later LCC stages (and other management techniques).

- *Step 7.* Have the client read collections of sentences, mixing the four levels of oral opening. Two examples are offered below.
  1. We haven't been to Chicago in years. I wonder what Clark street looks like now. I bet my old apartment on Deming is a high-rise now.
  2. Would you get me some tomatoes, a hot pepper, three turnips, and a dozen eggs? Oh yes, on your way home, would you pick up my dry cleaning?

  Make up six or so of these short paragraphs. Instruct the client to read each paragraph at a different oral opening level. Have client judge adequacy, while the clinician monitors. Inadequate production mandates repetition of the entire sequence. When done, go back over the paragraphs and have the client read them aloud again, but with a different opening level on each sentence:
  - First sentence at Level 3
  - Second sentence at Level 1
  - Third sentence at Level 2
- *Step 8:* Select a general paragraph of 150 to 200 words. Underline about 50 words where stuttering would be more likely (initial word, stressed word, longer word, key word, etc.). Have client read aloud, using LCC on underlined words, at a preselected oral opening level. Have client judge. Monitor, record, and play back to evaluate. If client finds a word poorly done, add two words to try in a new paragraph; if clinician deems any word poorly done (client had accepted), add four words in a new paragraph.

- *Step 9.* Set a time factor of 5, 10, or 15 minutes (or longer) for speech delivery. Require LCC on initial syllables of the first two or three words after each pause for breath. Mark each series as acceptable or unacceptable, based upon preset criteria. If ratio of acceptable to unacceptable falls below 10:1, add another minute of talking time to the duration target.
- *Step 10.* Take cumulative list of stuttered words (assignment following Step 6) and have the client read each word aloud, using one of the following behaviors:
  1. Read each word aloud with Level 1 or Level 2, or alternate words between the two levels.
  2. Read each word aloud, faking a stuttering spasm, pausing and relaxing, and then repeating that word with Level 1 or Level 2 LCC opening.
- *Step 11.* Have client make 10 in-clinic telephone calls of the "Do you have . . ." variety. They can be prewritten if desired. Use one or more of the following approaches:
  1. Use LCC 1 or 2 on every word.
  2. Use LCC 1 or 2 on preselected words, ignoring any stutterings unless they occur on the preselected words. If the latter occurs, make another call at once, using the same word again and moving to the next higher (wider open) LCC level.
  3. Use LCC as desired. On any stuttered words, pause and use LCC as a cancellation (see chapter 8) on the previously stuttered word.

At this point, client is ready to start or continue transfer work (see chapter 9).

Final Comment on LCC

When exposed to LCC in 1951, the particular stutterer used it as a fluency reinforcement device (on every utterance) 15 years before it surfaced as a product of the behavior modification and fluency reinforcement advocates. Over the years I also have seen it used, and used it, as a symptom modification device in cancellation, pullouts, and preparatory sets. LCC probably has more efficacy than many believe, but has not been popular because it lacks the backing of an authority figure to publish findings and promote successes. I think it is less effective than Easy Onset (discussed next) because it neglects the respiratory and (mostly) laryngeal components of speech production. Whether a noticeable EO is more, or less, acceptable and effective than a noticeable LCC is open to speculation. Any judgments will have to be made by the client and the clinician working together.

EASY ONSET

Stutterers typically approach vocal tract modulations from a state of anxiety and hypertense physical function. A "relaxed stutterer" is an oxymoron. Tense musculature tends to result in fixations of structures; delayed onset of articulator movements; inappropriate speed of movements; and errors in the extent, duration, and strength of movements. There also is frequent distortion of the normal articulatory preparatory sets.

However, if the stutterer can initiate an utterance without excess tension, then the other abnormal states or actions cited above are less likely to occur. For generations, therapy efforts have been directed at easing the tension, relaxing the onset of utterance efforts. EO reflects these efforts. EO has been applied in one form or another for hundreds of years. In this era, it has been used in partial forms in symptom control therapies. For example, Webster's precision fluency shaping program (1980) used the gentle onset of phonation, whereas Schwartz (1976) involved EO ideas in his passive airflow and airway dilation. Individuals can change labels, rearrange sequences, alter criteria, and invent impressive names but a reduction in production effort and an increase in production timing still is EO. During the unpleasant confrontations between symptom modification and fluency reinforcement approaches in the 1960s and 1970s, EO was simultaneously praised as a new discovery and as an old, shopworn gimmick.

Van Riper (1973) wrote about the tactile and kinesthetic cues of the stutterer's speech mechanism acting to establish a trigger pattern for precipitating stuttering spasms. The clinician's task was to find some way to keep the sensory perceptions from triggering stuttering spasms. Perkins, Rudas, Johnson, and Bell (1976) suggested a discoordination hypothesis for stuttering, linking the complexities of coordinating respiration, phonation, and articulation production to the occurrence of stuttering. EO, aside from reducing the tension with which speech function areas interacted, also provided a time/rate lengthening factor that improved the speaker's opportunities to integrate neuromotor and psycholinguistic aspects of speech production (Perkins, Bell, Johnson, & Stocks, 1979; Starkweather, 1986). Along this line, Williams and Brutten (1994) compared stutterers and nonstutterers, finding that the former (in fluent speech) exhibited greater laryngeal and respiratory latencies (delays) than those exhibited by nonstutterers. EO might well minimize or compensate for these differences.

The mechanism of EO will change as practitioners change. In general, EO applications will involve the following three elements:

1. A moment or pause for relaxation prior to the formulation of the ensuing utterance
2. Usually, as part of (1) above, an inhalation to ensure adequate respiratory support and to promote relaxation
3. A relaxed release or utterance, structured toward gentle contacts (see LCC) and slowed movements of the articulators and vocal folds, as opposed to quick movements and hard contacts

How the elements are put together will vary.

EO has been, can be, and is used as a sole method in some stuttering management plans. As indicated earlier, EO also can be regarded as a controlled disfluency in some symptom modification approaches. It also is an inevitable side effect of relaxation therapies and of most respiratory reconfiguration approaches. It is found as one of the fluency inducing gestures (FIGS) in Cooper and Cooper's (1985) Personalized Fluency Control Therapy and in the Easy Speaking Voice (ESV) of Shine's (1980) fluency program. In this chapter, EO will be presented "as is." How it will be used is up to the individual clinician.

EO should not be used as a sole management approach. Even though this usage occurs fairly often, it rarely should. Even with a structured transfer program, I question total dependence on EO (or any sole method) except with select preschool children. In the mature stutterer, habituation of distorted speech patterns and associated behaviors is so automatic and deeply ingrained that the relapse probability with single solutions is very high.

As just indicated, there is a role for single-focus programs with young children. Many relaxation games for children lead easily into EO production. With adequate and intensive modeling by the clinician, children usually can learn EO quickly.

EO can be of value alone and as a precursor to other procedures, especially if there is a perceived need to provide early progress (and motivation) for the client. EO can be used as one part of a multiple attack on symptom patterns. This is exemplified in the next chapter when rate control is discussed, or earlier in this chapter with coverage of prolongation. Finally, EO can be used as a late addition when "something more" is needed to help clear up residual problems in a client who otherwise has made good progress.

Both LCC and EO often are directed at initial syllables or initial words in an utterance, because the majority of stuttering tends to occur there. At one time it was suggested that adults and older children tended to cluster spasms more on consonants, and younger children to cluster more on vowels. Wall and Myers (1995) summarize this situation quite well, by noting that young children tend to start utterances with "I" and with "and," and that this tendency shifts with maturation toward a greater use of consonants. Therefore, it seems that position, not phoneme, is more important. Wall and Myers also describe an EO (easy speech) process for children. A breathy, relaxed utterance of "I" or "I'm" is introduced, and later reduced. In addition to modeling, they also suggest unison speech to help with instatement. In the following acquisition sections, instructions will assume that clients are at least 9 or 10 years of age.

Easy Onset Acquisition

Preliminary Comments

I used these instructions in "classroom form" for 2 years, as a project in a senior class dealing with stuttering and in a graduate class on stuttering. About 160 students worked through them as "clinicians" and as "clients." Part of their report included criticisms and suggestions, which I generally have incorporated. In the original form, all phonemes and words were expressed phonetically, because I thought it would help the clinician keep track of what vowels were being worked on. A large number of comments argued against this approach because the student clinicians used my lists "as is" with their clients (usually roommates), and most roommates could not read phonetic symbols. After some head scratching, I decided to be consumer oriented and rewrite the lists. Some phonemes, especially some diphthongs, do not lend themselves well to nonphonetic expression. After a while, I gave up and tried just to have a good representation of vowels and assume that "spread of learning" would include any I did not include. As with other techniques, I will present EO as a solo technique and, near the end, I will taper off with a suggestion to refer to chapter 9 for general suggestions on transfer.

Acquisition Steps

The following steps are somewhat pedantic, taking things in rather molecular bites. Clinicians may skip or combine steps as desired, but such decisions should be for the good of the client, and not a surrender to impatience and a desire for quick results.

- *Step 1.* Explain two things to the client: (1) Rationale for working on EO, and what it is supposed to do. Assure him or her that initial exaggerations (model) will be shaped into adequate EO productions (model) that compare favorably to tense, distorted stuttering spasms (model). (2) The performances in breathing and relaxation that need to be checked on, in case one or both need attention before EO can proceed. Invite questions, discuss, model again as needed, and then go to next step.
- *Step 2.* Check diagnostic information for adequacy of the vegetative (nonspeech) respiratory pattern. If information is not available, check the respiratory section in chapter 1 of this book, and determine client adequacy. Do not worry if there is poor use of air stream now, because correct acquisition of EO behaviors should provide a foundation for appropriate use of the air stream in speech.
- *Step 3.* Stop to explain, and demonstrate, to the client the differences among the three types of vocal attack: hard, simultaneous, and breathy.

  Hard (glottal shock)—the vocal folds are tightly approximated and then forcefully blown apart (as in a loud "Ha!").
  Simultaneous—the most common type of vocal attack. As the vocal folds approximate, an easy air stream is released at the same time.
  Breathy—an audible release of air occurs before vocal fold approximation, and the released tone is breathy.

The clinician should explain these differences carefully, model several examples, and encourage the client to try and imitate the models. Explain how stutterers often overuse hard glottal attacks.

- *Step 4.* Provide the client with stimuli to repeat to begin EO production. Clinician models all productions at first and then drops out, modeling only to reinforce or correct. In every case below, the client is to prolong the initial /h/ into /hhhhhh/ as a voiceless production (do not anticipate the following vowel). Then the client is to easily "slide" into the following vowel. Do not allow an audible shift between /h/ and the vowel. The entire production is to be easy, relaxed, slightly breathy. If needed, go back and work on relaxation and practice the gentle releases, but do not allow too much breathiness.

heee	hih	ha	If not sure what one
ho	hoo	how	representation means,
huh	hoy	hay	make up your own

Listen for any combinations that are better or worse than the others in terms of EO quality, breathiness, loudness, and so on. Work on this until you are assured the client has a firm grasp of the concept and is able to produce consistently isolated consonant-vowel (CV) productions with EO.

- *Step 5.* Repeat Step 4 using the same vowels, but have the client utter two productions of the same CV pair (see below).

hee-hee	hih-hih	ha-ha
ho-ho	hoo-hoo	how-how
huh-huh	hoy-hoy	hay-hay

Pause and breathe between productions of the same pair, and take a breath before going to the next pair. Record and play back, comparing productions within and between pairs and listening for breath support adequacy, adequate prolongation, EO characteristics, and so on.

- *Step 6.* Repeat Step 4, using the same vowels, but have the client utter two productions of the same pair without pausing for breath. Record and play back, comparing productions for breath support adequacy, prolongation adequacy, EO characteristics, equivalence of the two utterances, and so forth.

- *Step 7.* Produce CV pairs on one breath, as in Step 6, but make each CV in a pair different.

he-(pause)-ho	hi-(pause)-he	hay-(pause)-ha	hoo-(pause)-huh
how-hi	ho-hay	hoy-he	huh-hoo
ha-he	huh-how	hi-hoo	he-heh

Record and evaluate as before.

At any point above, the clinician can insert performance criteria, generally in the range of 80% to 90% acceptability, based on intake of air sufficient for productions; air release equivalent for each production; air release adequate and without strain for all productions; comparable loudness and duration; and so forth.

- *Step 8.* Produce CV utterances with the aspirated /h/, followed by a vowel and terminating in continuant fricative. This makes it easier to produce a prolonged, breathy utterance.

his	has	haf	hif	hish
hus	hos	hays	hof	hesh
hes	huhs	hef	huf	hooz
hiz	haz	hav	hiv	hazh
hoz	huz	hiv	huv	hizh

As before, the vowels can be called anything; it does not matter. Notice that the terminations start as voiceless productions, and then switch to voiced.

Depending on the client, the clinician may very easily skip a number (or many) of the preceding steps. Likewise, steps may be shortened or eliminated, depending on where the client needs to start work. These steps are deliberately started on a very simple level, and progress in microsteps, which may be too simple and slow for some clients. Adapt as needed.

- *Step 9.* Repeat Step 8, but in each CVC (consonant-vowel-consonant) unit, terminate the unit by repeating the carrier vowel a second time.

hisi	hoso	husu	hese
hivi	hovo	huvu	heve
hini	hono	hunu	hene
hizi	hozo	huzu	heze
hasha	hosho	hushu	heshe

- *Step 10.* Repeat the previous procedures, but make terminating consonant a stop.

hip	hit	hid	hik
hob	hog	hod	hok
hag	hat	had	hak

hek	hep	hed	heg
hug	hut	hud	huk

Have the client work on making the final-position stop consonants a sort of moving production of the articulators, rather than hard stops. This production more or less combines LCC and movement.

- *Step 11.* Have the client drop the aspirated /h/ and substitute a variety of voiceless continuants, prolonging them and making them breathy before easing into the following vowels. If necessary, at first, start with the /h/, ease into the following consonant, and then finish.

fa	fai	feh	fo	fu	fee	fi
sha	shai	sheh	sho	shu	shee	shi
sa	sai	sheh	so	su	see	si
tha	thai	theh	tho	thu	thee	thi

(*Note:* At times lists will generate what seem to be real words. There is no problem with that. However, do not change the pronunciation— as in /thee/ above, do not pronounce it "the.")

- *Step 12.* Monitor closely to determine whether the /h/ needs to be inserted at first to ensure a relaxed, breath production.

va	vai	veh	vo	vu	vee	vi
zha	zhai	zheh	zho	zhu	zhee	zhi
za	zai	zeh	zo	zu	zee	zi
tha	thai	theh	tho	thu	thee	thi*

*Remember, this is the voiced /th/.

- *Step 13.* Repeat Step 11 and Step 12, substituting voiceless stops/ plosives for voiceless continuants used in Step 11 (pa, pu, peh, kee, ki, tai, to, etc.), and substituting voiced stops/plosives for voiced continuants used in Step 12 (bo, bi, gu, ga, dai, dee, etc.). Monitor closely because the client may tend to revert to old, distorted preparatory set configurations because there are more possibilities for loss of relaxation, hurried release, and so on. Copying the sound lists in Steps 11 and 12, there are 48 (2 × 24) productions in Step 13. When the client produces 20 out of 24 acceptable utterances (83%) in each group, proceed to the next step.
- *Step 14.* Develop a word list based on age, grade level, Jonah words, occupation, and hobbies for the client. Select words that can be used later to construct sentences. Have client utter the words in isolation.

Where needed, initial /h/ can be used at first. This will help the client prepare for later transfer work so that if, outside, he or she "gets stuck" he or she has practiced falling back to a more basic EO using the prefix /h/ to get started.

is	are	was	were	have	had	give	do
be	am	take	want	will	go	come	see
who	what	when	where	why	which	with	how
some	few	many	fair	big	little	left	right
I	you	me	they	he	she	them	us
may	can	should	would	water	milk	beer	juice
butter	bread	pizza	burger	hot dog	pasta	fries	milkshake

- *Step 15.* Shift to short sentence or phrase utterances, using as many words as possible from Step 14. Concentrate on using EO of first words, stressed words, and client Jonah words, and encourage client to drop EO where he or she thinks it "feels safe." Occasionally require a client to say every word with EO, just to keep skill and self-efficacy feelings up.

Who are you?	I will have a hot dog and fries.
Where am I?	Can I see that when you are done?
That is juice.	I will give you one more chance.
Butter my bread please.	Some friends have all the luck.
She is my friend.	This should replace pizza as food.
He left us alone.	What a waste of time for me and you.
Would you go there?	Such a waste of time for us all.
May I see that glass?	There is more in the trunk of the car.
I want a milkshake.	I'll see you about 8 or 9 o'clock.
Move to the right side.	Never look behind you on a dark night.

Add more sentences as needed. Pass/fail criteria are hard to set here, but the following are suggested:

-EO was not used there and it should have been.

-EO lacks slight breathy quality.

-EO lacks relaxation.

-EO lacks slight prolongation.

-EO does not move smoothly from one sound to next.

-Rate is too fast for effective use of EO.

One way is to simply mark for each error (only one error per EO effort) and set an allowable limit of errors per 10 sentences. When that limit is passed, stop and start the sentence list (or group of 10 sentences) over again.

- *Step 16.* Lengthen sentences to increase complexity of word combinations, need to pause for breath, appearance of Jonah words, undesired rate increases, and so on. Set a target of 100 sentences (or 50) with no more than two errors per sentence, as defined below.

  – One EO that should have been used but was omitted and one error

  – Two EOs that should have been used but were omitted

  – Two errors in production of EOs

The first two are very judgmental, and the client is allowed to argue. EO errors are the usual, cited before. When one of the three criteria cited above is met, an extra sentence is added. When extra sentences go over 10% (5 on 50 sentences, 10 on 100 sentences), erase all efforts and start the step over again. Ten illustrative sentences follow.

1. Where do I go to find the best watermelons, and who pays the bill?
2. Give me some idea of what you want, and I will do my best.
3. It is a pity that she is too young to try out for the pep squad this year.
4. Excuse me for interrupting, but it is time for me to go home now.
5. A long time ago and far away there lived a fairy princess and a mean witch.
6. Some people have problems with understanding the metric system, but it makes sense to me now that you have explained it.
7. Some stutterers talk in long sentences because they have found that once they get started it's easier to keep going than to start over.
8. Drop by some time and I will show you how to build a model airplane without using plastic or other modern stuff.
9. If you cannot see the reason for this, I doubt very much that you would be happy with a career in politics or any aspect of government.
10. Never think that you can get away with dishonesty all of the time, because sooner or later somebody will catch you.

The clinician may mix sentence applications of EO in three ways: (1) clinician underlines words that are to have EO applied, (2) client underlines words he or she thinks might need EO in "real life," or (3) client reads the sentence without advance preparation and applies EO as she or he goes along. All three approaches can be used.

- *Step 17.* Introduce spontaneous speech. Use questions that can be answered briefly, preferably using the words introduced in the questions.

> Clinician [models EO]: "Do you have apples and oranges?"
> Client: "No I don't have apples and oranges."

Make up about 50 sentences. Model every sentence. Have client re-use modeled words, if feasible. This approach will become less feasible as questions change or require longer answers After about 10 short-answer questions without any errors in the responses (keep working until client gets 10 consecutive acceptable responses), shift to open-ended questions, such as:

- Tell me the story or plot of the most recent television show you have seen.
- As a child, what were your favorite games?
- Describe the room we are in.
- Who is your favorite actor (actress) and why?
- Tell me a funny joke.

Have client evaluate recording of his or her efforts, and correct. After 5 or 10 questions/answers, instruct the client to pose 5 or 10 questions. Demonstrate good and appropriate use of EO in answers. Have client evaluate and comment on clinician's performance. Do not try to be perfect. It is best if there are omissions and errors for the client to catch. If clinician feels the need to save face, warn the client in advance that deliberate omissions and mistakes will be made.

- *Step 18.* This is a checkup step. Four speech activities follow. Record each one, but do not play back until all four are completed. Follow the evaluation recommendations at that point. Have client read a 150- to 300-word paragraph that contains underlined words that would be good EO targets. Then give client a different 150- to 300-word paragraph, unmarked, for client to read aloud, using EO where it seems appropriate. Ask client limited-answer questions, instructing him or her to use EO as if it were a group situation with strangers. Give client a topic to speak on for 3 minutes (approximate), as if he or she were giving a talk before an audience, using EO appropriately. Play back the recordings and evaluate them with the client, concerning:

- Overall judgments of EO quality (relaxation and gentle onset, slight breathy quality, slight prolongation, easy blending of initial onset to the rest of the word)
- Specific words (make a list) where EO either was unacceptable or borderline
- Specific words where EO probably should have been used, but was not
- Common factors (word position in phrase, initiating phoneme, Jonah word, monitoring fault, "fatigue" with EO, etc.) on unacceptable or omitted EOs
- The number of unacceptable EOs in each of the four speech modes, subjectively balancing to see where more problems occur

The clinician is to avoid doing the analysis and instructing as much as possible. Push the client to perform all of the evaluations and problem solve for solutions and possible corrections.

Easy Onset Repair

EO Repair is a concept and a practice related to the symptom modification technique, cancellation (consult chapter 8 for a full explanation). Here it is used to build self-monitoring, evaluation, and self-efficacy in using EO. Any control technique, whether it is symptom modification or fluency reinforcement in nature, can be used incorrectly, used unsuccessfully, or fail to be used when needed. Thus EO Repair can be used with any of the modification techniques. In this instance, failure in EO is not to be accepted and left behind as a failure. It is to be canceled, as explained in the next step.

- *Step 19.* Explain the concept of EO Repair to the client. Tell the client that it is to be used in either of two circumstances:
  1. No EO was attempted and there was a stuttering spasm (failure of monitoring, control, or prediction).
  2. EO was performed or attempted, but client slipped into a stuttering spasm.

  Note that a poor EO, if successful, is accepted in this step. Nothing succeeds like success. In either instance cited above, the client is to stop immediately after the flawed word is completed, pause, inhale and consciously relax, and then repeat the word with a slightly exaggerated EO production. Demonstrate EO Repair by pseudostuttering failures (see chapter 2), and then repairing the "failure." Have client perform pseudostutter and Repair (about 25 to 30 practice efforts, each).

By now, the client should be ready for transfer work. Home assignments should be started by about Step 4 or 5 (see chapter 2 concerning assignments). Start other transfer work (see chapter 9) to out-clinic use after this step. Use the fear hierarchy concept described in chapter 4.

Easy Onset Summary

East Onset is presented here as if it were going to be the only control technique used and is not associated with any other management procedure. It can be shortened and simplified to the extent that the clinician desires. However, I would warn against untoward simplification. Easy Onset is not just easing up on onset aspects of production. It is a complex adjustment of respiration, phonation, articulation, speech rate and timing, auditory-tactile-kinesthetic monitoring, anxiety control, and self-confidence (as are nearly all techniques). Often, it is rather easy for some clients—as long as it is in the clinic. However it often falls apart completely when self-efficacy becomes the issue. Common sense and ethics require careful management.

WHISPER SPEECH

Whisper Speech, as a technique, needs to be specified because many people misuse the term. Zemlin (1998) stated that, in whispering, the two arytenoid cartilages are slightly abducted and their vocal processes turned in toward midline. This toeing in creates a small opening between the cartilaginous margins of the vocal folds. This space or chink is greater than the abduction space between the membranous margins of the vocal folds. Air rushing through the open area creates the friction sound of whispering. Some individuals show slight vocal fold vibration, and some show none. Properly speaking, a whisper has no harmonic characteristics, no fundamental frequency, and minimal capacity for change. It uses air much more quickly than during usual fold vibration, and one must breathe more frequently. Obviously, during a whisper the speaker shifts his or her vocal fold patterns away from the usual, which may help explain its fluency support. That the whisper is a simpler neuromotor task than typical phonation is not questioned, and research (Perkins, Rudas, Johnson, & Bell, 1976) reporting that stuttering during whispering fell well below stuttering by the same speaker in ordinary speech production should not astound.

The fluency effect of whispering may relate to motor simplification. Starkweather (1982) thought it might involve aspects of slowed rate and increases in the duration of vowels and consonants. For many years, only "quacks and charlatans" (supposedly) used Whisper Speech. It is found today in a number of reputable management programs, including Shine's (1980) use of Whisper Speech in the acquisition of the ESV.

In most therapies where it has been used, Whisper Speech is not really the true lack of vocal fold vibration described earlier, at least not for very long. An absolute whisper, especially with children, may be fun to play with in therapy. However, Whisper Speech generally leads quickly into a very breathy, soft, monotonous (or stereotyped) vocal pattern. This is partly due to a desire to move toward a more natural sounding speech pattern. Also, the modified whisper usually is more relaxed than a pure whisper, uses less air, can be heard more easily, and should be less of a strain on the vocal area. Few directions for Whisper Speech are needed, but the following should be borne in mind:

- Reduce utterance length sharply, shorten phrases, and increase frequency of breaths.
- Do not suggest or allow projection with a whisper voice. Loud whispers are counterproductive (tension) and abrasive.
- Use the whisper voice to compare words and phrases uttered in normal voice and in whisper.
- Use whisper voice, if desired, to show that the client can speak without stuttering.
- Use whisper voice as in the first item in a move into another fluency or control mode, limiting whisper to early learning steps.

CONTINUOUS PHONATION AND BLENDING

A person can eat for social reasons, for taste, for nutrition, and for other purposes. Even if one purpose is paramount, most of the other effects cannot be avoided. EO generally involves some level or degree of prolongation, prolongation "always" has an element of continuous phonation, and continuous phonation usually involves a certain degree of blending. All of the foregoing will serve to reduce rate. All factors, including rate reduction, will have an effect on respiratory patterns and frequency and on airflow. When I read about airflow therapy contrasted with rate reduction therapy, I am aware that, to a significant degree, different parts of the same structure are being viewed. Continuous phonation is no exception.

I have used continuous phonation for many years, yet find very little about it in the literature, journals, or texts. Pindzola (1987) describes it in her program. Curlee and Siegel (1997), in describing the Computer-Aided Fluency Establishment Trainer (CAFET) program, cite both continuous phonation and blending. Continuous phonation has been incorporated into some electronically programmed, computer-based sequences. This is an impossible application for most SLPs because of the cost of equipment and the need for special training. I used continuous phonations in the 1950s as part of pullout strategies. I also used it in pseudostuttering as variations in a pseudostuttering program. Continuous phonation can be used in concert with LCC, or it can be used in the kinesthetic and tactile intensification efforts involved in the strong articulator movement control method (see chapter 7).

Definition and Description

Continuous phonation, for purposes of this book, is a process in which the production of one phoneme/syllable merges, without interruption, into production of the following phoneme/syllable. All surds (voiceless sounds) tend to become sonants (voiced sounds). A word, whether it is "feather" or "sphygmomanometer," is uttered as one continuous production, subject to breath availability. *Blending* uses exactly the same definition, but the term generally is used to describe a continuous phonation *between* words, on the terminating sound of one word and the initiating sound of the word following. Some persons use the terms, continuous phonation and blending, as synonyms. Others have different preferences. I will not separate them in this brief section on acquisition.

Rationale

Continuous phonation and blending (hereafter referred to as continuous phonation [CP]) have a foundation in several effects created by application:

- It changes or eliminates dysfluency triggers involved with certain articulatory postures (see "Preparatory Sets," chapter 8).
- Profound changes in prosody stress, inflection, and so on will eliminate or reduce other dysfluency triggers or loci.
- Tactile and kinesthetic feedback is increased, and the stutterer can be practiced in monitoring these avenues rather than concentrating on auditory feedback, which is associated with stuttering.

We know that stuttering is more likely to occur on stressed words, stressed syllables and words, nouns/verbs, adjectives/adverbs, and so on. CP tends to change or minimize these cues or landmarks. Finally, as with many techniques, CP is a distraction factor, a different mode of speech, that will facilitate fluency. Hopefully, the induced fluency will be used to learn and channel new motor patterns and positive attitude changes.

Acquisition Steps

- *Step 1.* This step helps the client understand the concept of continuous phonation and blending. Have the client read the following word pairs aloud, producing each word separately without exaggeration.

Some more	Six cents	Half full
Let's see	For rent	Row over
Barrier reef	Ten nails	Mirror red
Mechanical failure	Reference library	Felonious assault
Never-ending story	Mississippi River	Transcendental meditation

  Record and play back, noting (slight) separations between each word in a pair. On the longer words, note the stressed syllables.
- *Step 2.* Take the previous list and have the client practice saying each single word, prolonging each phoneme. (Theoretically, CP can be done without prolongation but, practically, they are inseparable.) The sounds *sssum* or *sssuuum* are not desired; *sssuuummm*, where each sound receives an approximately equal duration, is the goal. Repeat this with other words. When the client reaches the multisyllable words, make sure she or he takes a breath when it is needed, and not when it is proper for continuity.
- *Step 3.* Still using same list, have client utter each pair of words, extending the CP to blend one word into the next. Record and play

back, listening to make sure each phoneme receives similar treatment. Reject any production where one word in a pair receives greater stress than the other, or any syllable in a word receives greater stress (or duration). (*Note:* On longer word pairs, inhalation and airflow patterns must be dealt with.) On the 15 pairs of words, work and repeat until 12 of the 15 pairs on 15 consecutive productions are generally acceptable. Awareness and voluntary control are being targeted, not an outcome form of production. Proceed to the next step when the client can go through the list of 15 pairs three times with no more than 30 errors of omission or inadequacy (because the 15 pairs generate about 180 syllables and around 360 phonemes, 30 errors is a fairly high standard).

- *Step 4.* Move to reality-based utterances. Any sentence with more than two errors must be repeated. Keep count of errors, and if the error total reaches 15 or more, pause to problem solve, and start the sentences over again. Use 10 sentences, three times (same sentences). Evaluation criteria are as follow:
  - Equal stress
  - Equal duration of prolongation
  - Blending within words
  - Blending between words
  - Adequate phrase breathing

  Eleven sample sentences are offered below (1 for starting practice; 10 for practice).

  1. Hello, how are you?
  2. Glad to meet you.
  3. My name is _____.
  4. Where is the restroom?
  5. How much does that cost?
  6. My telephone number is _____.
  7. What time do you open?
  8. Where will I find your _____?
  9. I don't really know that.
  10. This needs more salt and pepper.
  11. I can do that without any trouble.

- *Step 5.* Repeat the procedure and criteria from Step 4 (but not the sentences). Ask short, closed-end questions, having the client answer using the same words as much as possible. The clinician models continuous phonation and blending in her or his questions.

1. Did you see that kennel club special on television?
2. Do you stutter when you read aloud?
3. How far is your home from here?
4. Do you often use postponements when you stutter?
5. Have you ever taken a roller coaster ride?
6. Have you used word substitutions at all today?
7. Are horses smarter than pigs?
8. How many times a week do you use the telephone?
9. Do you often stutter when saying your own name?
10. What time do you usually go to bed at night?

Be sure to watch for respiratory insufficiency on longer sentences, and have the client practice phrase breaks. Set a pass criterion of no more than one error per sentence, repeating any rejected sentence until criteria are met.

- *Step 6.* Discuss turning CP into an intermittent, where-needed procedure. Identify where in the previous 10 sentences the client would have been likely to stutter. Look for Jonah words, longer words, key information words, initiating words of a phrase, and so on. Run through the 10 sentences from Step 5 again, but leave it to the client to use CP where it "feels best." Discuss the outcomes, and compose additional sentences, if useful, on which to practice.

- *Step 7.* Formalize the finishing activity above. Present new, longer sentences and tell the client to use CP as it feels best. Record and play back for evaluation. Question use/nonuse of method, but focus mainly on how well it is done, when used. Ten illustrative sentences follow.

1. We have not been able to decide on a single cause for stuttering.
2. Female stutterers generally have milder symptom patterns than males do.
3. A significant number of "stuttering" children outgrow their stuttering, without formal therapy.
4. The telephone generally is the stutterer's most feared situation.
5. Many years ago, most clinicians thought that stuttering involved a change in the child's handedness.
6. Some psychiatrists still believe that stuttering is caused by too early toilet training.
7. Many mild and moderate stutterers are reluctant to do anything in therapy that will "advertise" stuttering.

8. Stutterers' intelligence scores distribute the same way as do the IQ scores of nonstutterers.
9. Some research suggests that the fathers of stutterers are more perfectionistic and demanding.
10. We have not found a significant relationship between psycho-neurosis and stuttering.

These sentences are longer. Practice until the client is comfortable with what feels like "appropriate" use of CP, and the clinician agrees.

- *Step 8.* Provide the client with a printed paragraph. Underline the word(s) where CP would be most appropriate (based on knowledge of the client and his or her stuttering characteristics). Have the client read aloud. Record, play back, evaluate, and discuss. Then give the client an unmarked copy of the same paragraph, and have him or her read aloud with the following direction, "Use continuous phonation and blending wherever they would be of greatest value to you if you were reading this paragraph to a group." Record, play back, evaluate, and discuss. Repeat if needed.

- *Step 9.* Ask the client questions, instructing him or her to talk for about 1 minute, or until the signal to halt is given. Have the client use CP as it feels best. Develop questions that are open ended. Six are offered below, but the clinician will want to develop more so that the client will have about 30 minutes of actual talking time.
    1. Assume I am a layperson. Please explain prolongation and blending to me.
    2. If I gave you a 2-week, expense-paid vacation, where would you go and what would you do?
    3. What is your favorite sport, and why do you like it?
    4. Tell me about the best pet you ever had.
    5. When you first attended school, what were your stuttering experiences?
    6. Tell me about the worst movie or show you have ever seen.

    Terminate each answer after a minute or so. Interrupt if little or no CP is used, or if it is poorly done. As a penalty, have client restate the entire answer, and add 1 minute more to the 30-minute target.

- *Step 10.* Have client practice CP on 10 prewritten telephone calls. Criterion is zero stuttering on 8 of the 10 calls (reset other criteria as seems best). When communication or social stress is introduced, add

EO or Bounce or some other initiating form of controlled utterance, as necessary.

As in the earlier section of this chapter on LCC, the client is ready for transfer work (see chapter 9). The clinician should employ a talking rate, a difficulty sequence, and a fear hierarchy level that is appropriate to the particular client and the particular situation.

SUMMARY

LCC, EO, and CP are closely linked, or can be. In my opinion they are best used as transition techniques, rather than as terminal targets for acquisition. However, they can be valuable when linked to additional therapy targets in fluency reinforcement or symptom modification methods. They also can be helpful in working with several forms of dysarthric speech and in some types of dyspraxia. In chapter 6, additional techniques—ones that can either augment, replace, or incorporate those presented in this chapter—will be discussed. I would stress that effective use of any of the techniques will rest on the self-monitoring skills of the speakers. If monitoring is not singled out and developed, then any of the control methods in this chapter will, at best, be used in a haphazard and incomplete fashion. The capacity to monitor effectively is vital, here and elsewhere.

REFERENCES

Cooper, E.B., & Cooper, C.S. (1985). *Cooper personalized fluency control therapy, revised.* New York: Slosson Educational Publications.

Curlee, R.F., & Siegel, G.M. (1997). *Nature and treatment of stuttering, new directions* (2nd ed.). Boston: Allyn & Bacon.

Froeschels, E. (1950). A technique for stutterers—"ventriloquism." *Journal of Speech and Hearing Disorders, 15,* 336–337.

Perkins, W., Bell, J., Johnson, L., & Stocks, J. (1979). Phone rate and the effective planning-time hypothesis of stuttering. *Journal of Speech and Hearing Research, 22,* 747–755.

Perkins, W., Rudas, J., Johnson, J., & Bell, J. (1976). Discoordination of phonation with articulation and respiration. *Journal of Speech and Hearing Disorders, 19,* 509–522.

Pindzola, R.H. (1987). *Stuttering intervention program (SIP).* Austin, TX: Pro-Ed.

Riley, G., & Riley, J. (1984). A component model for treating stuttering in children. In M. Peins (Ed.), *Contemporary approaches in stuttering therapy*. Boston: Little, Brown & Co.

Schwartz, M. (1976). *Stuttering solved*. New York: McGraw-Hill.

Shine, R. (1980). *Systematic fluency training for young children: A fluency training kit*. Tigard, OR: C.C. Publications.

Silverman, F.H. (1996). *Stuttering and other fluency disorders* (2nd ed.). Boston: Allyn & Bacon.

Starkweather, C.W. (1982). Stuttering and laryngeal behavior: A review. *ASHA Monographs #21*. Rockville, MD: American Speech-Language-Hearing Association.

Starkweather, F. (1986). The development of fluency in normal children. In H. Gregory (Ed.), *Stuttering therapy: Prevention and intervention*. Memphis, TN: Stuttering Foundation of America.

Van Riper, C. (1973). *The treatment of stuttering*. Englewood Cliffs, NJ: Prentice Hall.

Wall, M.J., & Myers, F.L. (1995). *Clinical management of childhood stuttering*. Austin, TX: Pro-Ed.

Webster, R. (1980). Evolution of a target-based behavioral therapy for stuttering. *Journal of Fluency Disorders, 5*, 307–320.

Williams, D., & Brutten, G. (1994). Physiologic and aerodynamic events prior to the speech of stutterers and nonstutterers. *Journal of Fluency Disorders, 19*, 83–112.

Zebrowski, P. (1991). Duration of the speech disfluencies of beginning stutterers. *Journal of Speech and Hearing Research, 34*, 483–491.

Zemlin, W.R. (1998). *Speech and hearing science, anatomy and physiology* (4th ed.). Englewood Cliffs, NJ: Prentice Hall.

CHAPTER 6

Control Methods for Fluency Reinforcement and for Symptom Control—II

- Overview
- Unison Speech
- Rate Reduction via Cognitive Control
- Shadowing
- Delayed Auditory Feedback
- Rhythm Procedures
- The Bounce
- Summary

OVERVIEW

Rate control is one of the oldest and most widely used management procedures in therapy of stuttering. It also has been used on accent reduction, dialect reformation, and so on. In stuttering therapy, rate control usually takes the form of rate reduction (i.e., slowing down). Research has been done in the area of rate acceleration (Kalinowski, Armson, Roland-Mieszkowski, & Stuart, 1993) but it is too recent for me to feel comfortable in advising clinicians on its uses. In most rate reduction therapies, clients are asked to slow down, are given slow models to emulate, may be trained to monitor and evaluate rate and use this information to achieve slower target rates, or may be subjected to various instrumental influences to encourage or force a rate reduction.

Three approaches to rate control are discussed: coerced rate control (unison speech), cognitive management of rate by clients, and instrumental rate control (such as delayed auditory feedback). These specific approaches are by no means the only ways to achieve rate alteration. Further, the particular approaches and steps within each approach are not the only methods of application.

UNISON SPEECH

Rate control can be achieved in a variety of ways—simple or complex, inexpensive or expensive. One of the simpler, less expensive methods is that of choral speaking or unison speech, where one person provides a vocal model that the other speaker follows by speaking simultaneously the same material being uttered by the model speaker. The model controls or manages rate or other aspects of production. The clinician must be able to consistently produce 30, 60, 90, or more words per minute (wpm), or model other controls. If rate is the target, as it is here, the clinician also will need to be able to sample client rate. Sampling is done most easily in 5-second segments of client speech, counting the words (or syllables) and multiplying the result by 12 (7 words in 5 seconds would equal 84 wpm). This method is favored over straight wpm or syllables per minute (spm) measures, because the clinician can avoid pause time delays when trying to assess actual word, or syllable, rates. If used frequently, the clinician will find that she or he can do the 5-second counts and calculations mentally during therapy and have immediate data for recording, evaluation, reinforcement, and so on. Unison speech can be used simply to induce fluency for various reasons. It usually is used to instate some other behavior. In this instance, rate control is targeted.

Rate Control via Unison Speech

One cannot say when choral reading or unison speech was first put into use. Surely, for educational applications, it has been in use for thousands of years. Slightly more recently, in 1937, Johnson and Rosen reported on the favorable effects of unison speech, noting that 17 of 18 stutterers were fluent during its use. Some 42 years later, Ingham and Packman (1979) reported that unison speech performances were related to a substantial reduction in the percentage of words stuttered. Apparent increases in wpm speech rate were found to be accounted for by reduction in the percentage of words stuttered.

Orientation

Unison speech generally is used with a reading-aloud performance. Thus, many clinicians do not use it outside of probe applications in diagnosis and assessment. Culatta and Goldberg (1995) recommend unison speech as 1 of 10 items to use in screening stuttering apart from other fluency disorders. Supposedly, unison speech will have little or no fluency induction effect on nonstuttering fluency problems, but it will reduce or temporarily eliminate the dysfluencies of stutterers. Silverman (1996) discussed unison speech in assessment, in differential diagnosis, and in therapy management. I have used it in all three aspects.

A number of clinician have used unison speech over the years (Falck, 1969; Gregory, 1968; Ham, 1986; Van Riper, 1973). However, there has been a tendency to dismiss unison speech as an effective technique, because of transfer inadequacies and lack of flexible uses. Silverman (1996) commented that fluent speech in unison speech would revert to stuttering at almost the instant that the unison speech activity was terminated. This phenomenon often is true if the clinician does not utilize unison speech for anything other than a temporary induction of fluency.

Unison speech has a number of applications that extend beyond just reading aloud in concert with another person. Some, but not all, of these applications are suggested below.

- differential diagnosis, where certain fluency problems do not respond well to unison speech
- in diagnosis/assessment activity, as a client demonstration of fluency induction possibilities
- practice in prosody alteration, initially or after the acquisition of certain controlled speech modes
- practice on various pause times or slow-downs in rate reduction, phoneme blending, continuous phonation, Bounce, or other methods
- practice in varying pause times on cancellations, preparatory sets, and pullouts, especially for clients who rush speech

- as a brief, initial activity in every management session to practice a particular target, or to remind the client of targets
- repair or penalty procedure when a client missed or performed poorly
- practice on specific utterances that are likely to happen for a client
- following solo modeling by the clinician, paired practice on pseudostuttering (faking), or negative practice
- as a way to model reinforcement or practice specific fluency induction modes initially

There can be values in unison speech that reduce or negate the transfer problem when the method is used with children. If age-appropriate adjustments are made, using unison speech to practice easy speech or other methods may show spontaneous and significant out-clinic transfer. Finally, unison speech (as suggested earlier) is best supported by solo modeling on the part of the clinician before it is used, unless the clinician is going to use pretaped stimuli for *both* purposes, modeling and unison practice.

Unison Speech Methodologies

Unison speech usually is practiced one on one, but it can be done on a group basis. When group work occurs, the clinician will have to organize time to attend to different group members to ensure adequacy in their performance. For finer differences, it may be necessary to break individuals out for quick checks and modifications. The simple structure of unison speech is that the client produces speech that coincides with and replicates the speech of the clinician when both persons are verbally producing the same material. Methods to achieve the basic concordance are varied, and can include the following:

- Face the client, sit near to him or her. Read loudly while the client also reads aloud from a copy of the same material.
- Sit by client's dominant side. Have client use nondominant hand to close off ear on that same side. Tilt your ear to within 3 or 4 inches of client's unoccluded ear (may cup hand around client's ear to channel sound). Speak more loudly than client as you read.

- Use a toy or real stethoscope, with earpieces inserted into client's ears and stethoscope bell or cone near clinician's mouth. Read aloud into the stethoscope bell, while client reads aloud. Be sure to check loudness comfort first; adjust to client comfort.
- Employ any electronic amplification system with earphones. Check for client comfort.
- Prerecord printed material on audiotape and play it back through earphones (or speaker), telling client to match and keep up with what he or she hears. Prerecord the same material several times at different rates, or with other differing characteristics.

Implementation of Unison Speech

Usually, skill acquisition goes from micro to macro. In unison speech I tend to reverse this process because I think the continuity of ongoing production is important to the client in the adoption of various production modes or changed behaviors. Single words, short sentences, and other micros offer too many start-again points at a time when the client is still uncertain about what or how he or she is supposed to do. On that basis, the following steps are suggested:

- *Step 1.* Give a printed (not small print) copy of a paragraph to the client and tell him or her to read it over silently. When client is done, ask if there are any words he or she cannot pronounce with confidence, or any words he or she does not understand. Be sure you can respond to both needs.
- *Step 2.* Instruct the client to listen silently while you read the passage aloud, solo. Be sure to model rate, onset, prolongation, or whatever you will ask client to do in the unison reading. If needed, model some individual phrases in the paragraph. Query client to ensure that targets and methods are understood.
- *Step 3.* Tell the client you and he or she will read aloud together, and to try and follow your verbal signal, not his or her own. Arrange whatever physical method you will use. Place recorder or microphone on the side of the client *away* from you, so his or her voice will be emphasized on tape. Start tape recorder and begin reading. Do not stop or start over; keep reading until client gets in step with you (or until it

becomes obvious that you must stop, reexplain, and demonstrate). Make any adjustments in your loudness, distance from client, and so forth as you go along. When finished, leave the tape running and say, "Let's do it again right now, just the same way. Ready?" Repeat the process. At the end, stop, rewind, and play back. Discuss. Compare both productions in terms of target of matching your speech. Listen for any stuttering. If present, discuss reasons.

If the purpose of unison speech is to provide some fluency experience for the client (to provide a model), a target, or some motivation, the clinician now would want to move on to the next activity. However, if unison speech is being used to acquire a particular skill, then subsequent steps are needed. For example, if it is being used to teach the client some of the modes available, the clinician might proceed with the instructions in the following step:

- *Step 4.* Tell the client, "After the first sentence, I will suddenly slow down for several sentences. Listen closely and follow my lead. Ready?" After the first sentence, drop to a very slow, prolonged utterance of 40 to 70 wpm. Stay at that rate for several sentences, jump back to a normal rate for two or three sentences, then shift to moderately slow (90 to 110 spm), then to normal rate, and finish a last sentence at the initial very slow rate.

At first, the clinician may need to pause slightly to switch rate modes and increase vocal loudness slightly to remind the client to follow the lead. If necessary, repeat Step 4 until the client is able to follow changes. Then instruct the client that, in the next step, different kinds of production modes, not just rate, will be changed and he or she will have to listen closely and change quickly. The paragraph in Step 5 is marked with nine mode changes. The duration of any mode and the specific mode can be changed as desired.

- *Step 5.* Read the following paragraph, adhering to the mode changes indicated.

  [normal mode] The average stutterer usually cannot remember when he or she first started to have trouble. [very slow] Actually, the trouble usually begins before he or she reaches school age. By first grade, stuttering usually is fairly well established. [whisper] When the child compares his or her speech to that of other children, he or she often feels it is his or her own fault. [normal mode] Guilt feelings only make things worse, and the stutterer builds up anxiety and tension. Awareness and anxiety tend to increase tension in the speaker so that any struggles become even stronger and spill over into the rest of the body. [very slow] It is possible that the rest of the body may become involved with abnormal movements and postures. [moderately slow] While these changes occur, the stutterer grows a bit older and meets more people and expeiences greater anxiety and tension. [prolongation mode] Strangers often are surprised by stuttering, and they do not know how to react to it. Their reactions may tend to disturb and upset the stutterer. [fast rate mode] Why do some people make it so hard for stutterers? [normal mode] Probably just because they are people and the stutterer has to expect what he or she gets and not much else. . . .

The preceeding paragraph can be extended as long as desired, and other modes can be added or substituted as desired. It does not necessarily teach a wide range of modes, but it stresses the idea of varying speech production, listening closely to self, and allowing the clinician to sample the effects of several different modes. If the clinician is capable, she or he also can insert pseudostuttering, Bounce, Easy Onset, cancellations, pullouts, preparatory sets, and other variations.

Rate Reduction via Unison Speech

The following steps use a variant form of unison speech to instate control methods:

- *Step 1.* Explain and model rate reduction. After explanations and modeling, utter (solo) the first sentence of a practice paragraph. Have the client attempt to replicate that production. Use any one of the various production modes (very slow, slow, fast, prolonged, and so forth). Record and play back. Discuss and problem solve. Model another sentence using a different mode. Repeat routine. Do this several more times until assured of client flexibility and adequacy.

- *Step 2.* Use a paragraph of 100 to 150 words. With the client, read together, forcing a rate of 30 to 40 wpm, taking 3 to 4 minutes to produce the short paragraph. (Be sure to have practiced 30 to 40 wpm in advance, with prolongation, etc.) Record, with microphone on the "away" side. Play back and evaluate; problem solve. Repeat exercises until client can match production and rate.

Often, a client will object, saying, "I never talk this slow!" The clinician should explain the need to learn control and variation at such slow levels and reassure the client that he or she will not be expected to use such slow rates in out-clinic speech.

- *Step 3.* Repeat Steps 1 and 2. If results are adequate, have client read aloud a third time while progressively dropping loudness level to that of a quiet voice. If the client starts to slip, increase loudness, and repeat the passage until client can maintain rate stability.
- *Step 4.* Repeat Step 3, but fade out completely after about 9 or 10 words. Record and play back. With client, take 5-second samples at five points (at 30 to 40 wpm, should produce no more than three to four words [five to nine syllables] in 5 seconds). If rate is over 40 wpm on more than one, or over 50 wpm on any 5-second measure, repeat entire step, problem solving as needed.

Clinician has now established a slowed rate of 30 to 40 wpm and can now follow rate reduction procedures or continue using unison speech, moving from 30 to 40 wpm to 60 to 70 wpm, and so on. Another application of unison speech involves using it to teach a fluency reinforcement of symptom control methods such as Easy Onset (EO) or Bounce, as shown in Step 5.

- *Step 5.* Take any paragraph of about 300 to 500 words and have client read it silently. Resolve any pronunciation questions, and together read it aloud in ordinary unison speech production. Produce a new copy of the same passage where words most likely to be stuttered on (first one, two, or three words of a breath group, Jonah words or sounds, stressed words, etc.) are underlined. Model, solo, for the client how underlined words are to be produced—with Bounce, Easy Onset, a strong movement, or some other form of production. An illustrative paragraph follows.

> A common fallacy among parents is the idea that very young children are unaware of their own stuttering. This is a myth. Most children are very aware of every stuttering because they see their parents being aware.

- *Step 6.* Read through the preceding paragraph with the client using unison speech. Slow slightly before hitting a target word, and ease into it. Run through the paragraph several times in unison speech, and then ask the client to read it solo. Listen for particularly troublesome words or trouble areas. Have client do another solo reading, with a pass/fail target of no more than 10% missed or inadequate productions.

Unison speech can be used to help a client learn to pseudostutter, to imitate his or her own stuttering without avoidances or struggles, or to practice altering specific aspects of her or his usual stuttering spasms. Unison speech can be used as an occasional "how to do it" practice, as a primer activity to start each management session, as a problem solver for difficult points, and so on. It is applicable to clients of any age and at any stage or type of therapy.

Unison Speech Variations

Model Tape Preparation

Teaching and modeling unison speech may be easier if the stimulus material is on tape. This approach allows the clinician to function as a monitor and evaluator without the distraction of having to produce stimuli at carefully controlled wpm rates. The clinician is encouraged to produce four permanent cassette tapes, representing four different reading rates. These tapes can be used in other rate reduction approaches. The reading rates can be varied, but I suggest the following: 30 to 40, 60 to 70, 90 to 100, and 120 to 130 wpm. The clinician can select other rates or ranges as desired. Basically, the four rates are intended to traverse from extremely slow to slightly slow. To prepare the model tapes, the following items are needed:

- four audiotape cassettes of 30 to 90 minutes duration
- timepiece with easily readable dial face or numerals
- audio cassette recorder, preferably with extension microphone
- printed, double-spaced paragraph of 200 to 250 words

Actually, several paragraphs are desirable. One of 240 words is provided in Exhibit 6–1. The sample paragraph has been marked at five-word intervals to make it easier to count words (syllable counts vary from five to about eight). For the same reason, at the end of each line the cumulative number of words is presented. Also contained in Exhibit 6–1 are four paragraphs with lengths of 30, 60, 90, and 120 words, respectively. The 240-word unit can be used for all types of readings, or the special-length paragraphs can be selected for a particular time frame. The step sequence immediately following describes how to prepare master tapes for rate control in a unison speech program. As noted before, the tapes also can be used as rate control models. I strongly urge the clinician, if she or he makes the master rate tapes just mentioned, to make duplicate copies of the tapes and store them for future redubbing needs.

- *Step 1.* Use either the 240-word paragraph in Exhibit 6–1, and mark the 120th word, or use the 120-word paragraph. Position the timepiece for easy viewing, and read the 120 words aloud, slowing and prolonging production to finish the 120th word at just about the 60-second point on the timepiece. Redo several times until the goal of 60/120 is attained. Do not lengthen pauses. Remember, more pauses are permissible (and will be needed for breathing), but do not prolong them. Shorten phrases to match breathing needs; do not overuse any one-breath cycle. Prolong every vowel of every syllable; prolong every continuant and use EO to prolong stops and plosives. Use continuous phonation (see chapter 5) between sounds, syllables, and words.

Once the clinician can produce an acceptable rate, he or she should go back and double-check all of the production variables. It will not be easy, but it is unfair to ask a client to do something that the clinician cannot do. In practice, the clinician must pay attention to prosody, pronunciation, and other normalizing factors and avoid monotone or stereotype production. When secure in this effort, the clinician should progress to making the first tape.

Exhibit 6–1 Practice reading material

240-Word Practice Paragraph

The problem faced by many / stutterers is that they tend / to slow down too much /	15
when they are faced by / a difficult speech situation. When / that happens, the	28
tension can / be rather high and this / tends to increase the probability / that the	42
speaker will stutter. / Most people, when faced by / a new situation, will tend /	55
to become tense and uncertain / and this tension and uncertainty / will show itself	68
in our / speech. Anybody is liable to / pause, hesitate, grope for a / word, stumble	82
over a word / or find themselves repeating a / word or sound without meaning /	95
to have that happen. Some / stutterers, on the other hand, / develop a defense	108
device of / speaking as quickly as possible. / They do this apparently in / the hope	122
that, once they / can get started, they will / not be interrupted or stopped / by	136
stuttering if they go / fast enough. The poor listener / then has to cope with /	150
the stuttering and, between blocks, / try to sort out what / is being said in that /	165
rapid torrent of mangled words. / The next problem faced by / the stutterer is that	179
of / abnormal articulatory postures that distort / the actual production of spoken /	190
sounds and make it hard / for the average listener to / understand what is being	204
said. / All of the above make / it more difficult for us / to help the stutterer bring /	220
his or her speech down / to, or up to, the / speech rate that most people / use to	237
talk to others.	240

30-Word Practice Paragraph

Some cats like dogs, but few dogs like cats. This sad tale is why my dog left me. The cat liked the dog, but she did not like the cat.

60-Word Practice Paragraph

How can I tell you the truth when I do not know the facts? Few of us want to lie when we talk, but it can be hard when some part of the news is false and we do not know which part is true and which part is not. Do not think facts and truth are the same thing.

90-Word Practice Paragraph

Much as I want to go to the fair, I am short of cash and do not want to ask for a date if I am out of luck that way. Ann would, I think, go to the fair with me and pay her own way. She would like to pay my own way if she knew about it. When I go on a date I like to think I can pay and not have to ask her for help. That way she will think I have lots of cash.

continues

Exhibit 6–1 continued

120-Word Practice Paragraph

Who has not hurt their foot when they stepped on a nail, kicked a brick, or dropped a box on it? You want to yell very loudly and say a curse or two. This will not be wise if your mother or father is near. Swear words make you hurt less, but parents would glare at you and tell you, "Stop that kind of noise!" Now, your foot hurts, they are mad at you, and you just must not do anything about it. Now, if you have a dog, the best thing to do is let him lick your nose. Dogs do not care if you are dumb or smart. They just love you and let it go at that.

- *Step 2.* Take the first cassette tape. Position the microphone, start the tape, and let it run 5 seconds. Utter, "Rate control tape 120 to 130 words per minute." Wait another 5 seconds and read the 120-word segment as practiced. Rewind and play back several times to ensure that this recording is acceptabe as a model for rate, prolongation, continuous phonation, and so on.

The clinician might want to run forward 5 seconds and record a new 120 words in order to provide variety for the client. Several more 120-word productions of different paragraphs would be useful. At this point I suggest copying the tape and starting a new cassette for the next step.

- *Step 3.* Follow the procedures outlined in Steps 1 and 2 for the 120- to 130-wpm rate. Remember, it will be harder this time because of the drop in rate to 90 to 100 wpm, using 90 wpm as the target. Use longer prolongations, slower pace, more frequent breath intervals, and so on to achieve the 30-wpm drop. Again, try not to increase the length of pauses. When practice efforts are satisfactory, record on a new cassette, play back several times, and evaluate. Again, do this rate with several different paragraphs.
- *Step 4.* Prepare another tape as indicated in Steps 1 through 3, with the rate range falling between 60 and 70 wpm. Remember the injunction about control of production because it will be much harder to produce a worthwhile tape at this rate.

The clinician should strive to produce the best model tape possible. The difficulty of this effort, even for the clinician, underscores the need for a solid example for the client.

- *Step 5.* Prepare the final tape using the procedures in Steps 1 through 3, with the rate range falling between 30 and 40 wpm. Mark the 30th word on the long paragraph or use the 30-word paragraph in Exhibit 6–1. Forget about prosody; it is not possible. Watch the pauses, as before. When satisfied, record one or several passages.

The clinician is now ready to use model tapes in unison speech therapy. I must comment that the clinician also can just practice "live" until he or she can reproduce rate approximations on the spot and dispense with the tapes. It is much more flexible than being tied to a tape model, but it has the drawback of not having tapes to send home with the client for practice.

Instructions to Clients

The clinician must explain carefully to the client what he or she is to do, and why it is to be done. Unison speech can remind many of childhood games, and clients may not see a valid reason behind the "silly factor" they perceive. They need to be told that the purpose of unison speech is to eliminate the old motor-speech patterns while learning more effective control patterns. Clients should be advised that the method is temporary and that the initial steps will be so exaggerated that they will not, for any reason, want to use them in out-clinic speech. It is the later modifications of unison speech that will be aimed at creating acceptable speech patterns.

The client needs to understand the added behaviors needed for unison speech at a slow rate. The clinician should explain why longer pauses are not desired, as well as model the elements of Easy Onset, prolongation, continuous phonation, and shortened phrase length. Usually, it is not necessary to practice these extensively in advance because the client will be following the clinician's taped productions. Occasionally, some clients are so inadequate in self-monitoring and production control that a tangent teaching program on prolongation, for example, is needed. If this situation occurs, the clinician should refer to the appropriate sections of this book. When the client is ready, therapy proceeds to the next phase.

Unison Speech Rate Control Instatement

Phase 1: 30 to 40 Words per Minute

- *Step 1.* Use a printed copy of the 30-word paragraph taped, and have the client read it over for familiarization. Play the recording on speaker (not earphones) while the client reads it silently (lip movement allowed) at the same pace. Discuss what it sounds like (awful), reassure the client, and review the behaviors used to slow down and smooth production (prolongation, Easy Onset, and so on).

  Play the tape again, on speaker, while the client overtly and silently "mouths" the printed material. Have client apply all the methods requested, but in a miming mode. Again, review and discuss when the activity is completed.

  Switch to placement of earphones on the client, place the script paragraph in front of the client, and play the tape. (*Note:* It is helpful to have a second cassette unit available to record the client as he or she speaks.) Be sure that the output of the unit is loud, about 80 to 90 dB. Later, when assured that client is working well and used to the activity, drop the loudness level.

  This first effort usually will have more than a few errors. These mistakes typically are variations of going too fast, pausing too long, or speaking too loudly (Lombard effect probable [Ham, 1989]). The client may show a tendency to speed up within a phrase, then slow down, then speed up, and so forth. There also may be a problem of trying to have one breath serve for several phrase productions. Once the analyses, evaluations, repairs, and so on are finished, a renewed production of the paragraph is attempted.

  Run through the same 30-word paragraph. Stop the client whenever production errors occur. (This effort can take an entire therapy session or be accomplished in about 10 minutes, depending on the client.) Give client "cognitive encouragement" to motivate, as necessary. Take a "talk break" whenever frustration becomes too evident.

- *Step 2.* Prepare a typed list of questions and answers in advance. Using the list, ask the questions at a 30- to 40-wpm rate. Instruct the client to respond at the same rate. At 30 to 40 wpm, if words average 1.5 syllables, then wp5s (words per 5 seconds) will run about 5 syllables. Suggested questions/replies are offered below. Give the client a copy.

– Are you feeling better? I feel better now.
– Do you enjoy books? Yes, I enjoy reading.
– How much do you drink? Usually not a lot.
– How much is that ring? The ring is expensive.
– Is it time for us to go yet? I think it is past time to go.
– Where is your fuzzy hat? A bald man has it.
– Would you like a cookie? No, I am on a diet.
– Where did you go Tuesday? I went to a baseball game.
– Are you too tired to go? Yes, I just want to sleep.
– Are you afraid of cats? No, I just like dogs more.

Add other sentences as needed, or reverse roles and let the client ask the questions. Be sure to let the client criticize clinician productions as well as his or her own. Move slowly and evaluate each response, repeating as often as is needed. (This stage may go quickly or take considerable time, depending on the client. If the latter occurs, pay attention to client impatience and motivation.)

- *Step 3.* Ask questions that require short answers, but do not use a prepared script. Continue to ask questions that can be answered in three or four to seven or eight words. Listen for too many polysyllabic words in 5 seconds or for too few words or syllables in a period of 5 seconds. Monitor for noticeable errors, not split-second or one-syllable mistakes. Whenever a noticeable error occurs, stop the client at once and have him or her repeat the sentence. When satisfied with the basic rate of wpm, repeat this step, adding the elements of prolongation, Easy Onset, and any other elements to see if they are adequate. Set a criterion (e.g., in 10 sentences there will be no more than 5 instances where the rate slips noticeably away from 30 to 40 wpm and no more than 10 instances of significant slippage on the various production elements).

- *Step 4.* When proficient in Step 3, have the client meet performance criteria (adjust them as necessary) on longer sentences. Keep the same ratio of acceptable errors or establish new ones. Make up additional sentences as indicated.

  Use the following illustrative sentences that are designed to divide at the slash marks into two breath groups. Change breath pauses for individual clients as necessary.
  – I keep wondering where / we'll find an answer to these questions.
  – There is a feeling here / and I don't want it spoiled.

– Who can say that is true / and who will argue fact is fiction.
– Show me the horse you saw / and I will show you a nag.
– I can't agree that you are / more important than others.

• *Step 5.* (In this step, control is more or less turned over to the client.) Ask a question or utter a topic, and have the client respond with three complete sentences. Use the wpm rate and target production aspects as the performance measures. Record the activity. Provide 20 stimuli utterances, which should generate 60 utterances. When completed, rewind and play back. Have client evaluate; then evaluate the client's analysis. When 20 unacceptable events are agreed on, use the rest of the tape as follows: At each error, stop the tape, analyze, and discuss the error(s), and have the client repeat the entire sentence with zero errors. Proceed to the next sentence on the tape.

  Use the 10 illustrative stimuli below; supplement with nine more. Note the example that precedes this list.

  > What makes you laugh?
  > Seeing people doing foolish things.
  > Something that catches me by surprise.
  > A really funny play on words or a goofy definition.

  1. What were your favorite toys as a child?
  2. What does it take to make most people happy?
  3. What are good ways to ask for a date?
  4. What are your three most valuable possessions? Why?
  5. What public figure do you think is most important? Why?
  6. What is the ugliest sight you ever saw?
  7. When you travel, what do you pack besides clothes?
  8. Are cats or dogs smarter?
  9. Should all cycle riders be required to wear helmets?
  10. Why do women live longer than men?

• *Step 6.* Use a paragraph of the desired length from Exhibit 6–1. Control length to stay within client's ability and tolerance. Develop tolerance for rate control that starts out well on an utterance and speeds up as the utterance comes to an end. When deciding on an error, ask the client, "Should your rate have been under control at that point?" Either accept his or her evaluation or take time out for some discussion of what constitutes adequate performance. Be prepared to be flexible or demanding, as the situation and the client dictate. Use a subjective criterion (e.g., Is the client able, while reading, to maintain adequate rate control and to use production modes adequately?). Move to the last step in the sequence when the client meets the criterion after 30 minutes of accumulated time.

- *Step 7.* (In this step, there is a brief move to spontaneous speech, mainly to have the client feel sufficient control to do it.) For a period of 5 minutes of client talking time, ask questions that require generalized answers. Record the conversation, rewind the tape, and play back. Have client signal when he or she thinks that rate has gotten unacceptably fast at a point where slow rate control could have been important. Allow one rate error every 30 seconds (15 to 20 words) at the 30- to 40-wpm rate. For each rate error over that figure, add another minute to the 5 minutes required. If other production modes are being measured (pause time, prolongation, EO, and so on), decide the error allowance and penalty. When 5 minutes (plus penalty time) has been achieved, move the client to the next level. If the client can achieve 5 minutes without error penalty, move on. Otherwise, it's the initial 5+ penalty minutes (could total 5+1, or 5+75, etc.).

At each step, the clinician must have established criteria that have been explained in advance to the client. At this stage, there is no out-clinic work, unless the client is doing solo practice with a recorder at home. Each session should start with an appropriate number of minutes of practice in a Step 1 iteration of the original taped reading of the practice material in order to acclimate the client. Whenever review (or a penalty) is desired in later stages, the clinician can return to one or more repetition readings with the master tape. The client can also be assisted in recording a personal "submaster" 30- to 40-wpm tape and use it in therapy sessions or for solo practice sessions at home

Phase 2: 60 to 70 Words per Minute

As soon as the client has met the clinician's criteria for Phase 1, the next rate, 60 to 70 words per minute, is begun. Again, the wpm rates are arbitrary, and the clinician can rearrange the levels as desired.

The paragraph materials in Exhibit 6–1 can be used. As before, the client starts by listening to the new tape and slowly works into the adjustments needed to maintain an even rate. The clinician should monitor the client closely at first to ensure that she or he does not speed up too much past 60 to 70 wpm. Production discipline of every utterance is the rule at first. Prolongation, phrase reduction, continuation, and EO are still the hallmarks of adequacy. Note that the reduced phrases will be longer for 60 to 70 wpm than they were for 30 to 40 wpm. At 60 to 70 wpm, the client should be encouraged to use prosodic elements (inflection, stress, and so forth) in speaking. At this rate, prosody will sound exaggerated. However, starting prosodic elements at this point will make it easier at the next rate level where it will sound rather normal.

The clinicain follows the same progression of steps as Phase 1, making any adjustments suggested by previous experience. Material can be augmented, as demonstrated below.

> 30–40 wpm: How much do you drink? Usually not a lot.
> 60–70 wpm: How much water do you drink? Usually about a quart a day.

The client still may continue to do home assignments with the Phase 1 tape. When he or she is ready, the new tape is provided. When established criteria have been met across the sequenced steps, the clinician moves to the next phase.

Phase 3: 90 to 100 Words per Minute

This phase reflects a 40-wpm jump, instead of the 30-wpm jump from Phase 1 to Phase 2. There is no rigid rule on the spacing, and it may be set as desired. A fifth phase could even be inserted to reduce the intervals between successive wpm rates.

The first two rates were set deliberately low to alter the client's usual speech production patterns drastically, eliminate any postural triggers for spasms, and force the client to pay very close attention to the tactile and kinesthetic stimuli created by combining very slow rate with prolongation, EO, and so on. This third rate is closer to usual speaking rates and could become a "safe" or "fallback" rate when and if a client has trouble during speech.

In acquisition, the Phase 1 steps are followed, making the types of adjustments discussed in subsequent phases. In this phase, prosody becomes extremely important, and it should become one of the accept/reject criteria when judging client performance. The clinician should use material that requires prosodic flexibility (poetry, dramatic literature, humor). In the final steps, role playing can be used if it will help.

As soon as the client is able to hold a good, normal-sounding rate, out-clinic activities (with the clinician) and home assignments that have the client using this rate level with other people can be assigned. In this regard, material on fear hierarchy (chapter 4), outside assignments (chapter 2), and transfer (chapter 9) can be consulted. The client should be pushed on outside work, self-responsibility, and work habits.

Phase 4: 120 to 130 Words per Minute

This step is intended to be the last, but others can be added. It is close to the average wpm rate for many speakers. It probably is slower than the phrase rate for most stutterers and, therefore, negates or minimizes their trigger preparatory set patterns. Assuming that the previous steps have been followed, the following additions are presented for your consideration:

- Start with the Step 1 level for Phase 4. Keep the client at it until she or he is able to maintain a stable rate. Then move as quickly as possible through the other steps. Keep the accept/reject criterion around 90% for this in-clinic work. If the client falls below criterion at any time, penalize by dropping back to the same level Phase 3 (90 to 100 wpm) for a measured period of time. When the final step is reached, concentrate on solid instatement at the conversational level of speech.
- Start each session with 1 minute of unison speech model tape reading at Phase 3 level and 3 minutes of reading time at the Phase 4 level.
- Set a high premium on prosody in conversational speech practice, continuing the work from Phase 3. Discuss more flexible criteria and less frequent use of reduced rate with the client. Practice (with real or faked spasms) a sort of cancellation if a real stuttering spasm occurs by:
  - Stopping after the spasm and pausing
  - Inhaling, relaxing, exhaling
  - Producing the next five or six words at a Phase 3 level (90 to 100 wpm)
  - Continuing as before
- Expand out-clinic activities. Do a lot of out-clinic modeling, throwing in occasional pseudostutters and cancellations, as described in Phase 3. Experiment with dropping rate control when not needed, but rein-

serting it periodically. Push client to do 100% of the evaluation and consequation.

- Give intensive solo home assignments (see chapter 2). Follow the fear hierarchy (see chapter 4).

RATE REDUCTION VIA COGNITIVE CONTROL

Overview

Procedures to reduce rate through client cognition and self-control follow the same outline used for unison speech. Some clients need forced guidance, such as in unison speech, whereas others will need the stronger control of a method such as delayed auditory feedback (DAF). However, some clients can effect their own rate changes as long as the clinician is competent at altering his or her own rate, and as long as the clinician is effective in monitoring and motivating the client to work individually.

I present a less imitative, more self-directed approach to rate variation. The client is, more or less, told to slow down, provided with particular techniques that usually aid or require a rate shift, and begins practice. This approach may be very fruitful with clients who have shown acceptance of responsibility, skill in self-organization, and willingness to work hard. If such sterling qualities are not evident, the clinician can fall back on unison speech or DAF. Some clients do not favor rate reduction, the so-called "smooth speech" prolongation, and so on. However, Craig et al. (1996) wrote favorably about rate reduction use with their therapy groups of clients 9 to 14 years of age. Ramig (1984) reported securing rate reduction when clients (18 to 37 years) deliberately slowed production on either the initial phoneme or the initial syllable of a sentence. Packman, Onslow, and Van Doorn (1996) criticized prolonged speech (PS) rate reduction obtained by building from a starting slow rate of 30 to 40 wpm. They feel such a micro process has not been validated by research (which is true of many other techniques). Instead they point to fluency shaping programs where length of the utterance (or duration of utterance components) and not rate of utterance is emphasized. They argue that PS rate reduction can, in the initial stages, sound much less fluent than the stutterer's ordinary dysfluencies.

Cognitive Rate Control Instatement

- *Step 1.* Establish a baseline reading rate. Position the timing device where you and the client can see it, place a reading passage before the client, and have the recorder ready. With one eye on the timing device, turn on the recorder. The clinician then reads aloud to the client for exactly 60 seconds (finishing any initiated last word). Mark the terminal word. Rewind the tape and play back. Evaluate for quality, clarity, naturalness. If there are any doubts, redo the reading (same material) until agreement is reached that this is a good baseline tape. Save the recording.

Set the timer and tape recorder for the client, and signal the client to read aloud in his or her normal fashion for exactly 60 seconds. Count the number of words read; write that figure down. Rewind the tape and play it back. Mark the occurrence of each stuttering or each identifiable avoidance on the reading passage. Evaluate the quality, clarity, loudness, vocal quality, prosody, and so forth. Discuss whether or not this recording sounds typical for the client. Perform the wp5s rate calculation described in Step 3 at several points where *there are no dysfluencies or noticeable avoidances* and compare these rate figures to an overall wpm rate for the entire 60 seconds. Use this to help client see the effect of stuttering and avoidance behaviors on speech timing. Use the practice paragraphs in Exhibit 6–1 or any paragraph, as long as the minor effect of polysyllabic words on rate is considered.

- *Step 2.* Use this step for the client to experiment with rate and develop a sense for different rates. In particular, use this step to experiment with behaviors to slow rate down to the slowest rate desired and to guard against undesirable behaviors (e.g., slowing rate by extending pause durations, excessively increasing the frequency of pauses). Encourage desired behaviors (e.g., prolongation, continuous phonation, and so forth). Instruct client to (initially) prolong the production of all speech sounds, especially the continuants (s, v, f, m, n, r, z, etc.) and vowels. Have client drag the articulators and move through stops and plosives (p, b, t, d, k, g) rather than explode them or come to hard stops on them. Do not worry if client has difficulty with the latter group; problem solve later if difficulties interfere with particular techniques used. Ensure client does not speed up as he or she nears the end of an utterance. Work with client on her or his ability to calculate or be aware of self-rate in order to accentuate the client's sense of rate.

- *Step 3.* Provide rate-timing practice to enable client to experiment with all target rates, sometimes in quick succession. Use the four practice paragraphs in Exhibit 6–1. Record a reading, time it overall (total wpm average), and then collect 5-second samples from the recording. Use the following formulas:

$$\text{Total wpm} \quad = \quad \frac{\text{Total words spoken}}{\text{Talking time}} \quad \times \quad 60$$

$$\text{Sample wp5s} = \text{Total words spoken in 5 seconds} \quad \times \quad 12$$

Take two or three wp5s samples from a 60-second recording. Follow the overall practice sequence below.

–Have client read a 30-word passage aloud. Record. Play back and time (redo if needed). Calculate the total wpm rate. Take three 5-second word totals from the sample and calculate the wp5s rate. Compare the three wp5s rates to each other and to the total wpm rate. Discuss variations and other factors noticed.

–Repeat the preceding exercise at a rate of 60 wpm. Take four wp5s measures. Evaluate as before.

–Repeat the previous exercise, at a rate of 90 wpm. Take five wp5s measures. Evaluate as before.

–Repeat the previous exercise at a rate of 120 wpm. Take five wp5s measures. Evaluate as before.

Have one of the wp5s samples in each of the four preceding exercises include a stuttering to see what happens to rate when interrupted by dysfluency.

These exercises provide at least four baseline rates for different wpm averages. Moreover, client and clinician have practiced calculating overall and wp5s sample rates about 20 to 21 times. Next, it is important to establish rates for spontaneous speech and to continue developing analytical skills.

• *Step 4.* Perform this step in two parts: in the clinic and out of the clinic.

In-clinic: Stipulate the rate for each task. Ask the client to give directions to her or his house from the clinic. Record and play back. Take at least three 5-second samples for analysis. Compare against the baseline for that rate.

Give the client a longer, more open-ended topic, such as retelling a story from a book or movie. Record and play back. Take at least five wp5s samples, calculate, compare, and discuss.

Have the client make three telephone calls to friends or family. Record the client's side of the conversation only. Take three 5-second samples from each call, and calculate a wp5s for each. Compare and discuss.

Try to find one wp5s sample in each exercise that has a dysfluency in it. Compare all the different samples (about 19) to each other and to the base rate(s).

Out-clinic: Stipulate the rate for each task, probably only 90 to 100 and 120 to 130 wpm. Have client, solo, record three face-to-face conversations with friends or family. Tell client each conversation must last long enough to draw at least five wp5s samples (total = 15).

Have client make five telephone calls to strangers, and record his or her own speech. Tell client each call must capture at least 30 seconds of client speech. Have client perform a wp5s analysis on the first, second, and third 10-second segments (or a near approximation). Advise client to do all calculations in advance and bring them, along with the tapes, to the clinic for discussion.

Both the in-clinic and out-clinic steps should be repeated until the client feels (and is) proficient in monitoring and evaluating speech rates. A very significant desensitization component is involved in this work aimed at increasing the client's ability to be aware without becoming too anxious and tense. Part of every in-clinic situation should be devoted to continuing practice on the different rates; regular home assignments should continue.

In order to proceed to Step 5, the client must meet basic criteria. He or she must be able to read at the four basic rates with no more than 20% of the wp5s samples showing a deviation greater than 10 wpm above or below the target wpm rate. Also, in comparing client evaluations against clinician evaluations, the two must, on the average, be within about 20% of each other. Finally, the client should show an ability to switch from one rate to another, achieving a stable wpm rate within 10 words of the change point. With these (or other) criteria met, progress work should focus on spontaneous speech. The 30 to 40 and 60 to 70 wpm rates are relegated to brief reviews used at the outset of a session, or as penalties for production errors or omissions.

- *Step 5.* Use this step to have client switch back and forth between 90 to 100 wpm and 120 to 130 wpm. Do not require changes to be frequent or fast; allow the client to "set" each rate before there is a change. Label the 90 to 100 wpm rate as "SR" or "safe rate," and the 120 to 130 wpm rate at "PR" or "preferred rate." Ask the client to perform wp5s sample analyses to help her or him monitor speech rate while practicing switches during conversations and monologues.

Spend more time on the PR, but never let a session go by without a number of SR demands. Use role play, dramatic readings, out-clinic extended situations, and progressively increasing reliance on solo out-clinic work. Have client occasionally go back through an utterance and use PR or SR for 100% during a brief period of time.

Now, the clinician should concentrate on transfer independence as discussed in chapter 9.

SHADOWING

Shadowing, or tracking, may or may not be a relatively recent development. In choral, or unison, speech, the second speaker (client) tries to coincide his or her speech exactly with the first speaker's model. However, in shadowing, the client listens to the model and attempts to repeat the model utterance, lagging one or more syllables behind the model. Also, for best results, the client is not allowed to look at the speaker he or she is tracking. Fiedler and Standop (1983) apply shadowing by having the clinician begin with a list of short sentences spoken at a slow rate. The client follows the model production, lagging behind as noted previously. Once the client is able to perform adequately, sentences are lengthened and speech rate is increased. Progressively longer and varied material is used. Deliberate changes in tempo, inflection, pronunciation, and so forth can be used. The clinician can send home taped material for practice. Finally, television shows and live situations can be used for practice.

Cherry and Sayers (1956) popularized shadowing as a technique, with the label "shadowing" apparently applied by Marland (1957). She used the method with cluttering and stuttering children and reported good results. Marland suggested that shadowing simultaneously provided practice in an altered speech pattern, while forcing the development of new listening habits.

Freund (1966) reported use of shadowing in Germany prior to 1900, but whether it was the same shadowing that Cherry and Sayers used is not clear. Silverman (1996) stated that shadowing is the spontaneous speech equivalent of unison speech, noting an extensive use of shadowing in Polish therapy programs. Cherry and Sayers (1956) suggested that shadowing might compensate for inadequate perceptual awareness of stutterers by shifting their automatic auditory monitoring to external control of a different mode of speaking. There is, no doubt, an element of distraction in shadowing.

Research on Shadowing

Sergeant (1961) noted that speech intelligibility on phonetically balanced (PB) lists was only 68% at 102 spm and reached as high as 80% intelligibility only after intensive practice. Whether contextual material would have improved intelligibility is arguable. Walton and Mather (1963) reported successful application of shadowing during 48 sessions over a month, but achieved very poor transfer out of the clinic. They followed up with 38 additional sessions adding Wolpe's (1973) systematic desensitization therapy, with significantly higher transfer success. Kelham and McHale (1966) had shadowing used independently by three different clinicians and found equivalent results with an overall success rate of 74%. They noted that successful outcomes were more common with younger clients.

Ingham, Andrews, and Winkler (1972) indicated that most therapy reports of shadowing seemed to state a need for "something else" to help translate shadowing values into useful applications. A study by Öst, Gotestam, and Lennert (1976) compared metronome, shadowing, and a form of whisper-speech therapy. The metronome was most effective, and the reduction factor was about the same 14 months later. However, both shadowing and whisper speech (less effective at termination time) continued to show improvement after dismissal and, 14 months later, basically matched the metronome performance level. Fiedler and Standop (1983) felt there was value in shadowing, if only to make the client feel that her or his speech was amenable to alteration and external control. Bloodstein (1995) summarized several studies, covering a total of 60 stutterers (from 4 years to 43 years or older) and varying time lengths in therapy. Overall, about 70% to 75% of the clients were reported as becoming fluent or greatly improved as a result of shadowing therapy.

Shadowing Efficacy

Exactly how shadowing works, and how effective it is overall, is unclear. The fluency effect of shadowing has been attributed to sheer novelty, distraction, induced rhythm, intoning effects, prosody alteration, timing alteration, changes in auditory feedback, and other factors. Wingate (1976) suggested that stutterers follow the lead speaker without knowing what will be said next. Syllable rate, usually 75 to 150 spm, is well below a usual 250-spm rate. The intoning quality, the little stress on emotional content, and the irregular and detached phrases all contribute to fluency. Wingate (1969) felt the most important components were reduced rate, an emphasis on phonation and stress reduction, and a subordination of articulatory gestures. Some have felt that the most significant aspect of shadowing is that of a vocal intoning of speech, accentuating or "riding" the melodic pattern. Sergeant (1961) stated that a good sense of rhythm (he tested for rhythm sense) will improve shadowing adequacy. Overall, then, shadowing significantly alters the rate, prosody, coarticulation, blending, phrasing, and monitoring behaviors of the second speaker. Any of these changes can temporarily reduce or eliminate stuttering. The key word here is "temporarily," and it raises a question as to what will happen afterward.

Shadowing Acquisition

The steps presented are my own, used and adjusted over time. With each client, they have been altered. Clinicians are urged to consider revisions as needed. What follows is one way, of many, to shadow.

- *Step 1.* Explain shadowing to the client, emphasizing the following four uses:
  1. to shift and sharpen listening skills
  2. to learn the effects on fluency of changes in different speech production parameters
  3. to develop abilities to alter speech production parameters deliberately
  4. to prepare for later control techniques
- *Step 2.* Have prerecorded materials and demonstrate live shadowing on a sequence of the taped utterances. Stop often for questions and

comments. Repeat each modeling at three rates (see later for suggestions about rate), when the level of short sentences is attained. A suggested modeling sequence is

Three-word, one-syllable: hay, run, get; fed, big, sir
Five-word, one-syllable: hay, run, get, fed, sir; big, cat, for, hop, sing
Three-word, variable syllable: television, dumb, airplane
Five-word, variable syllable: gotcha, carrot, factory, running, sofa
Short, connected sentences: Have you gone to see it?

Record each stimulus three times in your prerecorded tape, each time using a different rate (e.g., 75 to 95 spm, 95 to 115 spm, and 115 to 135 spm). Stop and discuss losses of clarity, prosody, and so forth with the client. Repeat the rate variation on the next two modeling levels below.

Longer sentences: I won't be ready to go until Carol has cleaned up her room.
Discourse: Linda could walk in the woods and near Avon Pond for hours at a time and enjoy herself without anybody else there. However, she was, at the same time, one of the most social people I know. Carol never had any great desire to be alone, but she was not social in the general sense. She enjoyed a sensible conversation, but was less liable to chitter-chat just for the sake of talking.

The clinician does not have to be excellent at shadowing. She or he must know *how* to shadow, perform it basically, and point out her or his own errors to the client. At any rate, the client soon should outshine the clinician at shadowing.

- *Step 3.* Prerecord a tape with 50 three-word, one-syllable sequences, as demonstrated in Step 2. Insert a 5-second (approximate) pause between each trial triad. At the end of those 50 sets, pause and then utter, "Next, five-word sequences." Pause another 5 seconds or so, and then record 50 five-word, one-syllable sequences. The prerecording is done without the client. In-clinic, have the client go through both sets, after modeling and problem solving. When client produces 30 acceptable three-word sequences, move to five-word sequences. Three criteria are
  1. Zero stuttering
  2. "Adequate approximation" of model utterances (this criterion becomes more elastic as utterances lengthen, later)

3. Stays "near" in terms of lag time behind model (on short utterances, a couple syllables; on longer utterances, up to a couple words)

- *Step 4.* Prerecord a different practice tape with 50 three-word, variable-syllable utterances, and with 50 five-word, variable-syllable utterances. Make sure that all three spm rate factors are represented on this tape. Apply and evaluate as in the prior step. As you begin this step, send the Step 3 tape (or a copy) home with the client, with instructions to practice it for 30 minutes each day.

- *Step 5.* Send a copy of the Step 4 tape home for practice. Be sure it is the tape with spm rate differences. For Step 5, prerecord 50 sentences with a mix of spm rates: about 10 at slowest, 20 at midrate, and 20 at the fastest rate. Mix them up. Apply same judgment criteria as in Step 3, but be more flexible on the third criterion. When 30 of the 50 sentences meet the three criteria, turn the playback unit off and provide 10 sentences, *live voice.* Tell the client not to look at your face as you talk (ever again) during such practice. Do not apply set criteria here; just use the 10 sentences as an opportunity to look for difficulties and problem solve them.

- *Step 6.* Send home a copy of the Step 5 tape for solo practice. Suggest that the client look for television newspersons or commentators who are slow and pompous in delivery. Have client try to shadow for several minutes each evening. For in-clinic work, prerecord 30 longer sentences, with 5 at slow rate, 10 at medium rate, and 15 at the fastest rate. Use same acceptance criteria as in Step 5, but the magic number is 20, not 30.

- *Step 7.* Send home a copy of Step 6 for solo practice. Prerecord a practice tape with at least 20 three-sentence strings for in-clinic use. For example,

> The heart of politics is compromise. If you can avoid a rigid position, do so. Only when you are flexible can you hope to win.

In each string, deliberately slow down, and then speed up, the rate. Use the acceptance criteria from Step 3. Allow two error counts for each sentence string; if more errors occur, the string must be repeated. Cycle twice through the 20 sentence groups. Have the client shadow a good target on television as part of the daily home assignment program. Instruct client to continue until she or he has accumulated 5 minutes or 10 errors, whichever comes first.

- *Step 8.* Send home a copy of the Step 7 tape for solo practice every day, and repeat the television shadowing assignment. Have a series of friends or colleagues record six short paragraphs on tape. Try to mix topics, speakers' sex, mild dialect variations, and so forth. Use materials that are read or spontaneous. For example,

> I really enjoyed my date last week. Uh, Linda has never been, she's never seen a real hockey game. You know, ice hockey. Well first off, she nearly froze her, she nearly froze to death, but she really loved it, the game I mean. Once she got used to who did what, where the puck was, you know, she could follow stuff. I don't think she liked the fights and blood, but maybe she did.

Allow five errors per discourse, depending on length and complexity of the material.

- *Step 9.* Send home a copy of the Step 8 tape for solo work every day. Ask the client to watch a panel or talk show on television and try to shadow the irregular, staccato conversations there. Ask for a report. Bring one or more videotapes to clinic—tapes representing different speaking situations. Have a mix of ordinary conversations, dramatic shows, arguments, comic delivery, and so on. Have the client work on these for a combined practice and pleasure activity in clinic. Try the fragments with the client watching and not watching the television screen.

I usually end shadowing at this point, by blending the heightened awareness and speech control into one or more of the fluency or symptom control methods, preparatory set approaches, or tension reduction efforts. At times, I have not gone beyond Step 5 or Step 6 before shifting away from shadowing. Occasionally, I have *started* at Step 5 or Step 6.

DELAYED AUDITORY FEEDBACK

DAF results when a speaker's voice is delayed in its journey to the speaker's ear. The technique was discovered many millennia ago when a cave man yelled in an empty cave. It was discovered again, for the umpteenth time, in 1953. Since that latter date our profession has used DAF. Regardless of the name applied, use has waxed and waned over the last 45 years. Today it is waxing, although under attack here and there.

DAF originally was envisioned as an opportunity for normal-fluency speakers to study "stuttering" under tightly controlled conditions. Subsequent evaluation disclosed that the fluency disturbances of DAF differed in significant ways from real stuttering (waning period). Later it was tried as a reward or punishment (waxed) in fluency therapy, but it did not hold up (waned again). Then, in the 1960s it was used as a coercive modeling device to instate fluency by its effects on rate and prolongation (waxed).

Recent History

Watts (1971) reported a restrained use of DAF. It was introduced in the initial therapy session and used until the client found his or her "best" delay time. This delay was used to generate the model for slowed rate and prolongation necessary for fluency. After that, DAF was used only to begin subsequent sessions, or if fluency interruptions favored a brief return to DAF.

Other clinicians, before and after Watts, used DAF as a complete therapy program (Adamczyk, 1994). Although I present it as a complete sequence here, clinicians are urged to consider limited or special uses of DAF as well. Perkins, Rudas, Johnson, Michael, and Curlee (1974) found that rate reduction alone produced good dismissal levels of fluency, but maintenance was better when the therapy program added control of phrasing, prosody, and breathstream management for the clients. This finding was echoed 2 years later by Wingate (1976) who stated that DAF is effective in what it does—slow speech rate, increase vocal intensity, reduce the prosodic stress contacts, and so on. However, he felt DAF by itself was not to be considered an adequate form of therapy intervention.

Another aspect of DAF, noted earlier, is the variability of client responses to, and the effects of, DAF. Fiedler and Standop (1983) noted that stutterers' responses to DAF are individual, and the most effective delay times vary from person to person. In addition, speakers' sex and age appear to affect delay time effects. In 1955 I noticed that mild severity stutterers were disrupted by DAF, whereas severe stutterers were assisted (reduced stuttering) by DAF. Wingate (1976) suggested that stutterers' auditory capacities in sound localization, auditory dominance, and so forth were different, or at least inconsistent, when compared with nonstutterers. Wingate's review of early DAF development and use is rather thorough and informative. Curlee and Siegel (1997) provide a brief but concise summary of comments about DAF. They suggest that DAF may actually impede development of self-control by the client, unless this aspect is worked on specifically after DAF therapy. However, the authors note that DAF use with clients for whom other rate reduction efforts have been unsuccessful may be its biggest value.

A special application of DAF, as chips and digital processors have developed, has been the "prosthetic" DAF. That is, the speaker wears a portable DAF unit, feeding into his or her ear. In 1976, Wingate described efforts to develop a portable DAF unit as being worthless and inappropriate. Twenty years later, Kalinowski, Stuart, and Armson (1996) stated that use of prosthetic DAF units appears to be viable as either an adjunct, or an alternative, to a regular therapy program. I am not satisfied. When I release a client with a prosthetic aid, but agree we must work with all systems that may aid a particular client until our profession can point to a better dismissal/relapse for general therapy of stuttering.

In terms of efficacy and effect, there are different points of view on DAF. Delaying the auditory return of a verbal signal is significant only for the variable of speech prolongation. Also, some have suggested that a DAF unit is not mandatory for that purpose. First, I disagree that prolongation is the only functional variable concerned in stuttering reduction by DAF. I agree that it is *possible* to achieve DAF-like effects without a DAF unit. Shames and Florance (1980), among others, made this point for years. However, the human tendency to feel a need for mechanisms to do what humans can do for themselves cannot be ignored. If DAF support is not available, it is 100% feasible to do it alone. Second, aside from the support value of a DAF unit, the issue that prolongation is the only value of DAF can be debated. Some, myself included, argue that the direct rate reduction effect provides more time for both neuromotor and psycholinguistic planning and formulation. Extending beyond that, Kalinowski et al. (1996) questioned the effectiveness of sheer alteration of motoric targets, such as rate, over the actual auditory alterations of DAF. Rate reduction, itself, may not favor naturalness in speech. I have felt DAF supports fluency via rate reduction, prolongation, altering coarticulatory patterns, changing preparatory sets, shifting the speaker's fundamental frequency, reducing and redistributing prosody factors, creating a new auditory picture of self, changing emphasis on tactile and kinesthetic feedback (as opposed to auditory feedback), and creating a feeling of support in the speaker. Whether these aspects are primary, or secondary, is not important if they exist.

Orientation to Delayed Auditory Feedback

Introducing a temporal delay in the return of speech to the ear of the speaker may have a dramatic effect. The person may stumble, "stutter," speak loudly, drone a stereotype pattern, shift pitch, make articulatory errors, and completely lose a train of thought. However, stutterers (particularly moderate to severe ones) often find an immediate, and significant, improvement in their fluency. What instrument can produce these effects?

Technical Aspects of DAF

A number of DAF units are on the market. For years they were tape recorders where the record and playback heads were both moved online, and then separated. What was recorded was then immediately played back some seconds or fractions thereof later. New units use microchips and digital technology to destroy and reconstitute an oral signal with a preset delay on the return of that signal to the speaker's ear. Retail prices range from a few hundred dollars to several thousand. DAF units come as table-top models, in-the-pocket devices, and behind-the-ear prosthetic models. Basic components include:

- *Microphone*—usually voice activated to reduce ambient noise. It helps if there is a low-frequency filter. For table-top sets, the microphone should be on a boom attached to the earphone headset (this helps keep the microphone a constant distance from the speaker's mouth). On body-worn units, the microphone may be of the contact variety.
- *Earphones*—many DAF units come equipped with fragile and inferior headsets. The ear cushions may be extremely poor in terms of their ability to mask outside noise. Some clinicians reject these headsets. Others argue that the client should attend to the DAF signal, and the poor quality of many headsets is not important. I understand the latter, but agree with the former. Our clinic's last table-top unit (about a thousand dollars) had the microphone boom break and one earphone detach from its holder in the first year. Insert earpieces also can be used.

- *Delay unit*—significant differences seem to exist between table-top and body units. Regarding table-top units, most clinicians prefer a visible on/off switch that does not "pop" when activated and a loudness setting (usually incorporated into on/off switch) with an amplification capacity to raise an input signal to about 95 dB. The unit should have a delay interval selection marked in millisecond intervals. The interval spaces can vary anywhere from 1 ms to 50 ms (usual), in a range from 0 delay to 300-ms delay, or higher. Body units often have only one delay interval. Kalinowski et al. (1996) reported that a 50-ms delay was generally optimal for positive DAF effects. However, they noted that there could be considerable variation of response among clients.
- *Wires/cords/batteries*—these components tend to be taken for granted. Length, strength, flexibility, and insulation of wires should be examined. The clinician should look at how secure connections are. Do table-top units have carrying handles? If batteries are provided, how many of what kind are needed? What is the usual battery life?
- *Special*—other features need to be examined. The clinician should ask, Is pitch shift or octave shift provided? Can "on" and "off" periods of DAF and normal auditory feedback (NAF) be preset? Is there a masking circuit? Any other "bells and whistles"? These features are not necessary for DAF use, and I would prefer a top-quality, simple DAF unit to a bell-and-whistle special.

DAF Implementation

Client Preparation

The clinician should explain to the client the reasons for using DAF and the target (i.e., self-control, not machine-control, of speech). The clinician then puts on a headset, with delay at 0 and volume at neutral and explains what will happen.

> When you talk, this microphone [point] will return your own voice to these earphones [point]. Two things will happen. Your voice will be a lot louder than normal. Also, your voice will be delayed so that it sounds like an echo [if needed, take time to

remind client of echo experiences]. Let's try it first to set the loudness.

The clinician then helps the client settle the earphones fully over each ear (be sure the client's hair is swept to one side and earrings do not pinch. The ms delay should be set at 0. Then the client reads aloud while the clinician turns the volume slowly up to 90 to 95 dB (on most units, 95 dB is liable to be well below the 95 dB setting, be careful). The clinician advises the client:

> As I turn this up louder, tell me if it actually hurts. You do not have to like it, but I do not want you to be hurt.

The clinician negotiates and notes an agreed-on loudness level. Then the clinician removes the headphones from the client and dons them, saying:

> In a moment I will turn the delay switch up so you can see and hear the effect of DAF if you fight it.

With loudness set at 90 to 95 dB, the clinician turns the delay interval up to a level known to be effective and reads aloud from a passage. The clinician reads just long enough to create a sample, stops, turns down volume and DAF, and says:

> Okay. Now I want you to try. One thing, be sure and listen to the earphone signal. Do not try and ignore or listen to your voice leaking around the earphones. Pay close attention to what you hear. Ready?

This step may take a number of attempts, mixed with laughter or irritation, confusion, and so on. Once in a long while, a client will instinctively adapt to DAF by slowing down, for example. However, usually the clinician must take the client through the following six ideas, frequently modeling for him or her (with or without the headset on):

1. Keep voice at a normal loudness level. Do not get too loud.
2. Slow rate so that speech rate finally matches the DAF delay. Do so by using prolongation, pause control, phrase control, and continuous phonation.

3. Use prolongation on all sounds at first. [Model and practice until idea is clear.]
4. Remember, the number of pauses will increase because prolongation/ rate changes will require more frequent breathing. Do not make pauses last longer.
5. Remember, phrase length should decrease as DAF effect increases. Phrase length will depend on the number of syllables, duration of prolongations, and adequacy of air supply. Adjust on an individual basis.
6. Keep phonation continuous as part of prolongation.

Depending on the client, previous therapy experience, and clinician experience, DAF acclimation may take anywhere from 10 to 15 minutes in one session to several complete management sessions. Delays usually occur because the client "fights" or ignores DAF, or the client has significant trouble acquiring one or more aspects of prolongation, pause control, breathing, continuous phonation, and phrase control. Each of these aspects of production is covered elsewhere in this book. Clinicians should check for the extended description of the technique and how it is performed.

The following four steps are used to prepare the client for DAF:

- *Step 1.* Fit the client with DAF accoutrements and give the following instructions:

    Do not talk until I signal. Then read these words, one at a time, putting a pause of about 3 or 4 seconds between each word so you can hear the word repeated in the headset. Then read the next word and pause, and so on. Ready?

    Place the following words (or any list) before the client, turn delay and volume up, and signal.

    one --- four --- three --- five --- ten --- eight --- two

    Correct any Lombard effect on loudness. Double-check earphone loudness comfort, and ask for questions or comments. Then give the following explanation to the client:

    This time, read the words without pausing, except for air. Just try and make your utterances exactly match the ones coming back to your ear. Remember, listen to the signal. Do not ignore it or try to fight it. Ready?

Have the client read the list below.

one-four-three-five-ten-eight-two

This exercise may take time and a number of repetitions, or the client may acclimate almost immediately. It may be necessary for the clinician to model a number of times, each time emphasizing a different aspect (rate, phrasing, breathing, pauses, prolongations, continuous phonation, and so forth).

- *Step 2.* Continue to adjust prolongation, continuous phonation, and so on into appropriate breath/phrase units. Emphasize that client will have to break utterances into inappropriate linguistic and/or phono- logical units. Have the client practice on the following utterances without a headset, using all the slowed-speech modes designated. Have client take a pause-breath at each slash mark.

  Revolutionary tel/ evision is here now.
  What an incredi/ ble answer you gave/ him.
  No one is free to/ evaluate mon/ keys but the men.
  Such unbeliev/ able stories must be/ lies or legends.
  Give me your starving/ birds and this new seed/ will work fine.

When the client has practiced the utterances several times, replace the headset and tell her or him that when the DAF is activitated he or she is to reread each sentence out loud and fine-tune productions. When that is satisfactory, instruct the client to read the sentences below, inserting pauses where they seem to be appropriate, based on the practice efforts.

  Give me liberty or give me a better salary.
  The Irish have a beautiful way of speaking.
  No one is more aware than I am of the problems around here.
  Such a rare treat is found only when one has been very good.
  I wish I knew why things happen the way they do accidentally.

Listen very closely for inadequate air, words or word parts that were not prolonged, any failures in continuous phonation, pauses that are too long, too loud a voice, a rate that ignores DAF pacing, and so forth.

Be very precise, explaining the need (at this stage) to control every utterance. Repeat as many times as needed to produce a good production pattern. If further practice is needed to set a pattern, move to Step 3. If further acclimation practice is not needed, move directly to Step 1 of the DAF production sequence (next section).

- *Step 3.* Identify the area(s) requiring further definition, discussion, modeling, and trials of prolongation, phrasing, or other aspects. Model on the list below, and have the client go through the list with, and without, DAF.

television	arrangement
difficulty	automobile
representation	indestructible
How are you?	I don't have any.
He has a headache.	I can see him now.
That just isn't true.	I want you to take your time.

Record the DAF efforts, play back, and evaluate. Repeat modeling if needed. Go through the entire step a second time, if needed.

If DAF worsens a client's dysfluencies (frequency or severity), it may be due to the mildness of the problem. However, it might be due to a cluttering problem (Peters & Guitar, 1991).

DAF Production Acquisition

After completing the preparatory steps, the client may be well on the way to acquisition. She or he should at least be adjusted to and familiar with its effects and what is expected during its use. A progressive, step-by-step sequence for acquisition follows. Suggestions for bypassing many of the steps will be made, especially if the client acclimates quickly and effectively.

- *Step 1.* Set DAF to 200 to 250 ms at 80 to 95 dB. Inform the client that this step has three levels: reading, monologue speech, and conversational speech. Remind the client of the production targets. Inform client that the pass criteria are 5 minutes in each of the three speech modes (total of 15 minutes) with
  - Zero stuttering

– No more than 10 clinician-determined errors on prolongation, continuous phonation, breath groups, etc.

Repeat the entire mode if the client stutters. Add 1 minute of practice time for each two "other" errors over 10. Take the time to play the tape back to the client, pointing out all errors and problem solving if needed, before exacting penalty minutes. Then go to the next of the three speech modes. Use any printed material for the *reading* mode. Cue *monologue* material with question cards or pictures. Use any topic for the *conversational speech*, basing the timing on the client's speech.

Repeat Step 1 completely, employing the same criteria. However, have the client make the judgments, guided by the clinician, on the tape playback. Use the same penalties.

In Step 1 a 250-ms delay typically will result in a 35 to 45 wpm rate. In the process the client learns to move through most of her or his articulator contact points so that glottal stops, plosive pops, and tight contacts are eliminated or minimized. Vocal pitch shifts downward, and a stereotypical pattern of falling inflections (this will change in later steps) occurs. This step should bring about extended speech times with zero stuttering, basic acquisition of some fluency or symptom control techniques, a significant increase in tactile and kinesthetic awareness, a shift in auditory monitoring patterns, and an increase in evaluation skills. Hopefully, desensitization has occurred as well. When Step 1 criteria have been met, the client can move to Step 2 or jump to a subseuqent (shorter delay interval) step.

- *Step 2.* Set the DAF unit to 250 ms and keep the loudness level high (unless the client will follow the delay interval easily). Don the headset and briefly model the speech patterns at 250 ms. Then turn the DAF setting to 200 ms and again produce some output, directing the client to notice the differences. Record both actions, and play the tape back for the client, pointing out production changes (ask the client first).

   Transfer the headset to the client, set the unit at 250 ms, and repeat the two activities just recorded. Record and play back for analysis by the client. When completed, move to having the client accumulate criterion time, using the same criteria as in the previous step. Change the time intervals and penalty allowance as follows:

Reading	3 minutes	Zero stutter, six "other" errors
Monologue	6 minutes	Zero stutter, 12 "other" errors
Conversation	Same	Same

When criterion time (plus any penalty time) has been met, have the client remove the headset and read the 3 minutes of material over again while trying to duplicate the rate, prolongation, and so forth. Record and play back. Do not penalize directly, but look for slippage faults and discuss what needs to be done.

When Step 2 criteria have been met, the client can move to Step 3 or jump to a later (shorter delay interval) step.

• *Step 3.* Don the headset and move the delay interval to 150 ms. Demonstrate (record and play back) the faster rate to the client. (The wpm value here will be around 90 to 100 and could be a viable production target for the client if he or she was in an out-of-control situation where minimal rate reduction, prolongation, and so forth was not resulting in control adequacy. Most will agree that this rate is better [a little] than moderate or severe stuttering.) Emphasize that this step is not a final target, but a viable way to regain control and then shift up to a faster controlled rate.

Phrase length will increase and breath support will need checking. *Prolongation* will continue as the core method, but the client should start dropping it when it is not needed. *Continuous phonation* is treated as prolongation. *Prosody* moves near the top of the priority list. There is an emphasis on "naturalness," although somewhat exaggerated at this wpm rate. As rate, prolongation, and continuous phonation are reduced or changed, the clinician may feel some need for introducing Easy Onset. Finally, self-monitoring and self-correction are major targets at this step.

Set the overall target at 30 minutes of accumulated monologue and spontaneous speech (perhaps 10 and 20 minutes), divided into 5-minute segments for criterion evaluation of live speech and recordings. Have client perform all evaluations, subject only to the clinician's corrections. Use the following criteria for evaluation:

– Zero occurrence of stuttering in any 5-minute segment
– More than 10 occurrences, in any 5-minute segment, of failure to use any rate control or other controls when *they should have been used*
– More than five occurrences, in any 5-minute segment, where controls were used, but they were incorrect or ineffective

Wipe out all accrued time for a 5-minute segment if stuttering occurs, and add 1 minute to the 5-minute segment for each occurrence beyond the maximum 10 allowances of "other" factors. Model what should have been done when/if the client's judgment is challenged. Add a reward factor if desired (e.g., "If you go 4 minutes with zero stuttering and no more than five 'other' errors, I will knock off the last minute of the 5, each time!" [potential of 6 minutes off from 30]).

Have the client remove the headset and continue talking (monologue or conversation) for about 5 minutes when the time target has been reached. Ensure client maintains the rate and other criterion aspects of this step.

When the Step 3 criteria have been met, the clinician can move to Step 4 or jump to a later (shorter interval) step.

- *Step 4.* Don the headset and reset the delay interval to 100 ms. Have client accumulate three 15-minute periods of a monologue and conversation mix (proportions depend on the client), totaling 45 minutes. Ensure each 15-minute segment is preceded by a 1-minute warm-up reading (at that delay) in which no stuttering is accepted (start over) and no more than three errors of too rapid a rate or absence or inadequacy of controls such as Easy Onset, prolongation, prosody, continuous phonation, phrasing, or breath support are allowed. Wipe out the reading minute if more than three (subjectively judged) errors occur; start over.

  Time the 15 minutes of client talking activity approximately. Explain to the client that errors can be canceled if they are self-caught and corrected immediately by repeating the error word or phrase properly. Add 1 minute to the 15-minute total when misses total five, without correction. Add a minute to the total for any stuttering; no canceling is allowed. Periodically interrupt time accumulation to play back parts of output to discuss whether all elements were adequate.

Two aspects of production, Easy Onset and prosody, will be much more significant at this rate level. Regarding prosody, the client may still tend to use stereotyped inflection and stress patterns from slower rates (and his or her own pretherapy speech pattern). Easy Onset may be significant because the new rate (usually something over 120 wpm) will make it easier to slip back into old, habituated patterns of articulatory tension and abnormal preparatory sets. These possibilities bring two functions up to significance level: problem solving and the concept of safe rate versus preferred rate. Problem solving focuses on the areas just cited, stereotypy and preparatory set slippage, because the wpm rate is getting close to the old, habituated rate of the client. This rate makes it easy for old, distorted, and trigger patterns to reappear. Certain sounds, specific words or word classes, production postures and/or other factors may need to be worked on. As a result some changes may need to be made in the time accumulation areas.

Preferred rate refers to the possibility that this step's wpm rate may be the rate that the client will prefer to use when rate control therapy is completed. Some clients will find this rate too slow (a few, too fast), but it may be just right for some. Client and clinician should discuss rate and compare different rates. During in-clinic speech, without rate control, sample recordings of 5-second, fluent speech segments (ten to fifteen 5-second samples) to secure an overall picture of rate. If pretherapy diagnostic samples were taken and saved, they can be used. If the client feels it might be the best rate for her or him, make the third 15-minute segment a trial run effort without DAF control.

Safe rate is that rate of speech at which it is unlikely, or almost impossible, for stuttering to occur if the client performs it with accuracy and consistency. Safe rate can have a fairly wide range, from 70 wpm up to 110 wpm, depending on the speaker. References already have been made to both preferred and safe rates. The client usually does not like the safe rate, especially if he or she has been fairly successful thus far in therapy. The safe rate is too atypical, too slow, and reminds the speaker of what he or she would like to forget—stuttering. Preferred rate is a rate that sounds near average, perhaps a little slow, but not too different from the pretherapy speech rate (for most, not all, clients). In many clients it will be better than pretherapy speech because of improvements in prosody, eye contact, and other aspects of communication.

- Determine whether the client has been favorably impressed by this rate and has gone through the time periods with minimal penalties. Consider having a trial run of out-clinic use for the successful client, such as:
  - Brief conversations with several in-clinic persons
  - 10 short telephone calls
  - A joint trip to a store to investigate a purchase (e.g., buying a new television)
  - 10 at-home telephone calls, controlled for length, performed solo

– An encounter with three friends to demonstrate this rate and get their opinions (instruct client to use each production mode for several minutes)

Consider also the possibility of moving the successful client to transfer actions.

- *Step 5.* Don the headset and set the delay interval to 50 ms. Demonstrate for the client by shifting back and forth between 100 ms and 50 ms. Have the client try the same thing, if he or she is able to make the shifts easily.

As noted earlier, Kalinowski, Stuart, and Armson (1996) suggested that 50 ms is a possible starting or ending point for DAF instruction. I suggested some reservations about quick fixes, but agree that it may be worth the time and effort to test this possibility, *especially if the client is focused on the idea of a prosthetic (see earlier) DAF unit.* If not, the clinician should move on with this sequence.

No new criteria are set for this step. The judgment points (zero stutter, adequacy in rate, prolongation prosody, and so forth) still hold. What I leave to the clinician is how much criterion time, what penalties, and so on are to be set. There also should be a mix of out-clinic and solo homework time utilized. The client is a very known factor by now in terms of goals, adequacy, reliability, and self-evaluation. Thus the clinician needs to adapt therapy accordingly.

- *Step 6.* Have client analyze and practice both preferred and safe rate of speech control, first on an in-clinic basis, and then on out-clinic work. Practice quickly switching from one to the other. Note that some clients adopt the preferred role as their standard rate, whereas others keep it as a fallback. Keep safe rate alive (if only barely) for the reassurance it provides. Shift to transfer and maintenance activity.

RHYTHM PROCEDURES

Use of cadence, or rhythm, is part of unison speech, and many other techniques involve superimposed or altered rhythm (Ham, 1986). Fiedler and Standop (1983) reported on the haptometronome, where a small device delivers a timed vibration or tiny electrical shock to the fingers or wrist. Silverman (1996) commented on the behind-the-ear or eyeglass metronome prosthesis. He also reported on studies where clients were taught to use rhythmic timing (and prosody reduction) without prosthesis support. Wingate (1976) summarized rhythm therapy noting that (1) its effect is immediate; (2) its effect lasts as long as the stimulus is applied (no fading); (3) its effect is relatively unchanged whether the stimulus form is audible, visible, or tactile; and (4) its effect occurs with almost all stutterers although younger clients may show the best acceptance and improvement, and the least relapse. He also suggested that rhythm may be more acceptable to severe stutterers.

Efficacy

Anything that superimposes or imparts a controlled rhythm can replace or alter the rhythm pattern of either fluent or stuttered speech. Brady (1973) compared the effects of having stutterers read while involved (separately) with nine separate rhythm conditions. These conditions included walking and reading, with one syllable uttered per step; a foot tap on each word; an arm swing on each word; a hand wave on each word; accenting alternate syllables; using a traditional metronome; and so on. The traditional metronome and the walking condition seemed most effective in reducing stuttering. (In therapy with young children, I have used speaking in time with clanking-banging-ringing rhythm band instruments to very good effect. Everybody was fluent, but nobody could hear them talk!)

In 1976, Öst et al. compared metronome-conditioned speech to shadowing (see earlier this chapter) on 15 subjects, divided into three groups of five. At the end of the trial therapy periods, the metronome group's stuttering was reduced by about 44%, compared with 15% reductions for the shadowing group and 16% for the no-therapy control group. Some time later, in their extended review of published stuttering treatments, Andrews, Guitar, and Howie (1980) found things to criticize about rhythm therapy. They noted its quick, positive initial effects, but criticized the cadence quality and what they felt was considerable deterioration in control after therapy was terminated. They suggested that good results from rhythm therapy would require at least 100 hours of work, inclusion of prolonged speech and rate reduction, careful shaping of speech to re-normalize it, systematic transfer and maintenance plans, and expectation of and alertness for possible need for counseling therapy. Of course those comments can probably be made concerning at least 90% of the therapy approaches today.

Hayden, Jordahl, and Adams (1982) evaluated the speech initiation time (SIT) of stutterers and nonstutterers under unaltered conditions, under masking, and under a pacing tone signal. Both experimental groups improved SITs significantly when paced stimuli were used. This improvement was better than SIT scores under masking and normal auditory conditions. Stutterers were slower than nonstutterers under all conditions.

Christenfeld (1996) looked at the metronome in terms of its effects on a common avoidance or struggle behavior of stutterers: the filled pause. They also evaluated the effect of a metronome on the filled pauses of fluent speakers. In both groups, a reduction in filled pauses was found to occur. They felt the reduction was not just due to simplifying or slowing speech, but suggested that metronome use actually forces the person to pay more attention to physical speech production and less attention to linguistic formulation.

Curlee and Siegel (1997) have little to say about the desirability of metronome use and do not describe common procedures. They do feel, however, that light pulses could be used to replace or accompany audible signals. In particular, they report on several computer programs that can variably control cueing rate for utterance of verbal material on the computer screen and suggest other computer applications in paced speech.

Speech Normalcy Concerns

Although rhythm-paced speech probably offers the fastest therapy "fix," the highest fluency induction level, and the highest consistency effect, it tends to be an unloved method. The resulting speech, if not reshaped drastically, is so mechanical as to be less acceptable than many mild and moderate stuttering patterns. At the least it slows rate (usually), reduces intonation and stress, equalizes stress, reduces and equalizes loudness, and yields vowels with a longer duration than usual.

Howell and El-Yaniv (1987) evaluated the normalcy of metronome-based fluency. Judges rated the speech naturalness of stutterers from a just-completed 2-week intensive therapy program. The judged conditions were NAF, application of a click tripped on every syllable utterance, and a metronome click generated automatically every half-second. Results indicated that the syllable-generated click produced the most natural speech. Out of 100 possible judgments, the onset click received 81 "most natural" votes, the no-interjection received 19 best votes, and metronome received no votes.

The study reported on another dimension of measurement. All subjects had just finished 2 weeks of intensive therapy. Under NAF the average number of dysfluencies was 20.2 (range, 7 to 33); under the onset click condition, the spasm average dropped to 2.5, with 3 subjects reporting no spasms; under the metronome condition, the spasm average was 0.6, with 8 of 10 subjects reporting zero dysfluencies.

Too many therapy programs, especially behavior modification programs of the past 20 years, have simply instated rhythm effects to achieve a quick, low stuttered words per minute (sw/m) measure. They do little or nothing to normalize the speech effects created by the rhythm program.

Application of Rhythm Procedures

Preparation

As with all management techniques, it is wise to stop and ask yourself several questions before moving into a program sequence:

- Why have I selected this method, as compared with others?
- What is my target, terminal application, or transition to a next step in my therapy program?
- If this approach falters, will I:
  - Back up and try it again?
  - Move to an ancillary program and then return to the main program? If so, what secondary program?
  - Cancel and switch to a new approach? What approach?
- Am I going to combine previously learned or acquired capacities of the client? If so, what?

The clinician must have at least one answer for each of these questions. Some other aspects to consider include:

- Client's past exposure to musical training, various forms of dance, gymnastics, and so on (Any or all of these might suggest [not guaran-

tee] exposure to rhythm, timing, movement coordination, monitoring movement behavior, and so forth.)
- Client's gait, manual laterality, eye-hand coordination, reaction time, or other aspects of neuromotor coordination as evidenced by observation or direct information
- Client's physical writing and drawing skills (These may suggest a level of motor ability.)
- Effects of masking, rhythm, DAF, and so forth, as observed by the clinician, as well as client's attitudes toward different stimuli
- Client's personality (Brandon and Harris [1967] suggested that some personalities [e.g., sociable, independent, cheerful, dominant, etc.] respond less positively to rhythm therapy [syllable tapping]. Supposedly, the quieter, submissive, introverted, dependent types are more amenable to such therapies.)
- Client's age (Client ages younger than 8 years are positively correlated with effects of rhythm use.)
- Stutterer's level of severity (Those with higher levels of severity may be more accepting.)
- Client's type of spasm (Stutterers with spasms that are predominantly oral [as opposed to laryngeal] in location and that are predominantly repetitive [rather than stops or prolongations] may respond better to rhythm therapies.)

Final Probe for Rhythm Use

I recommend a final probe of rhythm effectiveness and client reaction. It will familiarize the client with basic skills, disclose any serious problems, and help the clinician plan subsequent therapy steps.

- *Step 1.* Display and demonstrate metronome to client. Model its use, using some of the activities listed in Step 2. Ask for any questions.
- *Step 2.* Instruct the client to follow directions. Set metronome at 40 beats per minute (bpm) and have client perform the following acts, with one movement on each beat signal (10 to 15 times each):
  - Tap fingers on table.
  - Nod head left and right.
  - Open and close jaw.

– Utter buh-buh-buh.

Shorten or lengthen this activity as desired. Answer any questions; resolve any problems.

• *Step 3.* Keep metronome at 40 bpm for each of the seven substeps. Instruct client to read the following words aloud, one per beat. Have client pause if he or she misses a beat, get back in rhythm, and then continue.

see	dip	cat	go	fin
do	bag	fur	who	put
be	in	at	or	fee
tack	hot	sing	tin	run

Repeat and model as needed.

Instruct the client to read the following words aloud, ensuring that one syllable falls on each beat. Have client pause for a beat or two if he or she makes a mistake, get back on track, and then start again with the error word.

future	brother	pebble	singer	detail
whimsy	cookie	candy	baseball	auto
fasten	rubble	bitter	heavy	broken
limit	stutter	manage	simple	yellow

Repeat and model as needed.

Instruct the client to read the following sentences aloud, with one word falling on each beat. Have the client start the sentence over again in the event of a mistake.

How are you?
Where is the cat?
See me go up now?
Give me a bit more time.
Let the dog in and go home.

Instruct the client to read the following sentences aloud, with one syllable on each beat. Have the client use the same repair as before if any trouble is encountered.

We dislike real butter.
No children are allowed outside.
Bill works 1 day a week at the church.

> Give me liberty or deposit more money in my bank account.
> Government interference is intolerable to liberal personalities.

Repeat, repair, and model as needed.

Instruct the client to read the following short paragraph, one syllable per beat. Have client use the same repair strategy if a beat is missed.

> Stuttering problems may occur at any age, but usually happen between the ages of 2 and 8 years. Some suggest that a family history of stuttering is a significant indicator for the prognosis.

Repeat, discuss, and model as needed.

Instruct the client to answer the following questions by using many of the question words (but do not make repeating a problem). Have client respond one syllable per beat.

> What is your name?
> What is your favorite sport?
> What movie have you seen most recently?
> Do you drive a car?
> Where do you live?

Repeat, discuss, repair, and model as needed.

Give the client five topics, and ask him or her to pick one. Have the client talk on that topic for about 1 or 2 minutes, using one syllable per beat. Record the monologue.

> • Discuss the job you desire.
> • How would you evaluate your educational experience to date?
> • Do you want to raise a family some day? Why?
> • Tell me a joke.
> • How would you evaluate politics and politicians?

Play back the recording, looking for "misses" where more than one syllable occurs per beat. Correct all errors by repeating the entire sentence (approximate) where the error occurred.

The clinician should discuss the client's overall reaction to metronome bpm control, accepting that 40 bpm is a terrible frustration (after completing the first couple of substeps the clinician can switch from 40 bpm to 80 bpm, if the client seems too impatient). The client should be assured that 40 bpm is not the final target. It is the orientation rate only.

- *Step 4.* Repeat Step 1, substituting 80 bpm for the previously used rate. Omit this step if a switch to 80 bpm occurred during Step 1. Feel free to omit any substeps deemed too "micro" to repeat. Add new substeps or lengthen or revise existing ones.
- *Step 5.* Repeat Step 1, substituting 120 bpm for the previously used rate. Modify as desired, as suggested in Step 2.
- *Step 6.* Repeat all of the Step 1 substeps. Put the unit at 40 bpm for about one third of the stimuli, at 80 bpm for the second third, and 120 bpm for the final third. Where there are only five stimuli, use 40 bpm on only one, 80 bpm on two, and 120 on the last two. On the monologue answers, start at 40 bpm for about 10 seconds, shift to 80 bpm for 15 to 20 seconds, and finish with 120 bpm. Do not interrupt the client's talking; just reset the unit as she or he talks. Warn the client in advance of the changes in rate.

The clinician should discuss the previous sequence with the client for the purposes of performance evaluation, exploration of the client's feelings, and addressing any problems observed or reported. The next step is to explore and negotiate an *optimal* and a *secure* bpm rate. The optimal rate, or preferred rate, may fall below 120 bpm (not often), or it may run as high as 160 to 180 bpm (usually not desirable). The client's usual (fluent) speech rate will need to be considered. A person who usually speaks rapidly (when not stuttering) will lean toward a faster bpm rate. However, the clinician needs to be alert for the client who has used extrafast or extraslow speech rates as an avoidance behavior.

Although the preceding steps employed metronome-regulated speech, the clinician can adapt the sequence to syllable tapping, haptometronome, or other rhythmic stimuli forms.

Instatement of Rhythmic Speech

Relative to the instatement material that follows, its use depends on whether rhythm is the sole therapy technique or part of an overall program. Note that the instatement sequence omits many of the microsteps and starts at the sentence level. This change reflects the practice effects arising from the preceding step sequences.

Stuttering may occur during these early steps but, if it is not too intrusive, it should be dealt with later. The clinician also should discuss the acceptability of dropping the rhythmic cadence when it seems to be acceptable, but it should not be targeted yet. The client should be told about upcoming home assignments and their importance (chapters 2 and 9). Finally, the clinician should let the client know that the issue of initiating the first word will be discussed at or around Step 11. The only performance criterion for this step is that the client must be able to maintain the secure and the optimal bpm rates with and without instrumental support for at least 30 seconds.

- *Step 1.* Confirm with the client the agreed-on optimal and secure bpm rates (see "Final Probe for Rhythm Use").

    Optimal—a bpm rate the client feels is near to, but slightly slower than, his or her usual rate.
    Secure—a bpm rate the client feels "guarantees" fluency, but is undesirably slow and mechanical.

- *Step 2.* Have client practice switching from the optimal to the secure rate, and back, while reading sentences. Reset unit after each sentence. Start with secure, then optimal, and so on. Have client read each sentence only once.

    Which one of you is responsible for this mess?
    Let's grab our hats and coats and get out of here!
    Television is a vast wasteland, but I like it.
    There is no doubt that many people do not like him.
    Can you give me three tens and four fives for a fifty?
    Certainly you can go skiing with me.

Add others as desired.

Use a performance criterion of no errors (rhythm break) on any sentence portion *where both agree it should be used.* Use penalty of repeating sentence in both bpm rates.

- *Step 3.* Repeat Step 2 but alternate starting role (i.e., if Step 2 started with secure, start with optimal here, and vice versa). Turn the unit off as soon as each sentence is uttered and have the client repeat the sentence using same rate. Turn the unit back on, reset unit to other bpm rate, and repeat the process. Repeat this sequence for each sentence. Record the whole activity and play tape back to compare aided versus unaided efforts. Use performance criterion from Step 2; however, have client perform all evaluations.

Recycle this step with a change: Have client produce first sentence, aided, on secure mode. Turn unit off. Ask client to repeat sentence using optimal mode, unaided. Reverse the procedure on the second sentence (i.e., optimal first, aided; secure second, unaided). Continue rotation through all the sentences. As before, record, play back, compare, discuss.

Before meeting with the client for Step 4, the clinician must find a quiet spot, turn the metronome on, turn the tape recorder on, and fill one side of the tape cassette with recorded beats at the secure bpm rate. Then the clinician must switch sides of the tape, and record the second side at the optimal rate.

- *Step 4.* Use longer sentences and utterances with multiple, short sentences. Mix the use of optimal and secure rates, but skew it toward about 60% optimal. Have client do all evaluation and consequation. Record, but do not play back unless there is disagreement about an evaluation or the desire to discuss a special problem. Establish a criterion wherein the client must repeat any utterance set (entirely) when there is more than one unacceptable behavior (i.e., "unacceptable" is any stuttering or failure to keep rate mode when it would be appropriate). Five utterance units are provided below; compose 10 more.

  When persons stutter, most of their undesirable behaviors are produced by their efforts not to stutter.
  Don't believe it! You never get used to it! Stuttering never quits. It's always there.
  She smiled happily at the dragon. "Oh, how nice! I've always wanted a fire-breathing dragon," she said.
  "A nod is as good as a wink," I said. "Not to me it isn't," he said. This discouraged me very much.
  In Germany, in the 19th century, one treatment for stuttering was to cut a wedge from the tongue—with no anesthetic and no antibiotic.

- *Step 5.* Repeat Step 4 but do not use the metronome unit during actual utterances. Have the client use optimal rate on segments that seem "proper." Turn the unit on for about 5 seconds before each utterance, turn it off, wait several seconds, then signal the client to produce the utterance unit. Or, turn the unit on when the client reaches the last three or four words of each unit, to see if the bpm pattern has remained stable. (I do not favor this variation because bpm drop areas tend to occur near the ending points of phrase units.) Record, compare, analyze, discuss, evaluate, consequate, as in Step 4. Employ same criterion.

At this point, or earlier if desired, the clinician should give the client the tape of secure and optimal bpm rates and copies of the stimulus material used in Steps 2, 3, 4, and 5. Next, a home practice schedule is scheduled. Although 10 minutes, three times a day (soon after arising, after lunch, and after dinner) is preferable, the clinician should settle for what the client will agree to. Afterward, at the start of every in-clinic session, the clinician must ask the client about homework. The key is to be interested, not perfunctory. The clinician can ask questions, design a log sheet, ask for a diary, or check to see if there is any spontaneous spread to general out-clinic speech.

- *Step 6.* Continue the home assignments. Have client answer questions in complete sentences. Record and apply as before. Cue the client's bpm response rate by asking initial questions in the rate mode indicated. Use the metronome to pace bpm rate of questions, if necessary. Instruct client to respond at the same bpm rate, but without unit support. Penalize any error (stuttering, not using mode when appropriate) by having client repeat the entire utterance twice, using the metronome 100% each time, once at the rate just used, and once at the alternate rate. Use sample utterances that follow; an asterisk indicates secure rate, and no asterisk indicates optimal rate.

      What is the day of the week?
      *What color are your shoes?
      Do you sing very much?
      When did you first start to stutter?
      *Who first noticed your stuttering?
      *Does anyone else in your family stutter?
      Can you drive a car?
      Do you ever try to avoid speaking?
      Who is your best friend?
      What is your favorite television program?
      Does it bother your family when you stutter?
      What kind, or kinds, of dogs do you like best?

*How often do you substitute words because of stuttering?
Do you believe in ghosts?
What is the best book you have ever read?
Have you ever been scuba diving?
Has anyone ever, to your face, imitated your stuttering?
What is your favorite food?
Are you very talkative outside the clinic?
*How old will you be on your next birthday?

- *Step 7.* Repeat Step 6, but reverse roles. Have client ask the questions (on the "stuttering questions" respond as if you were a stutterer). Answer in the proper mode. Do not use metronome on either question or answer. Instruct client to evaluate and consequate his or her question posing and your responses. Use same criterion and penalty as before. Send the Step 6 questions home, if a home assignment is needed. Direct the client to answer the 20 questions at the proper rate. Record, play back, and evaluate. Use same criteria as before.

- *Step 8.* Use same evaluation criteria as before. Repeat all aspects of Step 6, but instruct the client to expand his or her answers to several sentences (see below). Mark some items for secure rate practice, if desired.

    Step 6: What color are your shoes? My shoes are black.
    Step 8: What color are your shoes? Right now, they are black but I have brown and gray ones at home. Most of the time I wear jogging shoes.
    Step 6: Do you believe in ghosts? No, I don't believe in ghosts.
    Step 8: Do you believe in ghosts? No, not really. However, my grandmother did. When I was a little kid, she used to really scare me with some of her ghost stories.

Prior to Step 9, the clinician may need to deal with dysfluencies that occur at the initiation points of utterances, points where a rhythmic cadence has not been established yet. If it is not a problem on an in-clinic basis, it very likely will be in out-clinic practice. Accordingly, I suggest the clinician consult the section titled "The Bounce" in this chapter. The Bounce is a natural accompaniment to cadenced, rhythmic speech. It can be taught to the client, as described later, with an addition: The utterance rate for the Bounce can match the optimal (and perhaps also the secure) rate in use with the particular client. Practicing both is not a bad idea. Note that Step 9 easily may take more than one session.

- *Step 9.* Have the client talk on a series of topics provided by the clinician. Tell the client to talk as long as possible on each topic. Instruct the client to use the optimal rate on the beginning series of words for each phrase group and the optimal rate at any other point where, outside the clinic, stuttering might be expected to occur.

  Time the client's speech to accumulate approximately 15 minutes. Record for playback. After the first 3 to 5 minutes, stop the client and play back a minute or so of the tape to see if the rate is correct and stable. If not, wipe the time out and start over. In the new cycle, have the client pause at the end of every 3 minutes of talk while the unit is turned on and then continue talking. Leave the unit on for about 30 seconds and then turn it off without stopping the client. Any time there is a stutter, stop and have the client start the particular phrase over again, use the desired rate, and use a Bounce on the word that had been stuttered. Add 1 more minute to the target 15 minutes. Be sure that home assignments include practice on spontaneous speech. Have a significant other help as a listener, if possible.

- *Step 10.* Particular procedures will vary with specific clients, and with their degree of naturalness already present. Suggestions include having the client read aloud (and record) material such as
  - conventional paragraph material
  - newspaper editorials or letters to the editor, where feelings are expressed
  - various types of poetry
  - song lyrics (do not sing)
  - dramatic material
  - humorous material

  The client and clinician listen to playbacks and evaluate naturalness for:

rate	rhythm
loudness	prosodic stress
inflection	other vocal variations

  Self-evaluation is important, but the client may need clinician assistance at first. If the client has significant problems in sounding more natural, a repeat of practice material may be needed, with the clinician modeling and the client evaluating and imitating.

- *Step 11.* Perform transfer activity. Consult chapter 9 for specifics. Do not allow the client to use a lot of rhythmic speech patterns—only when truly needed. Do not use set sequences due to variables involved. Use the following sequence, if desired:

- Invite colleagues to participate in a conversation. Repeat as a home assignment.
- Pre-script practice telephone calls. Repeat as a home assignment.
- Use unscripted telephone calls. Repeat as a home assignment.
- Enter a few supervised situations outside the clinic, and plan solo ones with the client.

Use final therapy sessions on Step 11 to hear extended reports on solo work, problem solve, plan additional transfer work, and conduct brief out-clinic exercises, where needed.

I have found that many clients do not like rhythm-based speech. Of those who favor it, a majority switch to some other major approach before they complete the sequence of activity steps. Those who complete the entire sequence often choose to invest in a prosthetic or portable body unit device, and they seem quite satisfied. When I use rhythm techniques, my general assumption is that they will comprise only one phase of therapy—not a total program.

THE BOUNCE

History

The Bounce is credited to Wendell Johnson (Bloodstein, 1993) and probably was associated with early efforts to alter the abnormal preparatory set in stutterers' speech (see chapter 8). Since then, the Bounce has led a rather checkered life. Culatta and Goldberg (1995) proposed that the Bounce was one of the techniques promoted by Van Riper as part of the overall program of therapy developed at the University of Iowa in the 1930s. The other three symptom manipulation components were cancellation, pullout, and preparatory sets. Bloodstein (1993) stated that Johnson's approach differed from that of Van Riper (1973). Van Riper utilized a prolongation of a word's initial sound, whereas Johnson taught an easy, slow, relaxed, rhythmic repetition of the first syllable of a word. Beyond that, their approaches were much in accord until the 1950s. At that time Johnson became interested in general semantics and developed the diagnosogenic theory of stuttering. As noted, Johnson's theoretical development did not separate him from the Bounce. In his 1946 book, *People in Quandaries*, Johnson was still recommending the Bounce, as a voluntary stuttering, although he did agree to accept a simple prolongation if that was more acceptable to the stutterer. He really did not favor that approach, however.

In a brief summary, Johnson suggested:

- Have the client practice intensively while alone (mirror work preferred).
- Record all efforts and listen to them repeatedly.
- Introduce the Bounce into real situations, gradually using a difficulty hierarchy.
- Use the Bounce deliberately and frequently when it is not necessary. (The more fakes are used, the less often real spasms will occur. As time passes, faking can be reduced as avoidance behaviors are reduced.)
- Taper use of fake disfluencies. (The speaker will become progressively less dysfluent as the faking disfluency increases.)
- Encourage or require the client to increase his or her speaking frequency greatly.

Application—Preliminaries

Implementation strategies for the Bounce are as varied as those for cancellation or Easy Onset. Accordingly I would suggest that, in most cases, it will be counterproductive to enroll a fluency client and then go directly to Bounce therapy. To "Bounce" is to commit overt, very noticeable, artificial-sounding disfluencies. Strangers will notice its use, and friends are likely to feel that the stuttering has gotten worse. In another area, I question use of the Bounce until the client can function effectively in:

- Self-monitoring, analysis, evaluation (chapter 3)
- Avoidance reduction (chapter 2)
- General desensitization and relaxation ability (chapter 4)

If Bounce training is given to an unprepared client, he or she may reject it. If the client does not reject it, then he or she will probably use it as a postponement or starter device (that always is a very thin line with techniques). Clinicians will need to assess each client and decide how much preliminary work is needed—a few sessions or a few months.

Application—Acquisition

Presumably every clinician has a client who, however reluctantly, is willing to talk to people, able to fake stuttering, and can at least reduce his or her tension to manageable levels. This client should be told about the Bounce as follows:

> I want you to learn to control your fluency breaks. Instead of stuttering like this [model an imitation of the client's usual pattern], I want you to Bounce easily and quietly, like this [use the same word, but with an easy, quiet, relaxed, 2-3 Bounce production]. Isn't that a lot better? What is your reaction to this method?

It is important to deal with questions and explain about the progressive learning steps. The clinician should impart the four basic rules to the Bounce:

1. Always Bounce in an easy, relaxed, slow, even pattern.
2. Always use the syllable, not the sound (i.e., "se-se-set" not "s-s-set").
3. Do not use "uh" in the syllable, unless that is correct (*i.e., "se-se-set" but not "suh-suh-set"*).
4. Do not differentiate within a Bounce production (i.e., the last Bounce should have the same rate, stress, and rhythm as the first).

Good eye contact is a must on every Bounce. Eye contact is desired at nearly all times, but is mandatory on every voluntary disfluency. Poor Bounces usually are caused by one or more of the following:

- Hurried, uneven, tense Bounce
- Schwa (uh) vowel, where inappropriate

- Too few Bounces to set a relaxed pattern
- Poor eye contact (nervousness, embarrassment)
- Jerk or tension on the last Bounce; a pause after last Bounce
- Unwillingness to use Bounce

For each of the items above, the clinician should explain and model (where appropriate). The client really must understand the error factors. Then the clinician begins the step sequence. The initial step is designed to have the client validate his or her ability to produce words in an easy, relaxed manner.

- *Step 1.* Have the client read aloud the word list below until in-clinic production is satisfactory. Help client use a little EO, if needed. Note that the words vary in length, and that continuants are used at first. Augment the word list as desired.

sun	wash	shovel	damp	garage	cannon
for	where	thinner	cover	double	tiresome
here	some	warble	trouble	gargle	volume
shoe	fruit	frantic	zebra	devil	bitter
thin	how	hairy	cabin	village	pasture

  Make sure the client maintains good eye contact with self in a mirror while reading. Record the activity in order to sample and discuss items. Have the client practice the list until control over the word productions is evident. Give the client a home assignment to run through the 30 words three times each day (solo) until notified otherwise.

- *Step 2.* Use the word list from Step 1. Have the client read it aloud and Bounce twice on each initial syllable.

suh-suh-sun	fru-fru-fruit	deh-deh-devil
tie-tie-tiresome	etc.	etc.

Sort out how much of a first syllable to repeat (e.g., "frantic" could be "fra-fra" or "fran-fran"). Apply the evaluations suggested just prior to Step 1.

Use the word list from Step 1 again. Have the client Bounce five times before releasing each word. Record and play back. Have the client help evaluate, listening for:

–Variations in one set of rate, rhythm stress

−Poor prosody (i.e., monotone)
−Jerk on or pause after last syllable
−Inappropriate schwa use
−Adequate air supply (Bounces use up air, especially when occurring in a running sentence.)

Assign the two- and five-Bounce activity to be practiced every day at home, until replaced, if in-clinic performance has been satisfactory.

- *Step 3.* Go directly into reality practice. Compose sentences that relate to the client, and have him or her Bounce five or more times on each underlined word. Use the 10 sample sentences below; add 20 more.

My name is _____.	(Bounce on one item)
I live at _____.	(Bounce on one item)
My telephone number is _____.	(Bounce on one item)

Where will I find typing paper?
Politics is the art of the possible.
Can you help me with my project?
Will you call me at home?
How are you today?
Is this the bus station?
I want a bacon cheeseburger, large fries, and a chocolate shake.

Listen for continuity of the sentence (when there is enough length of utterance [later on], the client will want to slow speech rate slightly as he or she approaches the Bounce word; adequate breath support becomes significant then). Mark about half of the 30 utterances and assign for home practice. Tell the client to read them aloud twice every day. Do five Bounces the first time; do as many Bounces as "feels okay" on the second reading. Report on the results at the next session.

- *Step 4.* Use any paragraph, or write one (a partial one is provided below; add to it as desired). Model reading it aloud. Have the client read it aloud and Bounce the number of times printed above the marked words.

```
  7      5            3                     7
Some children don't  really just start to stutter.  They seem to
  5       3           7     5      3
think faster than they can move their tongues and jaws, so
  7          5          3          7        5
words get all scrambled up. When they realize their trouble,
        3
they become frustrated. [Complete, as desired.]
```

Record and play back, judging on the error elements cited earlier. Have the client do the evaluations. Compare the 7, 5, 3 Bounces with each other. Repeat, with modeling, any unacceptable sentences. Repeat the process three times. On the last run-through, move on and assign this as homework if errors are at 15 or less. Repeat if errors are above 15.

At this point it may be worth the effort to jump several steps to Step 8. It is possible if the client is pretty stable, is an externalized stutterer, and has fairly low sensitivity levels. If the client leans toward the opposite of those aspects, or if any clinician uncertainty exists, proceed to Step 5.

- *Step 5.* Work to turn the Bounce method over to the client. Instruct him or her to respond to questions in one or more utterances. Have the client Bounce where it seems right, and use a variety of Bounce numbers from 2 up to 6 or 8. Record and play back. Ask five questions, rewind the tape, and play back. Evaluate the usual error areas (cited before), failure to Bounce when indicated (if client can defend choice, accept), and failure to vary Bounce numbers adequately. Discuss the evaluations.

    Inform the client that the preceding exercise was practice and that four sets of 5 questions (20 in all) will be posed for her or him to answer. Remind client to maintain good eye contact on each Bounce word. Use same instructions and criteria. Record and have the client evaluate. Set an error/accept criterion list such as the one below.

    Failed eye contact—Repeat specific word twice, with bounces.
    Hurried, jerky bounces—Repeat entire phrase with 10 to 12 Bounces on error word.
    Pause after last bounce—Repeat entire phrase with 10 to 12 Bounces on error word.
    Inappropriate schwa vowel—Repeat three times with one Bounce each.
    Jerk on last bounce—Repeat three times with one Bounce each.

    Count the number of words Bounced on in a five-answer unit. Wipe out the five answers and start over if more than 50% of the Bounce efforts are at three bounces or less. Give the client two questions to answer, record, evaluate, and consequate at home as an assignment.
- *Step 6.* Repeat Step 5, but direct the client to make her or his answers run for 2 to 3 minutes. Otherwise, use same directions. Record as before. Evaluate, applying the Step 5 criteria to the last 30 seconds of

each answer (when client is most likely to be careless). Organize a home assignment similar to that used in Step 5.

- *Step 7.* Provide the client with a list of 20 topics. Have client talk about a topic until words run out; select a new topic and continue. Allow client to accumulate about 20 minutes of talking time. Have the client start over with the first topic, repeating topics as needed, if the topics run out. Direct the client to use Bounces on "appropriate" words, varying from two to seven Bounces. Evaluate on the usual criteria, and stop the client every time an error is committed (stop timing then). Have the client cancel the error and use a seven-Bounce effort to do so. Start timing again when the client resumes talking. Interrupt if a lack of longer Bounces is obvious.

    Give a home assignment. Have client explain the Bounce to a family member or close friend. Instruct client to talk for 5 to 10 minutes, using the Bounce when stuttering is anticipated. If stuttering occurs, try once to cancel with a Bounce, and then go on. Try to use at least 20 to 30 times in the conversation when it is not needed.

- *Step 8.* Move to out-clinic transfer work, as discussed in chapter 9. Follow the general progression of steps there. Add an Easy Onset style of production to jump-start some words initiating an utterance sequence, if necessary. However, let the Bounce remain, if possible. If a stuttering spasm intrudes, practice relaxing and turning the spasm into a Bounce pullout (chapter 8).

SUMMARY

This chapter presented several frequently used control techniques. Some were fluency oriented, and a few were symptom related. Possibilities for mixing and interacting should not be ignored. Overall, any of the techniques can make dramatic changes in a client's dysfluency frequency and severity. However, if not used in a context of client preparation and client motivation, they will most certainly fail, possibly distorting and intensifying the client's existing dysfluencies. Clinicians must know their clients and their needs and abilities.

REFERENCES

Adamczyk, B. (1994). Stuttering therapy with the "echo method." *Journal of Fluency Disorders, 19,* 147.

Andrews, G., Guitar, B., & Howie, P. (1980). Meta-analysis of the effects of stuttering treatment. *Journal of Speech and Hearing Disorders, 45*, 287–307.

Bloodstein, O. (1993). *Stuttering: The search for a cause and cure.* Boston: Allyn & Bacon.

Bloodstein, O. (1995). *A handbook on stuttering.* San Diego, CA: Singular Publishing Group.

Brady, J.P. (1973). Metronome-conditioned relaxation: A new behavioral procedure. *British Journal of Psychiatry, 122*, 729–730.

Brandon, S., & Harris, M. (1967). Stammering—an experimental treatment programme using syllable-timed speech. *British Journal of Disorders of Communication, 2*, 64–68.

Cherry, C., & Sayers, B.M. (1956). Experiments upon the total inhibition of stammering, and some clinical results. *Journal of Psychosomatic Research, 1*, 233–246.

Christenfeld, N. (1996). Effects of metronome on the filled pauses of fluent speakers. *Journal of Speech and Hearing Research, 39*, 1232–1238.

Craig, A., Hancok, K., Chang, E., McCready, C., Shepley, A., Costello, D., Harding, S., Kehren, R., Masel, C., & Reilly, K. (1996). A controlled clinical trial for stuttering in persons aged 9 to 14 years. *Journal of Speech and Hearing Research, 39*, 808–826.

Culatta, R.E., & Goldberg, S.A. (1995). *Stuttering therapy, An integrated approach to theory and practice.* Boston: Allyn & Bacon.

Curlee, R.F., & Siegel, G.M. (1997). *Nature and treatment of stuttering, new directions* (2nd ed.). Boston: Allyn & Bacon.

Falck, F.J. (1969). *Stuttering: Learned and unlearned.* Springfield, IL: Charles C Thomas.

Fiedler, P.A., & Standop, R. (1983). *Stuttering, integrating theory and practice* (S.R. Silverman, trans.). Rockville, MD: Aspen Publishers.

Freund, H. (1966). *Psychotherapy and the problem of stuttering.* Springfield, IL: Charles C Thomas.

Gregory, H. (1968). *Learning theory and stuttering therapy.* Evanston, IL: Northwestern University Press.

Ham, R.E. (1986). *Techniques of stuttering therapy.* Englewood Cliffs, NJ: Prentice Hall.

Ham, R.E. (1989). *Therapy of stuttering.* Englewood Cliffs, NJ: Prentice Hall.

Hayden, P.A., Jordahl, N., & Adams, M.R. (1982). Stutterers' voice initiation times during conditions of novel stimulation. *Journal of Fluency Disorders, 7*, 1–7.

Howell, P., & El-Yaniv, N. (1987). The effects of presenting a click syllabic-initial position on the speech structure: Comparisons with a click. *Journal of Fluency Disorders, 12*, 249–256.

Ingham, R.J., Andrews, G., & Winkler, R. (1972). Stuttering: A comparative evaluation of the short-term effectiveness of four treatment techniques. *Journal of Communication Disorders, 5*, 91–117.

Ingham, R.J., & Packman, A. (1979). A further evaluation of the speech of stutterers during chorus and non-chorus reading situations. *Journal of Speech and Hearing Research, 22*, 784–793.

Johnson, W. (1946). *People in quandaries.* New York: Harper & Row.

Johnson, W., & Rosen, L. (1937). Studies in the psychology of stuttering: VII. Effect of certain changes in speech patterns upon the frequency of stuttering. *Journal of Speech Disorders, 2,* 105–109.

Kalinowski, J., Armson, J., Roland-Mieszkowski, M., & Stuart, A. (1993). Effects of alterations in auditory feedback and speech rate on stuttering frequency. *Language and Speech, 36,* 1–16.

Kalinowski, J., Stuart, A., & Armson, J. (1996). Stuttering amelioration at various auditory feedback delays and speech rates. *European Journal of Disorders of Communication, 31,* 359–369.

Kelham, R., & McHale, A. (1966). The application of learning theory to the treatment of stammering. *British Journal of Disorders of Communication, 1,* 114–118.

Marland, P.M. (1957). "Shadowing"—A contribution to the treatment of stammering. *Folia Phoniatrica, 9,* 242–245.

Öst, L.-G., Gotestam, G., & Lennert, M. (1976). A controlled study of two behavioral methods in the treatment of stuttering. *Behavior Therapy, 7,* 587–592.

Packman, A., Onslow, M., & Van Doorn, J. (1996). Syllabic stress and variability: A model of stuttering. *Clinical Linguistics and Phonetics, 10,* 235–263.

Perkins, W.H., Rudas, J., Johnson, L., Michael, W., & Curlee, R. (1974). Replacement of stuttering with normal speech. *Journal of Speech and Hearing Disorders, 39,* 416–428.

Peters, T., & Guitar, B. (1991). Stuttering, an integrated approach to its nature and treatment. Baltimore: Williams & Wilkins.

Ramig, P. (1984). Rate changes in the speech of stutterers after therapy. *Journal of Fluency Disorders, 9,* 285–294.

Sergeant, R.L. (1961). Concurrent repetition of a continuous flow of words. *Journal of Speech and Hearing Research, 4,* 373–380.

Shames, G.H., & Florance, C.L. (1980). *Stutter-free speech, a goal for therapy.* Columbus, OH: Charles E. Merrill.

Silverman, F.A. (1996). *Stuttering and other fluency disorders* (2nd. ed.). Boston: Allyn & Bacon.

Van Riper, C. (1973). *The treatment of stuttering.* Englewood Cliffs, NJ: Prentice Hall.

Walton, D., & Mather, M.D. (1963). The relevance of generalization techniques to the treatment of stammering and phobia symptoms. *Behavior Research and Therapy, 1,* 121–125.

Watts, F. (1971). The treatment of stammering by the intensive practice of fluent speech. *British Journal of Communication Disorders, 6,* 144–147.

Wingate, M.E. (1969). Sound and pattern in "artificial" fluency. *Journal of Speech and Hearing Research, 12,* 677–686.

Wingate, M.E. (1976). *Stuttering theory and treatment.* New York: Irvington Publishers.

Wolpe, J. (1973). *The practice of behavior therapy.* New York: Pergamon Press.

CHAPTER 7

Additional Procedures

- Overview
- Time Out
- Respiration and Breathstream Management
- Chewing Therapy
- Strong Articulator Movement
- Utterance Complexity
- Stuttering and Singing
- Role Play
- Summary

OVERVIEW

The preliminary outline for this chapter called for the presentation of 14 management procedures. After evaluating history of use, needs for special equipment or special training, and similar factors, I trimmed the list to 9. By the time of printing, the total was 7. As a general comment on all chapters, I have tried to minimize the use of rare or expensive equipment, purchased (usually expensive) programs, and procedures requiring at least one intensive workshop to be minimally qualified. I also stayed away from computer programs that "do it for you." In addition, the amount of direct information needed to apply a technique served as a criterion for space allocation. Breathstream management will require some rather detailed steps, while Time Out (TO) is much less demanding for the practitioner.

TIME OUT

TO was "discovered" in the 1960s by behavior modification specialists as a mode of punishment in the learning process. I personally experienced TO in 1937 when my teacher made me stand in the corner for 30 minutes with my nose pressed to the wall. Since that time (and much earlier), not much has changed—just the labels and the explanations. In 1937, all punishment was "aversive" and was a punitive response to a perceived behavioral lack or lapse. However, punishment is now defined as any response-contingent event that depresses a particular response. TO falls into this latter definition.

TO Application

Typically TO is applied on a "If you stutter, then you must take a Time Out" basis. The use of TO is contingent on the occurrence of stuttering, and it is intended to depress that response. Martin and Haroldson (1979) compared TO to delayed auditory feedback (DAF), to masking noise, to a metronome beat, and to the utterance of "wrong!" TO was slightly more effective (by 1%) than the metronome (second best) in reducing stuttering frequency. Onslow, Packman, Stocker, Van Doorn, and Siegel (1997) noted a scarcity of research on the effectiveness of TO with children, and they evaluated its use with three school-age children. On each stuttering a red light was flashed, requiring the child to stop speaking for 5 seconds. One third (one out of three) of the children failed to show a clear reduction in stuttering, but the other two did. Whether this finding has relevance to the universe population of children who stutter remains to be seen.

James (1983) reported effective use of TO with adolescent and adult stutterers. James, Ricciardelli, Rogers, and Hunter (1989) reported further on TO, using it with 20 adult stutterers. TO was found to reduce stuttering frequency significantly and speaking rate significantly, with a few differing response patterns.

Flanagan (1986) summarized TO use (at that time). He raised very interesting questions about the complexities of using any form of punishment, suggesting that use had to be decided on an almost case-by-case basis. He also raised a recurrent issue in response-contingent punishment, from Skinner (1953), who wondered whether the use of punishment was more rewarding to the clinician than to the client.

TO Concerns

Response-contingent methods should be applied cautiously in preschool (and some early school) populations. These children may perceive TO as a disapproval and real punishment for their speech. Moreover, in diganosogenic terms, they may suffer increased dysfluencies resulting from such experiences. Older children and adults generally respond well to TO, but some express giggles or laughter (nervous embarrassment?), or sharp irritation. Shames (1975) and Siegel and Martin (1968) noted that contingent occasion stimuli, or punishment, depends on several factors to be effective:

- quickness of application
- duration and intensity of the punishment
- noticeability (inability of the stimulus to be ignored)
- consistency of application of the stimulus
- client history of responses to punishment

Any punishment can be perceived as aversive, or not. Electric shock, "Wrong," and TO will vary on the reactions they get. TO itself is interruption of speech with a nonspeaking time period, following a failed behavior or occurrence of an undesirable behavior.

Possible TO Application Procedures

- *Step 1.* Explain TO.

   When you are talking, if you ————, I will stop you, like this. You must stop talking until I give you the signal, like this, to start again.

- *Step 2.* Explain any associated occurrences.

   I will turn my head away; I will watch the clock; I will turn to the next person. You must shut your eyes. You must shut your eyes and take ___ easy, deep breaths.

- *Step 3.* Demonstrate the signal (e.g., hand gesture, clicker, bell, red light, toy horn, whistle, clacker, drum, "STOP!").

- *Step 4.* Model the unacceptable behavior. Have the client signal and be the therapist, and carry out the penalty behavior. If group therapy, have each client take a turn and fake a poor response and be penalized by another member of the group.
- *Step 5.* Indicate restriction (especially for groups) on grins, giggles, laughter, pokes, teasing, shuffles, and so on.
- *Step 6.* Establish procedures for record keeping, usually to measure TOs (stuttering frequency).

Costello (1980) described dividing a management session into a baseline period, followed by a TO period (signal to stop, 10 seconds of silence, clinician's head turned away). The last 10 minutes constituted a non-penalty reward period. With additional work on monitoring and attention to fluency control, the final reward period would be expanded as the number of TOs (frequency of stuttering) decreased.

- *Step 7.* Be consistent. When TO is on, apply it 100% of the time, but for a set period. Take some TO from TO. Arrange a schedule similar to the one that follows.

    Settle-down time . . . . 5 minutes of interaction
    Baseline measure time . . . . 5 minutes of work
    TO application . . . . 10 minutes
    TO break (but count spasms) . . . . . . 5 minutes
    TO application . . . . 10 minutes
    Ending, no TO (count spasms) . . . . . 5 minutes

    Adjust the time distribution as necessary.

- *Step 8.* Apply TO at once, on each occurrence, unless a cumulative count is being taken before the penalty (not a very good idea, usually).
- *Step 9.* Determine the intensity of the punishment stimulus. How strong or how aversive will the punishment be? Consider how the penalty is signaled, clinician's personal behavior of voice and facial expression and posture, and the aversive strength of the penalty (e.g., 5 seconds, 10 seconds, turn chair around, go sit in corner, etc.). Employ minimal aversiveness.
- *Step 10.* In a group, prevent any teasing and gloating by nonpenalized members. Create a special TO for group members who transgress.

The clinician should check individual responses. If the client (child or older) consistently shows a rise in spasm frequency or intensity immediately following a TO penalty, perhaps the penalty is too aversive or the client is too sensitive for TO to be a successful support method.

TO generally is used as a support vehicle for a primary management procedure. It can be a sole therapy method, but not often. It can be used in symptom modification therapy if a client fails to use a control method, for example. TO is viable at the very outset of therapy, or in final transfer stages. TO can be self-applied, but clients tend to be less consistent in applying it to themselves, and they tend to "fudge" the penalty duration. However, a conscientious client may transfer TO very profitably.

RESPIRATION AND BREATHSTREAM MANAGEMENT

Over the centuries, respiration has cycled to center stage (and off again) in stuttering. In the literature search for this section, I compiled hundreds of pages on the history and theories concerning respiration. Some data came from early in the century when stutterers, stripped to their underwear, were seated in an air-sealed, converted "steam box" (only the head protruded). Rubber hoses ran from the box to pressure tambours whose needles (early on) scratched lamp black–covered paper on a cylinder. Variations in air pressure in the steam box jiggled the tambour needles, which caused scratches in the lamp black. A filled paper roll was stripped off, dipped in fixative (usually shellac or varnish mix), hung to dry, and then analyzed.

Instrumentation today is exquisitely sensitive, can measure many variables, is almost instantaneous in data production and analysis, and tends to be hideously expensive. There also is the consideration that hanging cords, tubes, transducer attachments, and masks on the face, chest, abdomen, and neck and then saying, "Now breathe normally" is a functional oxymoron. Anyway, not one clinician in a hundred has ready access to sophisticated instrumentation, so the issue is moot.

For decades, theories of stuttering involved assumptions about respiration as a direct causative agent in stuttering. As a result, many therapies assumed a need to build things like respiratory vital capacity and to strengthen breathing patterns. In conversations with Van Riper, Johnson, and with other mature stutterers in the 1950s, I heard repeated stories of physical jerks and breathing exercises to promote deeper, more regularized breathing. Most of this activity had occurred, for those people, circa 1920s through 1930s. In the 1970s, and since, a number of new breath management programs have emerged that revisit the old targets, but come with a new rationale.

Stutterers often tend to display markedly disturbed respiratory behaviors, around and during moments of dysfluency. Nearly 30 years ago, Sheehan (1970) summarized many reports on stuttering and indicated that stutterers may display poor thoracic and abdominal movement balance, freezing of breathing musculature during stuttering spasms, quick and brief initial inhalations, shallow respiratory patterns when there are fluency problems, and so on. Sheehan also commented that there is no typical stutterer breathing pattern. A few years later Perkins, Rudas, Johnson, and Bell (1976) very succinctly structured one of those insights into the "discoordination hypothesis." By simply comparing stuttering occurrences during silent mouthing (no air, no voice), whispering (air, no voice), and ordinary utterances (air, voice), respiration was demonstrated to be part of the stuttering effect picture.

At the moment, our profession holds some opinions about respiration, breathstream, and stuttering. They include the following:

- Respiratory, breathstream anomalies do not *cause* dysfluencies in the general population of stutterers.
- Many stutterers, particularly as they mature, develop and display disturbed respiration and breathstream patterns when they stutter.
- A few stutterers, even as children, display disturbed vegetative (non-speech) breathing patterns.
- Correction or amelioration of disturbed breathstream control may provide a vehicle for other control measures, or it may embody a control measure itself.

In reaching these opinions, information about what behaviors may be observed in stutterers, usually during stuttering moments, has been compiled. These observations, in part, duplicate those made in chapter 1.

- erratic, inconsistent breathing patterns
- frequent occurrence of apnea (temporary failure to maintain breathing, after a normal exhalation)

- apneusis (noncontinuation of the respiratory cycle following inspiration)
- rapid, or frequent, inhalations that are too shallow
- clavicular or upper chest breathing (possibly related to the above)
- slow, prolonged inhalation (hyperpnea) that results in more air than is needed and may contribute to thoracic fixation
- reverse breathing
- opposition breathing
- extended exhalation before any speech attempt occurs
- speech on inhalation
- spasmodic, brief inhalations interrupting the exhalation phase of the cycle
- hard glottal attacks
- interruptions in speech because of glottal stops
- excessive release of air for phonation
- actual spasms of laryngeal muscles (laryngospasms)

Any breathing behavior can be used as a stuttering avoidance or release device. It is often assumed that these behaviors will disappear if the stuttering spasms are eliminated or at least minimized. In that process, many management strategies use a breathstream orientation. Occasionally, and regrettably, it is the entire program. Typically, breathstream management is used as a part of some combination of other techniques such as relaxation, slowed rate, Easy Onset, and Light Consonant Contact. According to Miller (1982), how much help simple airflow can provide apparently ranges from none all the way to total reduction of dysfluencies and effective naturalization of the accompanying speech.

Management of the Breathstream

Early in approaches to stuttering management, the breathstream was singled out as a major focus. In the early decades of this century, many regimens for stuttering included breathing exercises to increase respiratory vital capacity, to reduce or increase depth of inhalation and/or exhalation, and to originate breaths from various areas of the body, including the diaphragm. Today there are many breathstream programs. Some are well considered and thoughtful. Some, such as passive airflow (Schwartz, 1976) and regulated breathing (Azrin & Nunn, 1974), were regarded favorably at first, but did not hold up as well on replication and continued use.

Breathstream explorations include the Hollins program (Webster, 1980) and the Perfectly Mastered Breathing program (Tonev, 1994). Tonev stated that clients are taught easy inhalation and relaxation of the diaphragm and rectus abdominis muscles. Then they use a gradual rise of the diaphragm to support outflow of air and the release of speech sounds.

The literature on airflow and respiration is encyclopedic. After I present a few representations from within the last 20 years, I will focus on management suggestions.

Breathstream in Progress

Gronhovd (1977) developed a respiratory therapy called BRAT (Breathing, Rate, Airflow, Tension). The client assumes a supine position and is trained in deep muscle relaxation. This effect culminates in sigh productions followed by varied sighs. The client then moves to counting aloud, starting with one digit at a time and moving to four successive digits, while practicing airflow control, slowed rate, and Easy Onset, among others. Progressive steps take the client to connected speech, prosody, and naturalizing of speech.

Overstake (1979) has a longer and more complex application of breathstream control work. The client starts with a complete Jacobson-style deep muscle relaxation program (may take 3 to 6 months on a twice-a-week schedule). Then the client moves to block breathing where each segment of a respiratory cycle is the same. Timing is established from the client's relaxed cardiac rhythm. Then the block breathing is regulated so that the durations of inhalation-hold-exhalation-hold are identical, timed by those cardiac rhythm beats. Stability of the relaxed block breathing cycles may take months to establish. From that point, known as stabilization, the clinician begins to build speech production, starting with isolated vowels and moving slowly toward speech. Therapy usually finalizes with rate control, duration timing work, and prosody improvement.

Wolpe (1986) speaks favorably of the potential implications of Schwartz's work (1976). However, he noted (as have many) a lack of follow-up studies to verify, validate, and extend these approaches. Nevertheless, in evaluated regulated breathing, Waterloo and Gotestam (1988) measured an 8-month follow-up of dismissed clients. The regulated breathing treatment group's measures were compared with their own pretherapy measures and to a control group. Stuttering, in both comparisons, remained significantly lower in the later measures.

Wells (1987) suggested minimizing the upper chest and shoulder girdle area during respiration. The client generates repeated respiratory cycles, each one carrying a voiceless consonant, until the respiratory-phonatory-articulation (r-p-a) coordination is smooth and automatic. Then various vowels and voiced consonants are practiced, until these also show a smooth r-p-a coordination of relaxed, breathy releases. The client practices in various postures to vary the postural stress on the speech production mechanism. Finally, the client moves to words, to sentences, and then to conversation.

There are a number of instrumentation-based respiration management programs, such as the Computer-Assisted Fluency Establishment Trainer (CAFET) system (Goebel, Hillis, & Meyer, 1987). Some utilize pneumographs and strain gauges. Some, like the CAFET, are accepted, but I do not want to assume that the clinician has access to special instruments or can afford software programs. Although I have elsewhere pushed DAF, metronome, and other special-need programs, it is possible to achieve the same effects without the special instruments in each case.

Dembrowski and Watson (1991) evaluated visual biofeedback therapy with a single fluency client, finding that irregular respiratory events were reduced and phonation stability was increased. Bloodstein (1995) summarized at least 12 management studies on airflow or regulated breathing, and the results ranged from fair, to excellent, to very disappointing. Curlee and Siegel (1997) summarized, in tabular form, the approach called "tailored treatment." They suggested that breathstream management may be particularly appropriate when the client uses quick, shallow inhalations, or talks too long on one exhalation. To this, I would add the following:

- speech attempt on inhalation
- excessive exhalation before utterance initiation
- obvious fixation of the shoulder girdle (neck, clavicle, scapula, upper chest)
- visibly excess tension of the neck strap muscles during phonation (mainly the sternocleidomastoids and the scalene group)
- evidence of opposition or reversed breathing (see chapter 1)

The tailored treatment list includes some spasm behaviors often involved in breathstream problems: short, tense, silent spasms; excessive prolongations; many vocalized pauses; and so on. Respiration basically is an inhalation/exhalation and capacity process; breathstream management is modifying the force, duration, timing, and variation of air, with most attention paid to the expiration aspect. Probably, as in most techniques, factors of greatest significance are the projection and credibility of the clinician and the belief and motivation of the client. With these conditions met, breathstream therapy can produce excellent results; without their satisfaction, therapy fails.

Approaches to Respiration and Breathstream Management

Orientation

Management applications can be divided into vegetative breathing and speech breathing (or breathstream management). The first category assumes that, under all conditions of breathing for life, the client exhibits incorrect and/or inadequate breathing patterns. Thus speech breathing also is affected to varying degrees. On the other hand, behavioral anomalies in the respiration and breathstream aspects during speech do not automatically imply trouble in the vegetative patterns or even in the patterns that occur during fluent, nonstuttering speech. However, the idea that stutterers may have particular and subtle deviations in breathstream patterns during nonstuttered speech is gaining acceptance.

Vegetative Breathing

Disturbances in vegetative breathing usually should be corrected, or at least improved, if they are contributing to speech breathstream functions. More serious vegetative respiration problems should be referred to pulmonary and respiratory specialists. Correction of vegetative patterns is affected by age, and relapse to old breathing patterns is probable and fast in clients, especially those beyond the elementary years.

The first consideration in disturbances of vegetative breathing is determining whether the client needs a full examination and evaluation by a pulmonary specialist. There are no absolutes short of obvious cyanosis, a history of major allergies and respiration problems, and an inability to exhale steadily for longer than 5 seconds or to maintain a quiet, steady "ah" for about 10 to 15 seconds (see chapter 1). If no referral is made, it is assumed that the client's vegetative problem involves a need to inspire or expire more air in each respiratory cycle (i.e., increase the air supply).

With adequate respiratory ability but improper breathing behaviors or postures, the target is to work with the client to increase the quantity and duration of respirations. The first step is to explain to the client and significant others how respiration occurs normally and define the client's particular problem. One frequently cited explanation for children is the garden hose analogy advanced by Conture (1990). Conture develops another analogy in which a balloon (lungs) is to be inflated and held by thumb and forefinger near the opening (vocal folds). Conture suggests having the child try to release air by squeezing on the balloon globe while pinching the neck shut, and by relaxing the fingers to show how a tight larynx blocks air. With a little practice, the child can work on slow, fast, and easy releases of air. For older persons, textbook or commercial illustrations and clinician demonstrations can be used. At any age, the clinician should never assume the client really understands the dynamics and components of respiration.

A second phase for vegetative structure involves actual breathing exercises. The following procedure can be used as a whole, or in selected steps.

- *Step 1.* Have client lie supine, clothing loose and comfortable. Instruct client to place both hands on abdomen, thumbs just touching lower edge of connected rib cage (the ribs that attach to the sternum costal cartilage). Give client the following instructions:

  When I say in, I want you to inhale. Keep your stomach relaxed, and feel your chest rise. Hold it until I say out, then relax your chest and tense your stomach muscles. Ready? Okay. In-2-3-4, Out-2-3-4 (counting seconds), In-2-3-4, Out-2-3-4.

  Monitor by watching client's abdomen and thorax (or by lightly touching, if allowed). Repeat this cycle 8 to 10 times. Proceed to Step 2 if movements are correct. If there is jerking, discernible abdominal tension on inhalation, or thoracic fixation on exhalation, discuss the problems with the client, and work to balance and smooth the breathing. Model behavior if necessary (lie down while client rises and watches you imitate what he or she was doing incorrectly, and how it should be performed). Move to Step 1-a if, after explanations and demonstrations, there still is a problem.

- *Step 1-a.* Have client lie supine as before. Secure a mirror on wall or floor so that client can see his or her abdominal/thoracic area. Bring in two clean styrofoam or light paper cups (preferably 16 oz to 32 oz). Place one cup (empty) on the client's chest, just on or above the xiphoid (ensiform) process of the sternum. Place the second cup about 6 inches further down, on the abdominal midline. On inhalation, have client observe the thoracic cup rise, and the abdominal cup fall or stay steady. On exhalation, have client observe the reverse. Repeat the practice over several sessions until the client can stabilize her or his breathing pattern while supine.
- *Step 2.* Repeat Step 1 with the client standing, and with his or her back against the wall. Instruct client to place hands as in Step 1 (you may want client's eyes closed to focus on kinesthetics). Try several trial cycles. Call any problems to the client's attention and indicate change requirements. Practice until you think the new pattern is possible and understood. Practice supine and standing for several sessions and then move to home assignments. When Step 3 and Step 4 are learned, add them to Step 1 and Step 2. Have the client repeat the four steps 10 times (each), three to five times every day, 7 days a week. Provide a check-off calendar or record card.
- *Step 3.* Concentrate on timing of each element of the respiratory cycle, first in supine, then in erect, position. Time each stage to 3 to 4 seconds: inhale, hold, exhale, hold, and so on (a complete cycle will take 12 to 16 seconds). Count aloud, make a clock secondhand visible, use a metronome set at 60 beats per minute (bpm), or tape-record beats to play back to help client develop awareness, control, and initial equalization of respiration. At the rate of four to five cycles per minute, have the client perform for about 3 minutes, five to six times in a session. Add this exercise to the earlier home assignments, or replace them with it.
- *Step 4.* Have client lie supine. Move away from even-paced cycles of Step 3 toward more typical vegetative and speech breathing (shorter inhalation and longer exhalation).

  When I signal, I want you to take a fast breath in, like this . . . then shift immediately to slow, easy exhalation, like this. See how much longer it takes for me to breathe out? I'll do it again. Don't breathe in real deeply, and don't breathe out past a comfortable level. I'll show you again.

Shift the client to stand-against-the-wall practice after several minutes of supine practice. Repeat the process.

Then seat the client with her or his back against a straight chair. Impress good sitting posture on the client, explaining about thoracic compression. Repeat the breathing exercises above. Have the client repeat the exercise while deliberately assuming poor postures, and compare to good posture respiration. Give home assignment of 2-minute practices, each, of breathing in supine, erect, and seated posture. Try and schedule two to four times per day, every day.

- *Step 5.* Have the client practice a "happy sigh," while seated. Tell the client:

  Imagine you have just finished eating a fabulous dessert, and now you push your chair back from the table. Smile, take in a deep breath, and let it out as a loud sigh.

  Use this step at any time to remind the client of his or her respiratory status. At home, do this 25 to 30 times a day, preferably 5 to 10 times before lunch, another set before the evening meal, and the last set before bedtime.

Years ago, as an undergraduate clinician, I had to develop a whole list of blowing exercises using odds and ends of equipment and supplies. Later, for years, I was informed that blowing exercises were futile (and they often were). However, in recent years there have been efforts to retrieve the infant from the expelled bathwater, so a few suggestions are offered in Step 6. These suggestions are as much to focus attention on air stream as they are to increase or have any other effect on volume, rate, duration, and direction of the air. There also are excellent, expensive pieces of equipment available to help achieve these ends.

- *Step 6.* Watch for hyperventilation. Try all the following, and other activities like them, in advance to determine when light-headedness occurs.
  - Blow on plastic pinwheels.
  - With air stream, hold a torn piece of tissue against the wall.
  - Tie a cotton puff on a string and try to blow it "straight" for as long as possible.

- Blow out candles at various distances (if fire safe).
- Blow a table tennis ball back and forth on a table top (two or more persons).
- Construct a light cardboard ramp about 12 inches long and 3 to 4 inches wide, rising from table top to about 3 or 4 inches high at one end. Glue a coping or edge along each length side (about ⅛-inch high) to keep ball on ramp. Blow ball steadily (not one big puff) up the ramp.
- Blow party ticklers and other toys.
- Blow bubble pipes and circles.
- Play a wind instrument.

   Mix these activities with others for in-clinic use and home assignments. Score and record time of duration, distance, accuracy, and other measures. Use some as earned rewards for good performance in more prosaic exercises.

The foregoing exercises are intended to deal with basic respiratory inadequacies identified earlier. Very often such inadequacies are sufficiently minimal (and firmly embedded in lower brainstem programs for respiration) that basic correction is neither needed nor profitable. Used briefly, they can be used in correlation with breathstream management for speech, something that is usually more responsive to change efforts.

Speech Breathstream

   As noted in the previous exercise, these activities can be used as initial steps to speech breathstream management. Upper chest (clavicular) breathing, speaking too long on exhalation, exhaling significantly prior to speech, and so on can be either corrected or shaped and assimilated into a breathstream program. Actually, beyond those basics, I will recommend only one preliminary step.

- *Step 1.* Confirm the presence or absence of breathstream inadequacies during fluent speech. Move to the next management step if there are none (or none obvious). Determine whether "all" breathstream anomalies occur at or immediately around stuttering behaviors. Resolve through fluency replacement or symptom modification techniques. Use fluency management techniques if the breathstream anomalies are obvious during some aspects of fluent speech (however defined). (This is stated because most fluency techniques start with a 100% application, where symptom modification procedures target the areas immediately around specific words or speech attempts. Fluency techniques, or specific applications, usually will correct problems, or will highlight them for specific attention.)

- *Step 2.* Use procedures from various parts of this book, depending on what aspects of the breathstream you wish to modify or shape. In the following list of activities or procedures, a chapter source is suggested for each category.

> **Relaxation**—requires regularization and control of a relaxed, easy breathing pattern.
>
> **Slowed rate**—from DAF or other sources; as rate goes up or down, frequency and pattern of breathing will change.
>
> **Easy Onset**—classical accompaniment to breathstream change, and vice versa, involving controlled inhalation, immediate exhalation, relaxed and prolonged release; very useful with hard glottal attacks.
>
> **Continuous phonation and blending**—good for clavicular patterns, interrupted patterns, glottal attacks, and hard glottal stops.
>
> **Rhythm**—useful extension; assign a desired number of metronome beats to inhalations, exhalations, pauses.

All of the foregoing, plus other techniques, typically address breathstream as part of the overall management program sequence. In so doing, breathstream can take precedence over fluency or symptom management, an emphasis that I feel is of questionable value over the long run.

CHEWING THERAPY

Breath and voice chewing therapy for stuttering is associated with Froeschels (1952) and with other clinicians such as Kastein (1974). It has been applied to a wide range of speech disorders, including dysarthria, vocal paralysis, and dysphagia. The technique is based on the premise that speech is a secondary, or overlaid, function on the primary biological functions of the articulators and vocal tract—valving the lungs, respiration, biting, chewing, and swallowing. Stutterers who suffer tonic or clonic spasms of the jaw, lips, tongue, and vocal folds are still usually able to chew and swallow without anomaly. Chewing therapy depends on securing continuous movement of the jaw, lips, and tongue (plus vocal folds) feedback resulting with strong tactile and kinesthetic stimuli. The emphasis is on a continuous series of connected movements rather than isolated contacts with preparatory sets intervening.

In stuttering therapy, chewing is used to secure a release of the breathstream, along with movement of the articulators, that prevents the stutterer from shutting off air in a laryngospasm or from wasteful exhalations prior to articulator effort. The chewing motions required of the client prevent anticipatory, distorted trigger postures or preparatory sets. Articulation is emphasized as a series of continuous movements, not a string of isolated postures. The stutterer is taught first to become aware of chewing motions and to attend to their tactile and kinesthetic sensory signals. From this awareness, he or she can move to deliberate combination of the breathstream release with articulator movement, so that she or he is, so to speak, "chewing air." The client then can add phonation to this chewed breathstream and, in calculated stages, progress to the production of speech.

The suggested procedures are not those of Froeschels or related clinicians. The original ideas came from Froeschels' work and Kastein's experiments with methodology. The actual sequence is my adaptation of a number of different sources. It is only one way to approach breath chewing, but it can be varied in many different forms. Purposes of application also can vary, including those listed below:

- Demonstrate initial fluency (usually a poor choice).
- Increase tactile and kinesthetic awareness.
- Change or retime respiratory release patterns.
- Relax phonatory/articulatory system and resynchronize movements.
- Demonstrate to the client that speech variation is possible.
- Help break down habituated respiratory, phonatory, and/or articulatory preparatory sets.

I believe the overall technique is used best when configured as part of an overall program, fluency, or symptom, and not as a total management program by itself.

- *Step 1.* Discuss with the client the idea that chewing and talking are basically the same thing. Note that closing the lips in biting and chewing is like bilabial closure for /p, b, m/; that jaw movement for

/f/ and /v/ and in moving from low-back vowels to high-front vowels also are like biting and chewing motions. Compare lingual movements for sound formation to lingual shaping for a food bolus and oral transit motions in swallowing. Assign client to watch people chew, and make comparisons (privately) to speech movements.

- *Step 2.* Have the client initiate chewing while watching self in a mirror. Instruct to exaggerate the movements so the chewing is "savage," but not grotesque. Use chewing gum, crackers, and pieces of candy. Concentrate on sensory feeling of chewing and swallowing, particularly on tongue movements. Give a home assignment to practice exaggerated chewing (with or without props) in front of a mirror, three to five times a day. In each session, practice for 15 to 20 seconds, pause for 5 seconds, then repeat. Do this exercise 10 times.

In this stage, desensitization work may be necessary.

- *Step 3.* Direct client to take a breath and exhale slowly so the release is prolonged. When the idea is firm, tell the client to repeat the action, but to "chew" slowly as the breath is released. When that is acquired, bring the intensity of the chewing up to the "savage" level practiced in Step 2. Follow the time frame for Step 2, and give similar tasks home assignments.
- *Step 4.* Have the client add voice (some clients may already be making a sound when they chew). Remind client that phonation should be easy; let the "growl" come from the chewing effort. Model this activity for client after each client attempt. When client is capable, have him or her vary the pitch and loudness of phonation. If client is able, have him or her try to produce a range of notes or pitches. Add this activity to home assignment list.

These first four or five steps can be acquired in 1 session, or may take 10 sessions. The issue is the satisfaction of the client and the clinician. Home assignments can become longer and more complex as time passes. It is important not to get lost in the oddity or possible humor of "chewing"; the clinician must remember why it is being done and assess progress toward targets.

- *Step 5.* Ask the client to chew while she or he produces vowels, usually starting with low-back vowels. Chew one vowel per inhalation. At the end of the breath cycle, the client is to stop, inhale, release air, and then start chewing the next vowel. When the method is clear, accelerate the vowel (chew)—stop to add vowel (chew) stop—inhale, so that a second vowel is chewed on the same breath. Add a third vowel (chew) if there is adequate air. Have the client shift smoothly from one vowel to the next, on the same breath. The client's air supply will set the limit on the number of vowels chewed on one breath. As the vowels multiply, have the client vary his or her production pitch, inflection, and loudness.

- *Step 6.* Have the client produce syllables while chewing, starting with voiced continuant consonants (/m/, /n/, /v/, /z/, etc.). Add other consonants, using printed lists or verbal cues. Emphasize the movement through each consonant toward the vowel. Occasionally use CV (consonant-vowel) or VC (vowel-consonant) combinations that form simple words (e.g., as, is, am, in, zoo, me, my, knee). Provide client with a list of 10 groups of 10 words each for a home assignment. Have client read one of the 10-word units aloud five times a day, switching to another set every day.
- *Step 7.* Transition completely to words, mixing different consonant combinations. Monitor for those that need more work. Plan to increase each set by at least 50%. Use samples below if desired.

we	wet	weather	whether	westerly
you	yawn	younger	yourselves	yesterdays
be	but	butter	basketry	brontosaurus
awake	awaken	awakening	alphabetical	

How are you?	Fish for whales.
No way home.	Get up now.
Drop that rock.	I won't do that.
Where is my gray hat?	Look at that silly goat!
My speech sounds better now.	Chewing is pretty hard to do.

Add to the sample list. Assign Step 7 as homework. Use new material.

- *Step 8.* Continue the practice, but develop words and phrases that come from the client's personal life (e.g., client's name, address, telephone number, names of family members and friends, business phrases and terms, social label and phrases). Drop chewing to a level of mild exaggeration. If any word is stuttered on, the whole word or phrase is to be "canceled." Record and play back the productions; discuss the degree of naturalness and problem solve. Give home assignments that combine solo practice in previous steps. Have client use 10 of the words or phrases in this sequence each day with a mild chewing effort and report back on three things: how it sounded/felt, how client felt, and occurrence of stuttering on any of the efforts.

- *Step 9.* Switch from printed material to questions posed to the client. "Chew" questions and answers. When 20 or so efforts have been mostly acceptable, tell the client to listen for switches from regular speech to chewed speech and to follow the style used with his or her answers. Repeat the entire utterance in the chewing mode if any answer is stuttered. Give home assignment in which some other person asks questions (no chewing) and the client is to alternate chewing/ regular speech on the answers.

- *Step 10.* Start with about 3 or 4 minutes of chewing practice, developing a routine that starts with breath chewing, then voice chewing, then vowel chewing, and so on. Record and play back. Start over again if any segment is judged to be unsatisfactory. Adopt a 100% acceptable "warmup chewing" as a standard in subsequent sessions until no longer needed. Assign client the task of performing this routine at least once every day at home.

    Shift to monologue and conversational modes of interchange with the client when the preceding sequence is set and operable. As much as possible, talk about transfer, problem solving, further needs, and so forth. Have the client talk without speech chewing until the clinician signals (e.g., raises her or his hand) and then have client "chew" until the signal is discontinued. Automatically cancel any stuttering by repeating the phrase with chewing action strong enough to regain control. Continue this activity in consecutive sessions until the client has accumulated about 30 minutes of talking time (client time only) with 15 or fewer stuttering spasms, all canceled successfully.

- *Step 11.* Start in-clinic transfer work (e.g., telephone calls, invited persons in the room, role play). Set the same pass criterion, 60 instead of 30 minutes, as in the previous step.

- *Step 12.* Work through out-clinic transfer activities, as discussed in chapter 9.

Speech chewing eventuates sounding very much like a mixture of prolongation, continuous phonation, blending, and strong movement. Exactly which technique, or techniques, will predominate will depend on the individual client and the clinician. The whole chewing process is a some-what dramatic and exaggerated way to break down habituated preparatory set patterns and to facilitate a continuous coarticulation pattern of produc-tion. Where drama is not desired, a simple application of strong movement of the articulators may be feasible.

STRONG ARTICULATOR MOVEMENT

Strong articulator movement (SAM), or just strong movement, is not noted for widespread familiarity and use. I encountered it in 1953 as a graduate student with Van Riper. I do not know where he obtained it, whether it was part of his famous 5-year cycles of therapy, or what. In this book it follows chewing therapy easily and logically, and it can be used as a modified continuation of that method, or as a replacement. SAM is a combination of prolongation, blending, or continuous phonation, and increased tactile and kinesthetic feedback in a pattern of uninterrupted coarticulatory movements. The speaker "drags" articulators through their contacts so that there is a continuous movement rather than a series of contacts. The goal is fourfold:

1. Eliminate trigger points of stuttering spasms.
2. Modify or destroy the abnormal preparatory sets that are part of those triggers and create visible distortions of the mechanism.
3. Enhance the tactile and kinesthetic feedback for the purpose of reducing the habituated dependence on auditory feedback.
4. Enhance and increase the self-monitoring capacities of the speaker using tactile and kinesthetic feedback.

Because SAM exaggerates articulator tensions, some stutterers cannot withstand the tendency to allow certain articulatory postures to trigger stuttering spasms. However, for some clients, especially those who seem to be less influenced by preparatory sets, the SAM approach may be useful. I have found it particularly useful when the client's syndrome pattern is strongly repetitive, as opposed to prolongations and stoppages. SAM also can be useful late in therapy when certain sounds or triggers are harder to manage than others. Some clinicians have found it especially facilitating with clutterers.

- *Step 1.* Explain and model for the client the concept of producing sounds with a slowed, exaggerated movement. Start with continuants. Ensure movement is prolonged and continuous, with a physical "scraping" of the articulators. Note that voiceless sounds, because of the blending, acquire a vocalized quality.

Strong articulator movement can be used as a solo technique or after work on self-analysis, desensitization, monitoring, and relaxation. It can be used in other venues, as indicated earlier. It is particularly applicable as the voluntary disfluency to be used in the classic symptom modification procedures of cancellation, pullout, and preparatory set (see chapter 8).

UTTERANCE COMPLEXITY

Whether correcting w/r substitution (when phoneme /w/ is substituted for phoneme /r/ as in wabbit), building comprehension in a Wernicke aphasic, or developing swallowing coordination following laryngeal cancer surgery, progressive complexity is applied in speech and language pathology. The idea of progressive complexity in language utilization is centuries old. When I learned spasm cancellation in 1953, it started with single words, each word canceled in different fashion. From there, I built up to phrases, and so on. Situation complexity is similarly developed.

In behavior modification therapies, a late development—utterance complexity—has been expressed as either extended length of utterance (ELU; Costello, 1980) or gradual increase in the length and complexity of utterance (GILCU; Ryan, 1974). Although the persons cited did not invent these approaches, their names are particularly associated with the approach.

Length is just one way of increasing utterance complexity. The act of increasing length can be varied, so that two different methods of increasing length may, even with identical lengths, be at different levels or modes of complexity. The possible different forms of length and complexity are numerous. Some of the more obvious include:

- physical length—from number of phonemes, to syllables, to words, length of words, and so on. Usually, the greater the number of syllables and the number of words, the higher the stuttering frequency.

- internal length—the length and complexity of individual words within an utterance.

  > His name is Sam and he does not like cats or dogs when he meets them for the first time. (20 words; 20 syllables)
  > Considerable perseverance is significantly involved in cosmopolitanism. (7 words; 25 syllables)

- grammatical complexity—a concept best demonstrated by an example. "See Linda jump," is less grammatically complex than "That which may have been of concern without regard to that which I have observed before."
- vocabulary—"widespread" and "ecumenical," where one is often used, and the second rarely used (and probably incorrectly).
- phonemic complexity—the presence of combinations such as str-, st-, -ds, sph-, and so on.
- topic familiarity
- emotional level or content
- utterance environment
- specific persons involved

I will not present complete ELU or GILCU programs because the previous list of factors make a complete formulation too variable. Some rather simplistic samples are suggested, however. The individual clinician can add complexities and variations as needed.

- *Step 1.* Decide on the control technique (fluency or symptom type) to be employed. Borrow exercise steps from presentations on relaxation, Easy Onset, light consonant contact, Bounce, and so on. Use the abbreviated ideas in the following steps to expand, revise, and apply.
- *Step 2.* Read aloud the following words. Model any control technique being used in the reading. Have client repeat until production is acceptable.

see	zoo	vine	blue	leather
who	way	dog	street	fever
for	view	cat	bag	searching
she	chop	mop	clamp	million
so	the	get	bang	purple

Stop the client if a word is stuttered; model using the control technique, and have the client try again. If there is a renewed stutter, mark the word and move on. Add about 25 more words to the list above. Repeat this step if more than 5 of 50 words are stuttered. Model and practice until a 90% success rate is reached.

- *Step 3.* Repeat the word list from Step 2, but do not model each word. Tell the client:

    Read each word aloud. Use your ___ technique on each word if you wish, or not. However, if you stutter, stop and repeat that word twice using that technique.

    Problem solve if client stutters. Employ 90% fluent utterances as acceptance criterion. Use this exercise as a home assignment after client meets criterion.

- *Step 4.* Use the same procedure, but have client complete each column before moving to the next column. Add 10 more stimuli to each column (note increasing length of utterance in each column).

my pizza	Where is Ann?	She is with Ruth.
this way	Bill is here.	Go look for Ed.
her cat	Catch the cat.	Henry is my friend.
the bear	Shoot the deer.	Hunting is my sport.
get off	Few can go.	Barb came back home.
what car	I can drive.	Who has more fun?
look here	You must have!	Send me a box.
such people	Raise your hand.	Blue is this one.
give me	Drop the basket.	Raise your hands sir.
top dog	I'll take that.	Never come here again.

Run the first 20 two-word utterances, applying the same criterion of 90% fluency (36 of 40). Model each production, using the control technique on the first word only. If client stutters on the first word, repeat the effort as before. If the second word of the utterance is stuttered, treat it the same. If there are more than four stuttered words, repeat the entire list.

Run the 20 three-word utterances. Follow preceding instructions, except the 10% acceptability criterion would be six stutters or less.

Run the 20 four-word utterances. Do everything the same, except the 10% acceptability criterion would be eight stutters or less. As each segment meets the acceptance criterion, use as a home assignment.

- *Step 5.* Repeat all of Step 2, but do not model, unless necessary to repair client errors. When performance is satisfactory (90%), move this step to a home assignment role. Rearrange as desired.
- *Step 6.* Draw on the progressive steps of Easy Onset in chapter 5, or the progressive steps of other techniques in this book.

Additional applications of extended utterance can be developed according to the age and language sophistication of the individual client. One that I like to use, at all ages, is a recounting or telling structure, as described in Step 7.

- *Step 7.* Show the client a picture from a newspaper, magazine, or book (lean toward complex pictures, not sunsets over the ocean). Instruct the client:

  > Look at this picture. Keep looking. Now describe this picture to me, as if I have not seen it at all. Make your description last for at least 1 minute.

  Stop any stutters as soon as they occur, and problem solve (i.e., shorter phrases with more frequent breath, slower rate, Easy Onset, whatever fits). If there are more than two stuttered words in the 1-minute response, take the stimulus picture and ask the client a series of short-answer questions that have him or her talking for about 1 minute (cumulative). Problem solve if needed. Then, repeat the original request (same picture) for the client to structure a connected description. Have a total of 10 usable pictures (out of 15 to 20 available). Set final target as 20 one-minute monologues with no more than 2 stuttered words per minute (sw/m). Set a home assignment practice series. Record one and bring it in for evaluation and practice.
- *Step 8.* Use the same 10 pictures as before, but direct the client:

  > Tell me a story about this picture—what is happening? What led up to it? What will occur in the future? Talk for at least 1 minute.

  Do some coaching at first, as necessary. If the client is talkative, cut her or him off after about 2 minutes. Use same criterion as before, no more than 2 sw/m. Use same repairs (if breaking story down, just ask questions to elicit a bit of the story at a time). Try story again. Give home assignment as in Step 7.

- *Step 9.* Develop a combined, abbreviated version of the last four or five steps; that is, cut down on the number of items and duration lengths. Invite in, or visit, other people to listen to or participate in performance by the client. Use, for example, the following versions:
  - Step 3 revision: Visitor reads 20 words aloud for client to repeat.
  - Step 4 revision: Visitor reads five phrases aloud from each of the three lists, for client to repeat.
  - Step 5 revision: Client reads 15 phrases used from Step 4 but to several different persons, one person at a time.
  - Step 6 revision: Depending on what was selected here originally, apply with strangers present.
  - Step 7 revision: No revision at all. Just repeat with several different visitors.
  - Step 8 revision: No revision at all. Just repeat with several different visitors.

When feasible, the clinician should try to repeat segments of Steps 3 through 8 with a variety of persons, to a small group, to a class (it is assumed that most length-of-utterance clients will be younger), and so on. Home assignments can be carried out easily, involving family members when partners are needed.

There has been a tendency in the recent past to view GILCU-like approaches as complete therapy programs, without adequate client counseling, transfer work, or additional fluency support systems. The results often have been total relapse. Thus some clinicians today tend to shy away from such a simplistic linguistic orientation. However, as clinicians become too accustomed to the college-level vocabularies of their peers, it is important to remember that many clients, of all ages, might profit from paced development in a linguistic structure.

STUTTERING AND SINGING

It has been an article of faith that people do not stutter while singing. Indeed, Silverman (1996) states that if a stutterer does not become normally fluent during singing, then the person probably has a fluency disorder outside the category generally labeled as "stuttering." This is, of course, possible. However, several research studies in singing report significant decreases in stuttering, but not total abolition across the test groups. Stuart (1996), Colcord and Adams (1979), and Healy, Mallard, and Adams (1976) all reported stuttering reductions, not eliminations, during singing. Nevertheless, singing is one of the potent effectors of non-stuttered speech production.

Exactly why singing reduces stuttering is somewhat confused. Colcord and Adams (1979) reported increased vocal durations, as did Healy Mallard, and Adams (1976). Wingate (1976) suggested an increase in loudness as well as vocalizing of all sounds. Ham (1986) speculated that duration and loudness were significant, but also targeted melody, inflection, stress, rate, and other factors. Singing can be nursery rhymes, operatic arias, or monastery chants. It can be intensely rhythmic, or as smooth as silk. What people call singing can vary widely. I recently heard a tape of singing stutterers and I must say that none of them seemed able to emit vocal fold vibrations in other than aperiodic form.

Application: Clinician Preparation

I regard myself as modestly qualified to deal with singing. All members of my family were "musical." I studied piano and music theory, and I performed in vocal music in all types of venues. In my speech-language-pathologist (SLP) courses, there have been many students experienced and talented in music. There also were quite a few who were musically inexperienced, or downright inept. A key issue is whether the clinician can carry a tune in a bucket, or even *find* a tune in a bucket. The clinician does not have to be skillful in music, does not have to play an instrument, or have particular expertise in harmony, counterpoint, or other esoterics. It is best if the clinician can meet the subjective criteria suggested below for clients.

Application: Client Preparation

People vary in their awareness of, and ability to respond to, musical stimuli. Some will lack that ability to a marked degree. This fact might not obviate music as a distractor, as a novel mode of expression, or as an alternative rhythm (if the client can pick up on non–metronome-type rhythms). The first issue is auditory acuity. "Normal" hearing is not mandated. If the curve is better than 20 dB or so across the 500 to 800 Hz range (aided or unaided), then auditory reception is adequate. The following items are guidelines I have used. Six performance areas are assessed subjectively and scored, using a 5-point scale (5 = excellent, obvious musical ability; 4 = good, consistent, meets all my needs; 3 = skill present, variable, not impressive but adequate; 2 = present, poor, generally poor and/or inconsistent; 1 = absent). The performance areas I generally check are:

A. Client can sing a pitch range of about one octave. Note-by-note is best, but the seven- or eight-note range is what is important.
B. Client can listen to and identify notes. The client listens to a tape of paired notes (made or obtained by clinician). Second note is to vary (higher, lower) or be the same each time.
C. Client can imitatively produce pitch tones to match clinician (live) or any source on tape.
D. While producing a steady tone, client can vary loudness in response to clinician signals.
E. Client can recognizably produce or imitate a simple song such as a child's tune ("Mary Had a Little Lamb," etc.).

If either A or E are rated as 1, or even 2, then singing may not be a feasible approach. In general, an overall rating of 3 or better is desired.

The value of singing can involve increasing the amount of air available, or learning to better regulate the release of the airstream. Work may be aimed at rhythm and timing of speech. The coordination of breath, phonation, and articulation may be targeted. Singing can be used to help in the control and variation of rate, prolongation duration of (mainly) vowels, and the blending of continuous phonation from one sound to the next. Singing also can be used to introduce more (or show variations in) prosody, stress, and inflection. Music can be used in relaxation.

Singing and music applications in general tend to have their best chances with children, from about 3 years of age up to 8 to 10 years of age. At older ages, clients may reject singing unless they have a separate interest in and enthusiasm for it, outside of speech.

The recommended activities are not sequential, so the numbers do not imply that one must come before the next. The first group of activities is intended for young children. An indispensable aid is a set of children's tapes that have marches or nursery rhyme songs. The clinician must screen the music first, however. Some records, particularly from animated popular films, have scores the children can enjoy listening to, but are too complex melodically for singing at that age.

1. Marching—Have child march around the room to the accompaniment of a march tape (clinician marches too). Have child swing arms or nod head in time to the beat. If the room is suitably insulated, have child count cadence, beat on toy drums, click rhythm sticks, clang on triangles, and so forth. Coordinate movement and sound.

2. Rhythm—Use music with a strong beat, or live metronome or audiotapes of different rhythms. Have client (child, adolescent, or adult) tap, bang, and so forth in time to the beat (old computer mouse pads, or surplus carpet squares make handy sound mufflers). Provide models for the client to follow.

   In a game or a nongame format, ask questions and receive answers in varying rhythm patterns. Model utterances (e.g., number strings, sounds, unconnected words, or short sentences) for the client to repeat back in the same rhythm.

3. Singing—Use the huge inventory of children's records. Start with songs to promote relaxation, extend vowel duration, slow rate, and improve the timing and rhythm of utterances. Employ "sing along" breaks as a reward during more conventional management sessions. Use singing to support fluency. Consider the following example:

   > I am Joe;
   > She is Jane.
   > Here I run.
   > There she goes.
   > We climb a tree and pick a pear;
   > It falls down to the ground below.
   > I never saw the man down there.
   > Let's all run home!

Use these lyrics with the tune of "Three Blind Mice" or select any commercial song. First, have the client(s) read or repeat the lyrics aloud, without music. If there are any stutterings, comment interestedly but not critically. Suggest that going too fast, cutting words short, and so on might be causing the problem. Have the client repeat the lyrics as a song. Model or read lyrics line by line at first, repeating this activity several times before the client tries to sing the entire song as one unit. Note any differences and discuss.

Singing use with older children and adults typically will be restricted to four purposes:

1. reinforcement and motivation, showing that stuttering can be eliminated or reduced
2. practice in monitoring, emphasizing tactile and kinesthetic cues
3. practice in overtly controlling vocal output instead of letting unconscious habits run the speech system
4. experimentation with rate, rhythm, duration, stress, and so on

What one clinician identifies as "singing therapy," other clinicians might label as chanting, legato, intoning, mumbling, and so on. Several activity sequences follow that can be embellished by the creative clinician. Again, the numbering does not indicate a sequence to be followed.

1. Use an appropriate recording of vocal music for the client (avoid lyrics such as "Baby I love yuh, uh, oh, oh; Baby I need yuh, ooh, ooh" and other excursions into poetic heights). Have him or her read the lyrics to the song, no music or recording, as if it were everyday speech. Record. Play back. Listen one or more times and comment on anything that would "smooth" utterances and improve rhythm. Play the original recording; have client hum along with performer, keeping time. Play back again. Have client listen to and repeat (not sing) lyrics, keeping time and rhythm. Play back for client to sing along. Record client as she or he recites lyrics without any support. Play back and analyze for comparisons to first reading effort. Repeat this with other songs.
2. Develop or borrow a few bars of easy-to-follow music and record it, using your own voice and/or any musical instrument you can manage. Play the result several times to the client until he or she can approximately reproduce the tune. Have a list of 40 or 50 questions that can be answered in one brief sentence. Proceed in one of the following ways:
   • Ask/answer questions, using the musical refrain. Then repeat in nonmusical form.

- Ask/answer questions in plain speech. For any stutter, have client repeat the utterance musically, and then say again in plain speech.
- Using unison speech printed material, or other sources, perform the material together "in tune," then have the client perform solo in tune and then in plain speech.
3. Take published songs and familiarize the client with them. Have her or him listen to a line sung, and then try to duplicate it exactly in phrasing, duration, loudness, inflection, but *not* the song notes (a bit of intoning quality is acceptable). Emphasize the idea of variation of different aspects of speech production.

There have been therapies where stutterers were actually taught to sing their speech, and there is an amusing story about a fluency client who tried to call 911 and "sing for help" when his house was burglarized during the night. Only a few examples of singing therapy are offered here because there are so many variables of age, musical ability, facilities, and so on.

ROLE PLAY

Role play, which is a widely used technique, divides into two major categories. One form, psychodrama, is used in various forms of psychological exploration and counseling for neuroses and other problems. It also can be applied to analyze and assess the communication behaviors of individuals. The other role play, although linked to the first (however, some deny it), is less intense and aims to study, realize, and change superficial behaviors or to practice desired behaviors rather than to alter the basic personality adjustment of the individual. Keeping the two categories separate at all times is impossible. Sheehan (1970) wrote about stuttering and role therapy, but leaned toward a relationship to classical role playing, psychodrama therapy. He regarded stuttering as a false-role disorder, a role-specific conflict involving approach and avoidance (Culatta & Goldberg, 1995). That is, the speaker is trying to deny his or her role as a stutterer and avoid occurrence of the abnormality. Wall and Myers (1995) do not report any separate emphasis on role playing. In other words, whatever it is, role playing does not figure prominently in more recent therapy designs. This may be due to the increased reliance on canned or packaged programs of therapy or emphasis on data collection by accountability offices and authorities.

Role playing, as psychodrama, has been used extensively in psychotherapy for many years. As such, it is a complex and demanding procedure, beyond the training of most SLPs. However, playing a role is so inherent to every stuttering therapy that all SLPs are practicing it. When clinicians accept dysfluent persons and initiate changes in the way they speak, their interactions with their society are being affected. When clinicians alter avoidance patterns, teach self-analysis, and so forth, attitudes and adjustments outside of speech itself are being affected. Simply expecting a situation-avoiding, speech-avoiding person to speak differently, speak more frequently, approach situations and persons previously avoided, and to view self and anxieties and fears differently than before certainly involves profound shifts in role.

Role Play—Children

There are many different approaches to use with children. In children between the ages of 3 and 8 years, role play can serve very well as *play with a purpose*. Dolls, stuffed toys, and character dolls can be given pseudolife. Speech characteristics for such toys can be discussed, rehearsed:

> Big-Woof talks in a sorta growly voice and "woofs" a lot; Little Mouse is squeaky and whispery, and talks in real short sentences so the cat won't hear him and catch him.

A lot of ad lib speech is involved, because reality is not important and stories (at young ages) tend to be made up by fragments of action rather than by a steady script and scene development. The child has an opportunity to speak in different modes and to be different people. Fluency periods can be measured, fluency breaks counted, and other required data collections performed. The following ideas are suggested:

- Have client take a role that, at once or later, will be a favorable character, a winner.
- Ensure enactment durations are less than 5 minutes.
- Encourage repetitions, sometimes 8 or 10, of situations.
- Play a role, even if interlocutor, in solo therapy. Be the stage manager in group sessions.

- Do not permit stuttering. Depending on reaction of child, wait and repeat the whole scene with review and modeling of speech patterns, or (preferably) stop, back up, and repeat a part of the scene with some kind of repair strategy.
- In some situation repeats, experiment with changing roles, but not if child wants to stay with one character.
- Monitor to squelch (nicely) overexcited, unacceptable behaviors, or to reshape undesired story occurrences.

Hand puppets make excellent role-play representations, whether human, animal, or fantasy figures. They can develop unique personalities. One of my child clients transferred his stuttering to a hand puppet named Mort. The client scolded him, demonstrated "lazy speech" for him, and told his own mother that Mort "needed to practice some speech stuff at home." Fairy stories, comic routines, television shows, movies, poems, real occurrences—any and all constitute sources that can be utilized.

In children 3 to 6 years of age, role play can be the only management activity used to simultaneously reduce tension, promote relaxation, and practice fluent speech controls. Transfer and home practice usually are easy to arrange. All the child needs to do is use fluent speech repeatedly when it is easy and fun to do to receive favorable attention and reward in the clinic and at home. Performance targets are easy to establish and measure. Time out can be used and probably has more strength when the child is briefly shut out of enjoyable role play, than when he or she is simply isolated from more mundane forms of activity.

Role Play—Older Children and Adults

Role play can be an adjunct to many therapy forms, or it can be a total therapy program. It offers opportunities to reenact past situations, rehearse future situations, gain a better understanding of feelings and situation dynamics, gain a better understanding of others' feelings, and desensitize negative emotions. Organization of role play is widely varied. I recommend Fiedler and Standop's (1983) summary of important factors. Basic suggestions are as follows:

- It helps to conduct role play in a room other than the usual therapy setting. If not feasible, the clinician should rearrange the furniture to create obvious differences to help clients make a mental shift.

- Props are not absolutely necessary, except where they can make a direct contribution. However, the more props that are available, the more real the situation.
- Time frames or structural limits should be set in advance. How long will a scene last? What is the termination point? What is the desired outcome?
- The clinician should insist that participants stay in character throughout an entire sequence, unless the activity is stopped. If others are involved, they should stay in character unless the scene is terminated.
- After each scene presentation, the action should be suspended temporarily to discuss the appropriate elements relative to the original intent of the role. These elements may include, but are not limited to:
  - Stuttering behaviors during scene
  - Monitoring and control efforts planned and attempted
  - Understanding of the role and client's feelings about it
  - Perceptions of others' role efforts
- It often is profitable to follow a successful presentation with a role reversal (two persons only) or a role trade (several clients) so that a scene can be repeated a number of times. Role switches do not require that the "new" person imitate the way the prior person projected a particular role.
- A scene may be repeated a number of times, working for progressive variations. For example, a role play of a job interview could first focus on a stutterer as an applicant. Next, it could involve an impatient, overbearing interviewer. Then the stutterer and interviewer could switch roles. Last, the interviewer could be a stutterer and the applicant could be an insolent individual. The variations are endless.
- Audio and video (much preferred) recordings are highly desirable, especially where client is reenacting real experiences, or rehearsing for anticipated real situations.
- A strong rapport between client and clinician is very important and, in group situations, within-group bonding is a prerequisite to people being themselves.

Initially, role enactment situations (notice the switch from role "play") should be brief, allow the stutterer to play himself or herself, and involve situations where there is not a high level of role stress. If the client exhibits some stress, it often helps to repeat the scene and switch roles. For instance, if the scene was one in which the boss gave the client a "hard time," it might be wise to do role reversal and let the stutterer hand out grief.

After acclimation to role enactment, the client can be placed in a variety of roles. It is important to evaluate his or her comfort levels with the roles and stress levels and discuss any differences. When it seems appropriate, the client sould recall actual events for reenactment. Before undertaking this activity, the clinician should take time to describe and dissect the scene (i.e., who said what, sequences, mannerisms, and so on). After rehearsing the scene several times, the final product is performed and repeated while being recorded. Evaluation focuses on what needs to be added, shaped, or eliminated. Such situations usually profit from further repetitions with role switching, especially if a group production.

Role enactments can be about therapy, with the client taking the clinician's role. The stutterer's actual history can be used as well as his or her present situation. Role activity can be used to rehearse home assignments. They are especially useful in preparing for solo transfer activities, practicing repairs, and so on. Sometimes, worries or adverse feelings about therapy can be released through role enactment. A "role pool" can be established where the client is encouraged to find things in her or his real life that could profit from role analysis and practice. This pool can be drawn upon periodically and combined with other management target activities. A series of suggestions to stimulate additional possibilities follows.

- Stutterer is to apply for a job. Interviewer asks tough questions but stays away from speech. Later on, speech is added.
- Stutterer is to play self and clinician plays a door-to-door salesperson. Later on the role can be reversed.
- Client and clinician talk, from different rooms, using telephones. The situation can involve ordering a pizza to selling a reluctant person a product he or she does not need. Situations should increase in difficulty.
- Stutterer is to play self, while another person plays an employer interviewing workers for a possible promotion. Applicant's speech is then discussed, being realistic but kind.
- The client is to describe people he or she has known. In the process, the clinician tries to identify those with diverse responses to stuttering—

unbiased, cruel, sickeningly sweet, and so on. The stutterer is to act the roles of these individuals while the clinician takes the client's role. Later on, the roles are reversed.

- The client is to recall and describe past unpleasant experiences. The clinician isolates six and amasses detailed information. After a discussion of what went wrong, how client would have liked to have reacted, and what a favorable outcome might have been, the scene is re-created. First, the scene re-creates what actually happened. Then the scene explores what might have happened.
- With the client, the clinician develops a list of 10 to 20 situations met frequently by the client. Several are dissected, as before. Each is quickly (2 or 3 minutes) enacted to develop any additional details. Then several situations are repeated three times, employing the following variations:
  - Mild fluency problem; nice other person
  - Moderate fluency problem; startled, upset other person
  - Severe fluency problem; hostile, negative other person

  Later on, the roles are reversed and the three scenarios are reenacted.
- The client is to identify upcoming situations, either because they happen frequently or they are scheduled to happen, where the client would like to rehearse behaviors and controls that could make the situations effective and satisfactory.
- Role reenactment can be used to rehearse them and problem solve formal transfer assignments in advance.

Such role activity is not carefully structured psychodrama. It is not intended to be advanced as a method of psychoanalysis or psychotherapy, in the classical sense of the latter word. The focus is on attitudes, feelings, and behaviors specific to communication situations. The client is given opportunities to reexperience and restructure communication activities under controlled situations, while practicing management techniques developed and applied by the clinician. Role activity offers opportunities to experiment with behavioral changes before transferring them.

Stutterers and clinicians vary in their responses to role therapy. Many factors contribute to its success and failure. Although role therapy does not always work, when it works, it works very well.

SUMMARY

This chapter presented a conglomerate of related, distantly related, and unrelated management approaches. In moving between and among breathstream management, TO, role play, and other techniques, there is little commonality. Nevertheless, one of these methods may be "just the thing" for a particular stutterer. Although these techniques can work in isolation, it is more likely that they will be part of an overall management package that is designed to fit the unique characteristics of a particular client.

REFERENCES

Azrin, N.H., & Nunn, R.G. (1974). A rapid method of eliminating stuttering by a regulated breathing approach. *Behavioral Research and Therapy, 12,* 279–286.

Bloodstein, O. (1995). *A handbook on stuttering.* San Diego, CA: Singular Publishing Group.

Colcord, R.D., & Adams, M.R. (1979). Voicing duration and vocal SPL changes associated with stuttering reduction during singing. *Journal of Speech and Hearing Research, 22,* 468–479.

Conture, E.G. (1990). *Stuttering* (2nd ed.). Englewood Cliffs, NJ: Prentice Hall.

Costello, J.M. (1980). Operant conditioning and the treatment of stuttering. In W.H. Perkins (Ed.), *Strategies in stuttering therapy,* J.L. Northern (Ed. In Chief), *Seminars In Speech, Language and Hearing.* New York: Thieme-Stratton.

Culatta, R.E., & Goldberg, S.A. (1995). *Stuttering therapy, an integrated approach to theory and practice.* Boston: Allyn & Bacon.

Curlee, R.F., & Siegel, G.M. (1997). *Nature and treatment of stuttering, new directions* (2nd ed.). Boston: Allyn & Bacon.

Dembrowski, J., & Watson, B. (1991). An instrumental method for assessment and remediation of stuttering: A single-subject case study. *Journal of Fluency Disorders, 16,* 241–244.

Fiedler, P.A., & Standop, R. (1983). *Stuttering, integrating theory and practice* (S.R. Silverman, Trans.). Rockville, MD: Aspen Publishers.

Flanagan, B. (1986). Operant stuttering update. In G.H. Shames & H. Rubin (Eds.), *Stuttering then and now.* Columbus, OH: Charles E. Merrill.

Froeschels, E. (1952). Chewing methods in therapy. *Archives of Otolaryngology, 56,* 427–434.

Goebel, M., Hillis, J., & Meyer, R. (1987, November). The relationship between speech fluency and certain patterns of speech flow. Paper presented at the annual convention of the American Speech-Language-Hearing Association, Washington, DC.

Gronhovd, K.D. (1977). A comparison of the fluent and reading rates of stutterers and nonstutterers. *Journal of Fluency Disorders, 2,* 247–252.

Ham, R.E. (1986). *Techniques of stuttering therapy.* Englewood Cliffs, NJ: Prentice Hall.

Healey, C., Mallard, A.B., & Adams, M.R. (1976). Factors contributing to the reduction of stuttering during singing. *Journal of Speech and Hearing Research, 19,* 475–480.

James, J.E. (1983). Parameters of the influence of self-initiated time-out from speaking on stuttering. *Journal of Communication Disorders, 16,* 123–132.

James, J., Ricciardelli, L., Rogers, P., & Hunter, C. (1989). A preliminary analysis of the ameliorative effects of time-out from speaking on stuttering, *Journal of Speech and Hearing Research, 32,* 604–610.

Kastein, S. (1974). The chewing method of treatment of stuttering. *Journal of Communication Disorders, 12,* 195–198.

Martin, R., & Haroldson, S.K. (1979). Effects of five experimental treatments on stuttering. *Journal of Speech and Hearing Research, 22,* 132–146.

Miller, S. (1982). Airflow therapy programs: Facts and/or fancy. *Journal of Fluency Disorders, 7,* 187–202.

Onslow, M., Packman, A., Stocker, S., Van Doorn, J., & Siegel, G. (1997). Control of children's stuttering with response-contingent Time-Out: Behavioral, perceptual, and acoustic data. *Journal of Speech, Language and Hearing Research, 40,* 121–133.

Overstake, C.P. (1979). *Stuttering: A new look at an old problem based on neurophysio-physiological aspects.* Springfield, IL: Charles C Thomas.

Perkins, W.H., Rudas, J., Johnson, L., & Bell, J. (1976). Discoordination of phonation with articulation and respiration. *Journal of Speech and Hearing Disorders, 19,* 509–522.

Ryan, B.P. (1974). *Programmed therapy for stuttering in children and adults.* Springfield, IL: Charles C Thomas.

Schwartz, M.F. (1976). *Stuttering solved.* New York: McGraw-Hill.

Shames, G.H. (1975). Operant conditioning and stuttering. In J. Eisenson (Ed.), *Stuttering, a second symposium.* New York: Harper & Row.

Sheehan, J.G. (1970). *Stuttering: Research and therapy.* New York: Harper & Row.

Siegel, G.M., & Martin, R.R. (1968). The effects of verbal stimuli on disfluencies during spontaneous speech. *Journal of Speech and Hearing Research, 11,* 358–364.

Silverman, F.H. (1996). *Stuttering and other fluency disorders.* Boston: Allyn & Bacon.

Skinner, B.F. (1953). *Science and human behavior.* New York: Macmillan.

Stuart, A. (1996). Effect of instructions to sing on stuttering frequency at normal and fast rates. *Perceptual and Motor Skills, 83,* 511–522.

Tonev, P. (1994). Speech control, correction, and overcoming stuttering: A solution by Perfectly Mastered Breathing (PMB). *Journal of Fluency Disorders, 19,* 216. Abstract.

Wall, M.J., & Myers, F.L. (1995). *Clinical management of childhood stuttering.* Austin, TX: Pro-Ed.

Waterloo, K.K., & Gotestam, K.C. (1988). The regulated-breathing method for stuttering: An experimental evaluation. *Journal of Behavior Therapy and Experimental Psychology, 19,* 11–19.

Webster, R.L. (1980). Evolution of a target-based behavioral therapy for stuttering. *Journal of Fluency Disorders, 5*, 303–320.

Wells, G.B. (1987). *Stuttering treatment, a comprehensive, clinical guide.* Englewood Cliffs, NJ: Prentice Hall.

Wingate, M.E. (1976). *Stuttering theory and treatment.* New York: Irvington Publishers.

Wolpe, J. (1986). Systematic desensitization based on relaxation. In G.H. Shames & H. Rubin (Eds.), *Stuttering then and now.* Columbus, OH: Charles C. Merrill.

CHAPTER 8

Selected Symptom Controls: Cancellation, Pullout, and Preparatory Set

- Overview
- History
- Cancellation
- Pullouts
- Preparatory Sets
- Summary

OVERVIEW

The title of this chapter reflects the fact that most recent management techniques advanced as fluency reinforcement procedures were (and still are) symptom control procedures. By the same token, classic symptom control methods often have been adapted for use in fluency reinforcement venues. Cancellation, pullouts, and preparatory sets are stamped with a classic trademark in symptom therapy. Their development and application is discussed historically in the next section. Today, generic equivalents of all three have been in use for years, under new labels. Where modern programs discuss "repair strategies," we often find cancellations. Similarly, old-fashioned pullouts are frequently found in "modulation strategies" and "shaping behaviors." Finally, much of fluency reinforcement consists of taking preparatory sets and using them 100% of the time, on all words, instead of on targeted stutter-probable words. The specific techniques in this chapter are presented as an interconnected unit because they were developed over time as a unit. These techniques are

Cancellation—repeat, immediately, a just-stuttered word, exhibiting some management technique.

Pullout—regain control during a moment of stuttering and complete the word, exhibiting some management technique.

Preparatory set—establish control prior to the onset of a stuttering spasm and utter the word, exhibiting some management technique.

HISTORY

Beginning in the 1950s, a number of views coalesced in the idea that all voluntary motor behaviors (and many automatic ones) were built on a series of neuromuscular preparatory sets. For example, to take a bite of food there are complex, interlocking "programs" to set the height and angle of one's arm-wrist-hand, the level and angle of the fork, the tilt of one's head, the direction and focus of one's eyes, the degree of oral opening, and so on. If one's arm is too high, one's hand trembles, the head tilts too far, or the mouth is not opened at the right time to the right degree, there will be a food mess. The same was thought to be true of motor speech function (Ham, 1986). Stutterers, through anticipation, tension, apprehension, and avoidance, were thought to develop abnormal preparatory sets. Thus the therapy target was to modify the abnormal preparatory set back toward normal. Unfortunately, getting control of the preparatory set (or avoiding it) was what most stutterers were doing in the first place, so the proper use of preparatory sets around stuttering spasms was a very low-incidence phenomenon. Therefore, clinicians developed the concept of pullouts to back up failed or incomplete preparatory sets. A good pullout rescues a failed preparatory set. Unfortunately, some stutterers missed doing a pullout, did it ineffectively, or failed altogether, especially with very short spasms or when under tense, anxious conditions. Thus cancellation was seen as a last-ditch stand to retrieve lost adequacy and to exhibit control. Once all three concepts were developed, the acquisition steps were reversed so that cancellation came first, pullout followed, and preparatory sets came last.

This sequence is described by Culatta and Goldberg (1995) and Van Riper (1958, 1973). Van Riper generally is credited with the design plan for all three techniques, in terms of their final forms and their use in therapy. They are not immutable, and Van Riper constantly adjusted them and varied their applications. Actually he did not like the three labels and tried to use the terms pre-block, in-block, and post-block correction (Stuttering Foundation, 1993). Those terms are not generally used today.

The three techniques are used widely, as a triad, as a dyad, and singly. They appear in a number of fluency programs, as well as in symptom modification sequences. I lay out each technique as if it were going to be used as part of a triad, although it does not have to be. Each technique can be varied as desired, and the descriptions here may differ from other versions.

CANCELLATION

Peters and Guitar (1991) provide one of the better current summaries of cancellation. Moreover, they include cancellation in their program integrating FEB (Fluency Enhancing Behaviors) and MMS (Modifying the Moments of Stuttering). In both sections of their text, cancellation is presented very much as it was developed originally.

In 1993, Gregory and Hill recommended using cancellation with school-age children with a deeply entrenched fluency problem. However, they suggested its use after stuttering spasms that are persistent (do not yield to other controls). Prins (1993) did not discuss cancellation directly, but did seem to approach its principles in several activities. Cancellation is obviously a viable technique today.

Orientation to Cancellation

The concept of cancellation as a management procedure has had its share of controversy and (mis)interpretations. One of the interpretation problems may be that some people use cancellation as a free-standing technique, as a specialized problem solver, as a linkage with other procedures, or as part of a development sequence. My coverage involves the usage, but it does not deny the validity of the other approaches.

In the 1950s, cancellation was developed to be one part of a three-technique sequence, which was to be preceded by certain desired developments on the part of the client. Cancellation acquisition and use could be regarded as a therapy goal, in and of itself. However, it also was one step in a sequence. The word *cancellation* implies that some preexisting event or condition is to be revoked, neutralized, compensated for, or otherwise rendered nonapplicable.

Historical Background of Cancellation

Bluemel (1957) regarded the pause after a stuttering spasm, not repeating the stuttered word, as the canceling action. Wingate (1976), on the other hand, combined the cognitive function of the pause with the repetition of the word (in altered form). Yonovitz, Shepherd, and Garrett (1977) felt that the pause segment of a cancellation was the equivalent of a Time Out (TO) punishment. Van Riper (1973) suggested that cancellation attacked the self-reinforcing aspect of stuttering, wherein the anxiety reduction and physical relaxation immediately following a spasm was a reward for having stuttered.

Cancellation has been used in a variety of forms. Ryan (1971) used it to have clients "catch" stuttering and then to repeat the word with a prolongation on the first syllable. Shames and Egolf (1976) used cancellation progressively. The progression started with the client repeating the stuttered word, moving to a Bounce (three times) on the first syllable, and continuing the Bounce until the word could be released fluently. The mode used depended on the client's success level.

Before cancellation can be attempted, the stutterer needs to develop a high level of knowledge about her or his own stuttering pattern, in all its forms and variations. Gross aspects of spasm types, locations, eye contact, avoidances, and so on must be learned. Also, the subtler components of articulatory posture, laryngeal tension, tremor characteristics, and transitional cues need to be recognized. All of this information must be recovered and studied in a wide range of situations.

Tolerance for stuttering is an important aspect. The client must be willing to stutter. The client should have experience (during pseudostuttering work) with various ways of altering the stuttering spasm. Van Riper (1971) described the stutterer ready for cancellation as having more mental and physical ease when stuttering. Clients should understand their personal feelings about stuttering and about auditors. Functionally, the client should have a recent history of at least partial success in self-acceptance and control and should have started to realize that there is less need for the support and approval of the clinician or the peer therapy group (but it still can be a big help for awhile).

Before running through the development and acquisition steps, I want to restate the goal orientation I have for cancellation. I believe cancellation is a behavior that allows the stutterer to reject any prior loss of speech control and surrender to pressures to hurry speech; to reject the desire to avoid stuttering, and all struggles to release the stuttering spasm, along with any other inadequate behaviors such as loss of eye contact, poor auditory awareness, reduced or distorted social interaction; and to correct failures to evaluate all of the foregoing occurrences rationally. The word reproduction that follows must reflect all of the previous concerns. Management programs that have the client "just repeat the word" may be valid, but they are not "cancellation," as envisioned.

Procedures for Cancellation

Prerequisites

Drawing from the history of cancellation, it is not hard to establish and specify prerequisites. This process assumes the more traditional uses of cancellation. With those considerations, before starting active work on cancellation, a client should be:

- Aware (self-monitoring) of each stuttering, the moment it occurs, and be able to complete the spasm
- Able to stop immediately after a stuttering spasm, relaxing, not performing the following word
- Able to analyze, on the spot, each and every spasms in terms of
  - Spasm type/form and whether it changes at any point
  - Anatomical location(s) of spasm pressure points
  - Status of eye contact, auditor reactions, and so on
  - Spasm struggle behaviors, localized and overflow
  - Avoidance behaviors, specific and generalized
  - Overall tension level, speech mechanism and body
  - Feelings, if any, of anxiety, fear, anger, embarrassment, and so forth
- Able to decide exactly what has to be done to cancel the above, how much of it he or she is going to try and cancel, and what needs to be done to achieve the cancellation(s)

Table 8–1 summarizes suggested performance levels. Each percentage performance level has two percentage figures. In each pair, the first

Table 8–1 Suggested initial and final target percentages for preacquisition skills in learning cancellation

Abilities and Severities	In-Clinic Target	Out-Clinic Target
Awareness of spasm		
Mild level	75% (50%)	50% (25%)
Moderate level	90% (75%)	90% (50%)
Severe level	100% (99%)	100% (90%)
Immediate stop after spasms		
Mild level	50% (20%)	30% (10%)
Moderate level	80% (50%)	70% (30%)
Severe level	100% (70%)	90% (50%)
Accurate analyses of spasms		
Mild level	50% (20%)	30% (10%)
Moderate level	90% (50%)	70% (30%)
Scvere level	100% (70%)	80% (50%)

percentage is the final target for that setting or level. The second, parenthetical percentage, is suggested as a minimal performance level before real instatement work is reasonably attainable. The client can be a long way from 100% on some measures and still start on actual cancellations. As long as performance measures improve, work can continue. However, at some point, low measures (especially on moderate and severe spasm severities) will generate poor and error-prone performances on cancellation.

Typically, the clinician works simultaneously on both refining prerequisite skills and getting started on cancellation itself. Occasionally it may be necessary to suspend work on cancellations to focus attention temporarily on a specific subaspect of prerequisite skills.

Problems with Cancellation

Using cancellation therapy may not be easy. Bloodstein (1995) noted that cancellations were not just a mechanical rearrangement of the mechanical speech production system. They are not just a neuromotor sequence of events. Cancellations were a basic form of psychotherapy where the stutterer (often for the first time) confronts fluency, fights against anxiety and tension, and tries to restructure his or her approach to speech and (often) to social interaction. In the complex cancellation scene, certain immediate problems can occur.

- Some stutterers are inadequate, on a perceptual level, of being aware of, and being able to, evaluate spasms. Major focus on improving attending and evaluation skills may be required.
- Some stutterers are so emotionally traumatized by their own stuttering that major desensitization work is required before they can tolerate cancellation work.
- Some stutterers appear to have logical, cognitive problems with cancellation. They just cannot "see the point" of the method. This reaction often is a defense from fear or inadequacy, but still must be dealt with on its own terms.

Cancellation is irksome, temporally dragging, and anxiety producing. Basically, it requires the speaker to expand his or her time of fluency disruption by at least 100%. This requirement fails to generate client enthusiasm and, the milder the stutterer, the lower the enthusiasm tends to be. Sometimes it is necessary to postpone or drop cancellation with mild-to-moderate stutterers, bringing it in later as a problem solver for specific difficulties. However, it is possible to argue that the value of cancellations in therapy could be proportional to the client's resistance to it (i.e., the more the client resists cancellation, the more he or she may need it).

Another problem with cancellation is that the client often adapts to the therapy milieu and stops stuttering there. This creates an in-clinic learning problem, possibly before the client is ready to tolerate out-clinic pressures while trying to learn basic steps. In such cases, pseudostuttering is the best method for in-clinic practice, and both client and clinician should use it. The extra value is that it does not matter if a fake spasm turns real, because either can be canceled. Additional problem possibilities are discussed later.

Acquisition Sequence for Cancellation

The first two steps are drawn from the self-analysis section of this book (chapter 3). It might be assumed that every therapy program would go through that sequence, even pure fluency reinforcement programs. Unfortunately, it may not be the case. However, if self-analysis has been adequately addressed, acquisition can start with Step 3.

- *Step 1.* Have the client develop basic awareness of spasms through counting and classification. Focus on the following questions:

−Did you stutter?
−How many separate times?
−What word(s) did you stutter on?
Set in-clinic target percentages such as those shown below.

Severity Level	Awareness Percentage
Mild	50%
Moderate	85%
Severe	100%

Vary the percentages for individual clients, and set interim targets. Next, have the client identify the specific word(s) on which stuttering occurred. Do not let more than three or four spasms accumulate before stopping the client, and asking, "Which word did you stutter on?" Analyze spasm characteristics, based on skills developed in initial stages of therapy. Ask the client to start a behavior that will be critical in developing cancellation: STOP/GO (S/G) is sometimes used as a therapy technique alone. Have the client stutter, and then stop once the word is completed to test the client's desire to "run away" from dysfluencies and his or her overall level of self-control. Practice S/G, as indicated by client performance. Set target levels (e.g., 50%, 85%, and 100% for mild, moderate, and severe spasms, respectively). Set lower interim targets if client is better at awareness than she or he is at stopping. When the client can stop after a spasm, ask him or her to report on the
−word stuttered
−type(s) of spasm(s) (tonic, clonic, mixed, etc.)
−anatomical location of spasm (jaw, tongue, larynx, etc.)
−eye contact during spasm
−amount of speech mechanism struggle
−overflow struggle to rest of body
−breathing pattern, breath supply at end of spasm
−any and all avoidance behaviors

Have the client analyze each and every spasm; clinician provide suggestions at first. Use a discussion format, or a scoring form (see Exhibit 8–1), if desired. Add additional scorable items as desired. Use a 0/1 rating scale where 0 equals "missed it, or poor job" and 1 equals a rating of "fair to good."

Exhibit 8–1 Scoring form

Item	Rating
Word identification	
Spasm type	
Severity level	
Spasm location	
Eye contact	
Local struggle	
Overflow struggle	
Breathstream	
Avoidance(s)	

Set a target of all items multiplied by 1 for the overall target score, or the value of any one measure (such as awareness of eye contact) for a subitem target score. Or, set an acceptable score level, item by item.

In Step 1, awareness and analysis focused on the actual characteristics of a spasm and on the behaviors associated intimately with it. Step 2 logically follows Step 1, but some clinicians may want to put it "on hold" and merge it with Steps 3 and 4 where out-clinic transfer development can become involved.

- *Step 2.* Help the client move from self-only awareness to awareness of listeners and auditors. Consult the chapter 3 section on listener awareness, in particular the Auditor Evaluation List. Use the list with rating scale elements, or simply as discussion points for reaching "adequacy."

Step 2 above is used in cancellation more as a measure of client self-control and evaluation ability than as an intrinsic part of cancellations. However, it is an important capacity and should be developed.

- *Step 3.* Never embark on production of cancellations unless the client can produce the following:
  - Pseudostuttering to imitate own spasms
  - Pseudostuttering to imitate other patterns
  - One (or more) controlled disfluencies, such as Bounce, Easy Onset, prolongation, Light Contact, strong movement, and so forth

  Review disfluencies as necessary.

Some clinicians will, out of hand, reject pseudostuttering. That choice is regrettable because it is a wonderful tool in developing analysis skills, working on desensitization, exploring experimental alterations of dysfluency, and making the client feel more in control of his or her speech. Pseudostuttering aside, it is noted here with regret that some clinicians will utilize only one form of voluntary disfluency. This one-size-fits-all philosophy is even worse if it is used from client to client to client so that ultimately the ridiculous management approach is adopted that the client must fit the therapy.

- Have the client read aloud the word list in Exhibit 8–2, in word groups of 10, with 2 words out of each 10 produced with the
  - Imitation of client's own spasms
  - Fake of a different kind of spasm
  - Bounce, three to seven times
  - Easy Onset
  - Some other disfluency

  Give any directions desired concerning the form or severity of the pseudostuttering and the acceptance criteria.

  Have the client read aloud the first group of 10 words in Exhibit 8–2 using a fake of his or her real spasms on each word. Have the client read aloud the second group of 10 words using a different spasm fake. Instruct client to read the third group of 10 words using one of the selected disfluency modes. Repeat twice more using a different disfluency mode in each set. Rate each production in terms of acceptability; real

Exhibit 8–2 Disfluency review word list

Real Spasm Imitations		**Different Spasm Fakes**	
dahlia	daffodil	rosemary	fennel
petunia	begonia	basil	ginger
daylily	tomato	nutmeg	apple
cabbage	lettuce	watermelon	cantaloupe
carrot	asparagus	raspberry	grapefruit

Bounce		**Easy Onset, etc.**	
fiddle	violin	trousers	sweater
piano	guitar	stockings	overcoat
trumpet	sofa	underwear	airplane
bookcase	headboard	helicopter	propeller
countertop	bureau	hangar	bomber

Other Disfluency	
automobile	Pontiac
busfare	convertible
Hudson	Rambler
vehicle	catfish
dolphin	lobster

Mark each unacceptable production, and have the client repeat it until acceptable.

stuttering spasms are acceptable. Do not allow fakes that are tiny tokens and very mild.

- *Step 4.* Discuss the outcomes of the previous step and together decide what disfluency modes are most appropriate (feel "right") for the client. Review the elements of a good cancellation with the client, modeling and securing imitations from the client. When satisfied that techniques are understood, give the client five words (words from Exhibit 8–2 can be used) and instruct the client as follows:

On each word, fake a stuttering spasm; finish saying the word. After the word, pause, and analyze the spasm (out loud). Cancel the spasm by repeating the word with the disfluency form you think fits best. Summarize (aloud) what just occurred and evaluate the adequacy of the fake and the cancellation.

Evaluate the evaluation, using a recording of the effort. Add and correct as needed. Do not debate; encourage stutterer to develop her or his own evaluation standards. Repeat the entire process on four more sets of words, changing the cancellation forms.

When satisfied with the first five trials, provide the client with a list of 45 words that mix numbers of syllables and prominent phonemes. Have the client read the words aloud in groups of five:

photograph	bathtub	basket	wobble	camel
adventure	politician	ant	fare	shipping
colony	satellite	war	rascal	label
filibuster	merriment	cannibal	awful	elegant
into	vigilant	zero	drummer	flavor
thimble	tranquil	medicine	ringing	
hoop	carbon	grubby	ship	
three	moose	double	electric	
melody	nearby	owl	require	
whinny	gargle	inside	forever	

In each five-word group, instruct client to use only one of the three disfluency modes (no fake spasms). Record and play back the 15 productions of each disfluency mode for evaluation and discussion. Note any stuttered words, for future use. Assess the quality of each disfluency type; determine where improvements are needed in each type. Note any effects of phoneme types, combinations, stress points, and so on.

Drop one disfluency mode and add another, or combine more than one (e.g., prolongation plus Easy Onset).

- *Step 5.* Remember, frequent, extended practice is important. When Step 4 productions are stable and desired changes have been made, turn Step 4 into a home assignment. Revise as desired, design a recording and evaluation procedure, and arrange some degree of diary keeping for in-clinic reports. Have the client perform the following exercise every day:
  - Read three sets of five words aloud, using a different disfluency mode on each set.

– Read another three sets of five words aloud, faking stuttering on each word (no cancellation).
– Read a final three sets of five words aloud, using the disfluency mode most preferred.

Have the client report at each in-clinic session; keep this assignment running for 2 to 3 weeks on a daily basis.

- *Step 6.* Evaluate, ongoing, the Step 5 homework, and run through the Step 4 sequence one more time (this step may not be needed, but often is). Review the elements of a good cancellation before moving to Step 7.

- *Step 7.* Have the client fake a spasm, and then cancel it, on each of the 100 words. Negotiate with the client who does (part, or all of) the ratings.

depression	pneumonia	prosperous	breakfast	canal
relative	fatal	bucket	fiddler	basket
dinner	grimly	walnut	bubble	peanut
supper	stallion	asteroid	sample	overhead
paddle	television	radio	concerned	cigarette
cumbersome	faster	headlight	crabby	famous
measles	beaver	ladder	musket	elevate
slowly	captain	receive	surprising	canal
equivalent	forcibly	catastrophe	babble	rifle
lieutenant	decision	happiness	contempt	opulent
succession	taxable	tobacco	hesitate	quickly
circulate	minimal	captivate	estimate	alcohol
paddock	cancellation	exceptional	nominal	lumber
absolutely	accuracy	remember	compare	calculate
positively	tentatively	escapism	formulate	howitzer
timidly	cantankerous	intimidate	escapade	antler
felony	misdemeanor	politician	formulate	ambulance
whipcord	grinders	represent	adultery	graduate
leathery	advertise	homicide	miniature	gigantic
titanic	circumstance	division	corporation	formulate

- *Step 8.* Begin to establish a sense of the rhythm of communication, starting with shorter utterances. Key efforts to utterances likely to be used by the client. Use the three sets of five utterances below, with accompanying instructions, if desired. Rearrange as desired.

On each utterance, pseudostutter and cancel the underlined word, using Easy Onset cancellations:

Hello, my name is <u>George</u>.
<u>How</u> are you?
Give me a <u>Whopper</u>, please.
<u>Excuse</u> me!
<u>Good</u> morning.

On each utterance, pseudostutter and cancel the underlined word with a fake spasm, so that the cancellation fake is different from the first fake.

Can you <u>tell</u> me where?
Do you sell <u>mushrooms</u>?
<u>What</u> time is it?
The answer is <u>John Smith</u>
<u>No</u>, I don't.

On each utterance, pseudostutter and cancel the underlined word with three to five easy Bounces:

<u>Thank</u> you very much.
Is <u>Marjorie</u> at home?
<u>Biggie</u> fries and a shake, please.
<u>Who</u> are you?
<u>That's</u> not true!

Record and sample the playback for quality of fakes and of cancellations. After the first three sets, repeat the cycle, but rotate the types of cancellation forms requested. Rate performances again. Repeat a third time with a final rotation of modes. Consider the following factors during evaluations of the nine production sets:

– Realism of fakes, before or after
– Adequacy of disfluency modes (be strict)
– Adequacy of pause durations and relaxation
– Degree to which each cancellation actually "cancels"

When performance is adequate, move this step into the home assignment category.

• *Step 9.* Have client produce 50 longer sentences, each with more than one cancellation in it. Use the 26 (13 pairs) supplied here; compose 24 others to complete the list. Give the following instructions:

In each odd-numbered sentence you are to pseudostutter/cancel the underlined words. In even-numbered sentences, you are to select the same number of words as in the previous (odd-numbered) sentence for fakes/cancellations. Words selected should be ones you think you would stutter in everyday life.

Record utterances. After each odd/even pair, stop and replay to judge. Work to reach accord between clinician and client judgments, or at least to reach an understanding of the other's criteria.

1. <u>Hobbits</u> always seem to be invisible unless there is <u>food</u> on the table and <u>beer</u> in the glass.
2. Wizards have a habit of staring at you and twitching their eyebrows in an irritating way.
3. Children learn a lot in their <u>summer</u> <u>camps</u> and little girls are not <u>bothered</u> while they are gone.
4. Girls, when you can get them all together, seem to be very well organized.
5. The helicopter actually is a rotary-winged <u>airplane</u>, while the <u>"airplane"</u> is a fixed-wing <u>airplane</u>.
6. Jet aircraft were introduced by Germany, late in World War II.
7. The <u>Southern</u> <u>plantation</u> owners <u>destroyed</u> hundreds of thousands of acres with unwise cotton planting.
8. Tobacco farming is one the worst soil-destroying crops a farmer can raise.
9. <u>Turn</u> left on <u>Tennessee</u> Street and keep driving until you meet <u>Capital</u> Circle.
10. Mahan Drive is very puzzling in that it suddenly changes its name and is called Tennessee Street.
11. Stutterers <u>hesitate</u> to <u>pause</u> and, therefore, find themselves <u>pausing</u> when they don't want to.
12. Most stutterers do not like to look at their listeners when they are in the middle of a stuttering block.
13. <u>Government</u> troops failed, for the third straight day, to <u>keep</u> rioters off the streets.
14. Some countries would like to influence Central Europe, but want other countries to supply the money.
15. <u>Duke</u> <u>Ellington's</u> "Take the A-Train" is a favorite of most people who love <u>jazz</u>.
16. Gershwin's "Rhapsody in Blue" was originally orchestrated for the Paul Whiteman orchestra.

17. Most childhood <u>stuttering</u> is <u>easy</u>, <u>effortless</u> repetitions with low awareness.
18. In childhood, withdrawal from speaking situations is a sign of developing awareness of stuttering.
19. <u>Adolescent</u> stutterers are caught between a desire for help and <u>resistance</u> to ideas from adults.
20. Stutterers older than 50 years often seem to reduce their severity by not trying so hard.
21. The <u>president</u> of the United States is also <u>commander</u>-in-<u>chief</u> of the armed forces.
22. Congress generally acts as if the sitting president is an obstacle to good government.
23. Some <u>stutterers</u> actually will <u>walk</u> out of a <u>room</u> in order to <u>avoid</u> answering the telephone.
24. Female stutterers typically stutter less severely than will an equivalent male stutterer.
25. Charles <u>Van Riper</u> was the <u>speech</u> pathologist credited with <u>developing</u> cancellations.
26. Mild stutterers rarely are highly motivated to work hard on cancellation skills.

- *Step 10.* Provide short modeling statements that involve no more than one or two sentences. Have the client repeat the one or two sentences approximately (word accuracy is irrelevant). Instruct client to pseudostutter/cancel (hereafter called p/c) in each response. Do not stop for discussion and analysis unless a particular effort is quite unsatisfactory. After 5 to 10 utterance units, pause and discuss work up to that point.

  Set target as 50 responses, with any unacceptable evaluation adding from 1 to 5 more utterance units to the 50. Determine how many p/c productions are required for each unit (e.g., "Do 2 p/c productions in each sentence for the next 5" or "I will signal by holding up fingers, just before you start on each utterance"). Continue work until there have been 40 (or whatever) acceptable sentence units (not 40 p/c but 40 sentences), or a total of 70 acceptable productions (regardless of the number of sentences) out of 80 tries. Use the 10 sample statements below; add 30 or 40 more.

  1. Stuttering is more common in males than in females.
  2. Stutterers generally start to talk later than other children do.
  3. Many parents feel they may have caused stuttering.

4. Mustard on a hot dog is a very distinguished preference.
5. Some physicians used to cut wedges out of stutterers' tongues.
6. Most therapy does not 100% cure stuttering in adults.
7. Cotton candy is spun sugar on a paper cone.
8. Research fails to show any lack of intelligence in stutterers.
9. What we call "stuttering" is usually the struggle not to stutter.
10. Hamburgers must have dill pickles on them, never sweet pickles.

- *Step 11.* Have a supply of 30 to 50 topics based on knowledge about the client's interests, age, information levels, and so forth. Agree in advance that the client will talk extemporaneously on each topic until there have been X number of p/c productions (e.g., five to eight p/c efforts per topic). Record. At the end of each topic p/c group, ask if there are any unacceptable p/c efforts, evaluating both p and c. If both agree on acceptability, go on. If there is disagreement or agreement on unacceptability, play back for analysis and repeat entire discourse segment. Check on eye contact and other peripherals.

Transfer of cancellations, the next step, does not quite match the usual transfer program. The reason for this difference is that cancellations are not, by themselves, inherently motivating. Performance does not reduce speech interruptions directly. It is quite possible that they may increase overall fluency breaks. Client motivation, therefore, may not be high. However, the clinician must consider the stutterer's increased feelings of efficacy, increased desensitization, accumulated practice with dysfluency modification, and other indirect values. There also can be special applications, as I heard a client say, "Usually when I stutter once, I know two or three more are coming soon. . . . When I cancel the first block that seems to clear out those follow-ups from happening."

Some clients, especially mild stutterers, may resist transfer, and the resistance may be strong enough to lead the clinician to make cancellations an in-clinic preparation for pullouts and preparatory sets. It can always be called back as a repair strategy, later.

The following suggestions are offered for transfer activity. Because cancellation can be complex, these suggestions may be more direct than those made for general transfer in chapter 9.

- *Step 12.* Use any or all of the following 10 exercises for transfer activity.

1. Use a recorder. Read each word aloud, using the type of pseudostutter set out. After each fake, pause for 5 seconds and cancel with a relaxed production of the disfluency type in parentheses.

hello—short, easy repetitions	(Easy Onset)
where—hard, fast repetitions	(prolongation)
give—silent, tense stop	(Bounce)
Susan—tense prolongation	(relaxed prolongation)
building—stop and repetition	(Light Contact)
favorite—slow, hard repetitions	(Bounce)

2. Have client select 5 to 10 words that occur frequently in his or her speech. Have the client use each word every day for a specified number of days with a fake and any choice of cancellation mode. Instruct client to keep notes and report.
3. Have client make a specified number of telephone calls. For each call, tell client to write down enough advance questions or statements so he or she can underline three p/c words each call. Require client to keep notes and report.
4. Ask client to select a specified number of persons he or she knows to tell about the theory and production of cancellations. Tell client to demonstrate four or five examples to each listener. Have client keep notes and report.
5. Have client stop five strangers each day for a specified number of days and ask them for directions. In each situation, have client ask for the same information. Instruct client to p/c on a specified number of words, trying to p/c on the same words as much as possible. Ask client to compare situations, evaluate auditors, and keep notes and report.
6. Have the client go to three stores each day for a specified number of days and ask for information about the same products. In the first store, tell client to p/c four times, p/c three times in the second store, and p/c twice in the third store. Have client compare, check auditors, keep notes, and report.
7. Tell client to take a newspaper article and underline ___20 ___30 ___50 words he or she might stutter on if reading aloud to a group. Have client read aloud, doing a p/c on each underlined word, and record the effort. Have client play back and rate each p/c for p, for the pause adequacy, and for c. If more than 10% of ratings are unacceptable, tell the client the exercise must be repeated. Have client bring the paragraph to the clinic and demonstrate.

8. Have client repeat 7, but make all cancellations a pseudostutter of a different variety than was used in the fake. Tell client to evaluate tape for adequacy and realism. How many fakes slipped into real spasms?

9. Have client make ___5 ___10 ___15 telephone calls each day without faking anything. Cancel real spasms only. If any cancellations would be rated as "poor" or slipped into real spasms, add 3 more telephone calls to the total.

10. Tell client to make one 10-minute telephone call each day for 5 days to people he or she knows (one may be to clinician). Instruct the client to tell auditors he or she is working on his or her speech and tell them how. If there are no real spasms, instruct client to insert several p/c productions. Have client ask auditors how he or she sounded. Report.

Cancellation Summary

As noted earlier, cancellations can present problems in motivation and consistency. In high-anxiety stutterers they can be difficult to implement until sufficient desensitization has occurred. Nevertheless, they can be of great value in providing focus points for self-monitoring, evaluation, relaxation, and desensitization efforts. They also provide a valuable venue for learning and practicing different forms of fluency reinforcement or of symptom modification repairs. Value to preschool children is doubtful but, in one form or another, they can be used at any later age and severity level.

PULLOUTS

Pullouts can be attributed to Van Riper (1958). When stutterers had difficulty mastering preparatory sets, he developed pullouts to "save" them. A Stuttering Foundation of America publication (1993) describes pullouts as follows:

When you find yourself in the middle of a block, don't pause and don't stop and try again. Instead, continue the stuttering, slowing it down and letting the block run its course, deliberately making a smooth prolongation of what you are doing. In doing this, you will be stabilizing the sound by slowing down a repetition, or changing the repetition to a prolongation, or smoothing out a tremor, or pulling out of a fixation as you ease out of the block. (pp. 119, 120)

Bloodstein (1995) noted that much of a stuttering spasm's abnormal quality resulted from the speaker's efforts to struggle through the spasm. He found that pullouts often enhanced fluent completions almost immediately. The basic idea is that when a person stutters, he or she should regain control while the spasm is in progress and then complete the utterance in one of five variant forms:

1. Stop the spasm and start over (rarely used now).
2. Stop the spasm and try to finish fluently (also rare).
3. Stop-and-freeze, holding the spasm in midproduction, then deliberately relax and release the rest of the word.
4. Slow the spasm down, relax while doing so, and finish with a fake of the original spasm.
5. Slow the spasm down, relax while doing so, and finish with one of several possible controlled disfluencies.

Prerequisites

To a significant degree, pullouts and cancellations have the same prerequisites. However, because clinicians may skip cancellations for various reasons, pullout prerequisites are presented here. The importance of meeting these criteria cannot be overstated. Too many clinicians jump right into pullouts, guaranteeing failure and frustration for the client.

The seven suggested prepullout criteria are:

1. Tolerance for stuttering (desensitization), major reductions in avoidances, positive attitudes to communication
2. Complete and accurate information about and awareness of "all" of her or his stuttering behaviors
3. Skill in rapid evaluation of spasms (on a postspasm basis) at a minimum level of 75% adequacy on moderate-to-severe spasms
4. Ability to monitor personal signals of body tension in general, and speech mechanism in particular, and to relax
5. Skill at pseudostuttering, own patterns, and in general

6. Familiarity with several general forms of disfluency
7. Ability to demonstrate that S/G can be moved from postspasm to in-spasm capacity

In the 1960s and 1970s, at the height of fluency reinforcement, some behavior modification clinicians questioned pullouts, labeling them as part of the "stutter more fluently" failure game. More recently, Prins (1993) stated that criticisms of pullouts have been justified. Silverman (1996), on the other hand, stated that there is an inherent logic to pullouts in that their place of occurrence is where the stutterer's struggles cause the worst distortion of and interruption in ongoing speech.

Recent Applications of Pullouts

Culatta and Goldberg (1995) are representative of the mixed philosophy evident today, where many behavioral modification clinicians have learned the value of certain symptom modification procedures. They appear to mix the Bounce (see chapter 6) with cancellations, pullouts, and preparatory sets. Bloodstein (1993) stated that Van Riper organized cancellations, pullouts, and preparatory sets. Wendell Johnson, on the other hand, modified stuttering with a pattern that Bloodstein felt differed significantly from Van Riper's use of easy prolongation on the three techniques. Johnson favored a paced, relaxed repetition of the first sound or syllable (i.e., Bounce). Bloodstein suggested that Van Riper tried to control stuttering, while the Bounce moved the stutterer in a very different direction.

Peters and Guitar (1991) discuss pullouts in their excellent amalgamation of symptom modification and fluency reinforcement therapies. They present pullouts in much the same form as Van Riper did over a half-century before.

Most sources today assume that pullouts are to be used only with adult or near-adult clients. This is not the case. Van Riper (1973) suggested clinician-client unison stuttering with children to "pull" the client into pullouts. In another source, Luper and Mulder (1964) recommended both cancellations and pullouts for young children who were confirmed stutterers. Dell (1993) suggested blending parent counseling and working directly with the child. Dell stated that facing stuttering and the client's fears is probably the hardest part of therapy and requires some toughness on the part of the client. Dell follows the preliminary preparation recommended earlier in this section (self-analysis, desensitization, and so forth). When the child feels a spasm beginning, she or he is to keep the spasm going until, on the clinician's signal, he or she relaxes and eases smoothly into the rest of the word.

Description of Pullouts

Overall, pullouts can be used at most developmental stages of stuttering, and they can cross age groups. Generally, however, they are used with more mature stutterers, usually at moderate-to-severe levels. Returning to the earlier definition from the Stuttering Foundation of America (1993), pullouts can involve certain required and certain elective steps.

- Go ahead and stutter. Drop all avoidance attempts.
- Be aware of what is being done every moment.
- Analyze every aspect of the spasm as it happens. Be sure where the locus of tension is, the form of the spasm, and any overflow.
- Relax the tensions at the loci, in particular, and in the body, in general. Make sure eye contact is good and start to slow the spasm down or relax it.
- Continue the basic stuttering spasm until control is regained; the spasm is now a fake.
- Control the utterance so the word is finished in one of two ways:
  1. By continuing the existing stuttering until it becomes a fake that is slow, relaxed, and completely voluntary.
  2. By continuing the stuttering until it can be shifted into a voluntary disfluency such as an Easy Onset, prolongation, and so on.

As the speaker becomes more proficient, and confident, the elapsed time shortens drastically and pullouts occur quickly. In its most successful form, the pullout is practically indistinguishable from the final step, the preparatory set.

Clinician Preparation

In order to teach pullouts effectively, the clinician should be able to pseudostutter to a degree that she or he can accurately mimic the client's stuttering pattern. Also, the clinician should be adept at all of the various methods of controlled disfluency production. In this way, the client can be shown what to do, when to do it, and how to perform. The clinician should demonstrate possible and actual errors and then model the correct form.

Pullout Acquisition Steps—Preliminary

No learning procedure should be rigid. Accordingly, the clinician is urged to revise, edit, and amend the following acquisition steps, changing them for every client. Client cognition, severity, prior therapy, and so on will affect planning. The clinician should review the client's monitoring and self-evaluation skills and consider her or his pseudostuttering ability. Material used in the previous (cancellation) section also can be used here. I will provide the first word list and then refer to cancellation steps, or the clinician can develop his or her own lists and materials.

- *Step 1.* Have the client read the following 50 words aloud. Ignore (for now) the underlined words. On any stuttered words, instruct the client to try and STOP/FREEZE (S/F) during the spasm, for several seconds, and then finish the word. Then have the client stop and describe all the spasm characteristics (see the relevant self-analysis sections in chapter 3).

block	theory	fake	analyze	masking
spasm	Johnson	cancel	plan	blending
repeat	Iowa	pullout	revision	triggers
prolong	postpone	bounce	airflow	preparatory
avoid	retrial	clinic	attitude	unison
tonic	starter	transfer	feedback	legato
clonic	fluency	relax	airflow	shadow
stop	stutter	maintain	delay	modeling
pause	substitute	insight	onset	monitor
duck	analyze	evaluate	freeze	punish

If there are not at least 10 real spasms on the reading, have the client repeat the list and pseudostutter with an S/F on a word in each horizontal row (client's selection), analyzing and describing as originally requested. If an original spasm or a fake is not adequately described, model it the way it was done and have the client imitate it while checking self in the mirror. Have the client continue until satisfactorily done.

- *Step 2.* Repeat the above exercise, using the sentences (all 26) from Step 9 in "Cancellation." The client is to S/F and analyze any real spasms and fake a spasm with an S/F behavior on each underlined word of the odd-numbered sentences. On the even-numbered sentences, instruct the client to select the same number of words (from the previous sentence) to underline and fake on. On each fake, S/F and analyze. Apply same criterion and penalty as for Step 1 above.
- *Step 3.* Repeat the S/F analysis behavior, using three 3-minute spontaneous speech periods. Keep time and count for client. Set performance target as client being able to S/F on 75% of the spasms where stopping in time is reasonable (i.e., spasms under 3 seconds are almost impossible to use S/F on). If real spasms are too few, rerun the step with a target of about 10 to 15 fake S/F performances (3 to 5 every minute) in each period.

The clinician should pause at this point and try to answer two important questions:

1. Is the success percentage so low that there is a need to develop some of the prerequisite skills further?
2. What spasm duration length seems to be the break-even point for adequacy on S/F?

The last question revolves around the typical duration mix of spasms. Very often, by the time pullouts are reached, a client may be close to near fluency through adaptation and clinician-induced efficacy. Some clients may have reduced stuttering frequency by 90%, in the clinic, and spasms that do occur are brief tokens of the past. However, when the client walks out the door, he or she may revert to near usual severity and frequency levels. Answering the second question is important because if in-clinic and out-clinic levels are both quite low, then pullouts may not have been a wise choice. However, if out-clinic severity and frequency are considerably higher than the in-clinic levels, then faking for S/F will need extensive use before transfer is feasible.

- *Step 4.* Using the list of 50 words from Step 1, have the client utter the words, varying three or four different disfluency modes. Try for at least three, preferably four, different modes. Skip this step if client's disfluency control status is acceptable.

- *Step 5.* Repeat the three free speech 3-minute periods in Step 3. Instruct client to use a different disfluency in each period, using that disfluency on four different words in each period. If any real spasm occurs, use a good quality cancellation on each, with the disfluency selected for that period. Target "acceptable" productions of four words in each of the three periods.

- *Step 6.* Have the client make five telephone calls in your presence. Tell the client to use S/F on every stuttering spasm that occurs. Add another telephone call to the five:

  – for each call not producing at least three stuttering spasms
  – for each failure to use S/F when real spasms lasted long enough to use S/F, but the client failed to do so

  At the clinician's discretion, added telephone calls can carry direction to: "Fake four spasm in this call and use S/F on each one."

Interestingly, I have had clients tell me that making calls with a "desire" for stuttering made it less likely that they were going to stutter.

- *Step 7.* Go out of clinic with the client and observe him or her in five contacts. Model the first one or two while the client observes. Use same target, criterion, and problem solving, as in Step 5.

- *Step 8.* As homework, have client make three telephone calls and make three personal contacts a day for a period of 5 to 11 days. In each call or contact, tell client to use three S/F behaviors on real spasms, or add one more and make four or five fakes with S/F behaviors. Report to clinician. Utilize in-clinic time for a mix of home assignments, problem solving, and current in-clinic activity.

- *Step 9.* Have the client practice S/F in three telephone calls a day for a period of 1 week following the Step 6 description. In the clinic, review client out-clinic activities, problem solving, supervised out-clinic practice—whatever the client needs.

During this tune-up process the client should revitalize past skills, improve desensitization, and improve spasm prediction skills in terms of when he or she is going to stutter on what words. Now, clinician and client will want to negotiate short-term and long-term performance-level targets, such as:

Spasm Duration/Severity	Short-Term Target	Long-Term Target
Severe	75%	90%–100%
Moderate	50%	75%
Mild	0%–10%	10%–20%

Target percentages are, of course, subject to modification. Finally, client and clinician should look for words or circumstances that are particularly troublesome or conditions that seem to favor one disfluency mode over another.

Pullout Acquisition—Instatement

All of the previous steps may have taken 6 to 10 sessions or, because of client preparation, may have been been condensed into a couple sessions. As mentioned earlier, practice material can be borrowed from the section titled "Cancellation." To perform a pullout successfully, the client must do the following:

- As soon as a spasm occurs, let it be a signal to relax and slow down (not tense and push harder) and to move into an analysis mode. Start correcting any lost eye contact, facial grimaces, articulator distortions, and so on.
- When relaxation is verified, rate slowed, and other areas under control, continue the spasm into a voluntary fake of the real spasm.
- When the feeling of control is realized, let the fake spasm merge into a disfluency mode that seems appropriate, and finish the word.

The majority of this book sets out detailed step-by-step acquisition procedures for techniques. For a change, a hypothetical therapy session is presented:

- After session initiation, have client read aloud, faking spasms and pullouts on underlined words and pulling out on all real spasms. 3 minutes
- Play back and analyze. 5 minutes
- Have client present oral report on prior outside assignments since last session; instruct client to use pullout on all reasonable spasms. Evaluate reports and work on any problems. 10 minutes

- Have client present monologue discourse using pullouts. 5 minutes
- Have client place several telephone calls, pulling out on all reasonable spasms. If not enough spasms occur, require fakes and pullouts. 10 minutes
- Discuss home assignments to be done by next session. 5 minutes
- Depending on time, let client decide on task, or try for a few outside contacts, using pullouts.

Other activities that can be inserted into the work session include:

- Inviting extra persons in for conversation and pullouts
- Role playing of imaginary or real situations
- Engaging in extended spontaneous discourse with fake/pullout targets
- Undertaking prearranged, longer outside situations
- Problem solving with videotape

Pullout Problems

Pullouts combine a lot of different factors. They usually are extremely attractive to all clients except those with very mild stuttering. Because of technique complexity and client haste, the clinician should be alert for the following nine problems:

1. Missed spasms. The clinician should employ a reasonable criterion. If more spasms need to be caught, the clinician should discover the reasons and work on them.
2. Control loss. This problem results in a renewed spasm or a slip back into real stuttering. It may be caused by faulty analysis, poor relaxation, or hurried effort.
3. Hurried pullout. This problem is a reflection of control loss, and it is quite common at first. If it is a real problem, the clinician should insert cancellation as a penalty, so that hurry generates its own punishment.
4. Jerky pullout. This occurs due to incomplete relaxation of the articulators, and usually is hurried (the pullout) as well. Even if the clients slows the utterance down, old habits may generate a tension level that causes a jerky release rather than a smooth transition to finish the utterance of the word.

5. Poorly executed disfluency. This problem may be due to a desire to sound normal too soon, careless learning and practice (clinician fault), or need for different disfluency form.
6. Need for different disfluencies. Some clients may do well with one disfluency mode; others may need Easy Onset for certain phonemes, a Bounce for others, and so on.
7. Anticipatory pullout. It may occur when the client misjudges timing, relaxation, control, and so forth and tries too soon.
8. Token pullouts. These occur when client pulls out slightly but actually lets the spasm dictate. For some it can be an adjustment to reality, but usually it is a sign of inadequacy.
9. Special problems. Special problems require special work. Clinicians should not go with the "Time will solve" disclaimer. More likely, such failure pockets will undermine self-efficacy and ultimately destroy pullouts in general.

Transfer of Pullouts

Common sense should tell all clients, even very young ones, that they must "use it or lose it." Pullouts require constant use to be of value. Some broad suggestions include the following:

- Use outside, solo assignments regularly. Have client increase frequency of outside contacts, if appropriate. Set a daily target for number of pullout attempts, and negotiate a penalty for failures to meet the target. Work out a reasonable recording and report system.
- Use in-clinic exercises. Have the client fake spasms three to five times in a row, on the same word, delaying the pullout from a 5-second, 4-second, and 2-second fake.
- Go back in therapy history to look for struggles and avoidances that have been eliminated in the past. Deliberately introduce some of them to be "overcome" in a pullout practice sequence. Remember, one of the best ways to prevent recurrence of old behaviors is to maintain awareness of them through fake practice.

If extra practice is needed, any number of approaches can be used. Nearly all the in-clinic and out-clinic exercises presented for the cancellation technique can be reworded and used with pullouts. In addition, 12 suggestions follow that are demanding. The clinician may want to downsize some of them in terms of demand level. The items are intended for out-clinic work and are written from the perspective of the client.

1. Each day, set a target of ___ high-quality pullouts. When the target number is reached, stop and decide whether time-off for the rest of the day is deserved or if some things need further work.
2. Set up a mirror and a tape recorder. Make five telephone calls to strangers and one extended call to a friend. Use a pullout on all reasonable spasms. Afterward judge if further practice is needed.
3. Make a list of ___20 ___30 ___50 words that tend to give fluency troubles either because of phoneme combinations or word fears. Practice faking a spasm on each word, trying to make the fake turn real and then use a pullout.
4. Write a thorough description of your spasm pattern when you started therapy, and then write a description of your present spasm pattern. Produce 10 to 20 fakes of each type and practice pulling out.
5. Find a willing listener and explain the theory and practice of pullouts. Demonstrate different ways, simulate problems, and try to teach listener.
6. Make a list of 10 to 20 words with phonemes you are more likely to stutter on, plus 5 to 10 of your Jonah words. For the next 5 days, use each word at least once. Watch for spasms and chances to use a pullout.
7. Take a newspaper or magazine paragraph and underline at least 20 words in it. Read aloud and record. On each underlined word, fake a severe spasm that lasts 4 to 5 seconds before you relax and use a pullout. Play back and evaluate pullout quality.
8. For 4 or 5 days, try to keep a list of every word that you *could* have pulled out on, but did not. Then, set out to use each word three times over several days, faking a spasm and pulling out each time.
9. For 5 days, make a telephone call each day until you have had and pulled out on three spasms, or until you have faked and pulled out on three spasms. If you miss, or do poorly, add another telephone call for each time.
10. Over the next 5 days, plan to monitor your speech until you have collected (each day) ___10 ___30 ___60 quality pullouts. As soon as you reach your target, take the rest of the day off.

11. Call local schools and find out how to contact the parent-teacher group. Contact them (use pullouts) and volunteer to be a guest speaker on, "How To Help the Dysfluent Child in School." Before your talk, explain pullouts and tell the audience you will be trying to use them as you talk.
12. Set a 10-day period aside to work on pullouts. On Day 1, try to pull out of all spasms in 10 different situations (create them if needed); on Day 2, repeat this on 9 situations; on Day 3 on 8 situations; and so on down. If pullout goals are not met on "reasonable" spasms, or if enough situations are not generated, back up 2 days and continue.

Pullout Summary

Pullouts can be one step in an overall management program. They also can be the final target of therapy, without going on to preparatory sets. Pullouts have been adopted in some fluency reinforcement programs, usually when the "fluency" is insufficiently complete, or stable, to maintain a level of control that is acceptable to the client. Pullouts are as valuable and viable in 1999 as they were in 1939.

PREPARATORY SETS

To say that preparatory sets are used in therapy is to create the false impression that they are used only in therapy. Actually, preparatory sets (prep sets) are used on every sound and syllable uttered. They are used on every breath and every vocal fold adjustment preceding any phoneme. They also occur in one's fingers and hands as words are written. Every motor act is coordinated by a linked series of preparatory sets, which are a series of programmed adjustments in the organism to provide for a subsequent movement to occur in a certain way, pattern, duration, intensity, range, and so on. As we talk, it extends to facial expressions, eye contact, stance, and so on (i.e., body language).

In therapy of stuttering, clinicians generally are involved with abnormal prep sets (but not always). Fluency reinforcement therapy may try for a rather universal change in motor speech prep sets, and symptom therapy may focus on those around the moment of stuttering. The main target of such efforts is the abnormal, incorrect, distorted formation of the articulators that make up the prep set of a stuttering spasm. The stuttering does not distort or "abnormalize" the prep set; the stutterer does this in an effort not to stutter at all. Much of stuttering is what the person does in an effort not to stutter.

Most people have typical, and slightly different, prep sets prior to performance of a motor act. Before I say /r/ I may quirk the corners of my mouth a bit more than you do, or you may take a deeper breath before releasing /h/ than I do, and so on. Once speech is emitted we tend to move from one prep set to the next and changes (coarticulation) are affected by that which preceded and that which is to follow.

Stutterers also have preparatory sets. Research does not suggest that all stuttterer prep sets are abnormal; they do not have to be to act as triggers for a stuttering spasm. However, for many stutterers, it seems safe to suggest that they:

- Have more frequent and inappropriate prep set points.
- Form many prep sets that last longer than required and are at a higher tension level than is desirable.
- May generate prep sets that physically distort, or even negate, normal production of target phonemes/syllables.
- Create a stuttering spasm "trigger" where the occurrence of the prep set actually precipitates (or at least predisposes to) the occurrence of a stuttering spasm.

History

Preparatory sets date back to initial efforts to alter the initiating movements or the articulatory components of speech. Strange substances smeared on the tongue, props and pads under the tongue, clamps around the lips, and support collars around the head or neck all acted to restrict or alter the speech postures available to the speaker. More recently, elocution approaches to teach cultured, pseudo-oratorical speech patterns (round, pear-shaped tones) have been employed. The last few decades have seen the advent of fluency reinforcement therapy where (initially) the management program's drastic modifications of all production postures completely shifted and shaped all prep set patterns where the "fluency mode" was applied. In a very real sense, fluency reinforcement simply built on the concept of altering the prep set (normal or abnormal).

In Europe, Freund (1966) claimed credit for hypothesizing the concept of preparatory sets (circa 1932). The credit for organizing and applying them in a therapy construct belongs to Van Riper (1958). He defined the prep set with reference to stuttering and theorized that the prep set, itself, establishes, directs, and controls the response to the anticipated stimulus (for speech). Van Riper also suggested that because stuttering spasms vary, it makes sense to assume that prep set patterns vary. Moreover, stutterers, being individuals, can have individualized prep set patterns.

By the mid-1940s, prep sets were established in many symptom modification programs, moving away from a faked replication of the real stuttering spasm toward a slowed, relaxed, and prolonged disfluent pattern (this was what some fluency reinforcement enthusiasts called the "stutter more fluently" mistake). Van Riper believed that prep sets were intended to help the stutterer's efforts to try and get into the spasm and then out again with as little abnormality as possible.

Current Applications

There are many variations in prep set methods (Ham, 1986; Luper & Mulder, 1964; Ryan, 1971; Shames & Egolf, 1976; Silverman, 1996). I will settle for a prep set summary from the Stuttering Foundation of America (1993):

1. Anticipate stuttering. (There is an assumption that the stutterer is a good anticipator, but, as we have noted, there is disagreement about this.)
2. Pause before attempting the word, slowing the rate down to a complete stop. As you stop, identify tense areas and completely relax them.
3. Estimate the probable spasm pattern, the nature of the anticipated stuttering, based upon past study and experience with particular words, phonemes, stress levels, etc.
4. Plan how to correct or modify the usual initiation of the first sound or syllable.
5. Rehearse mentally, or actually pantomime, how the initiation effort will be performed. Most auditors will recognize that an effort is being made to overcome an obstacle.

6. When breathing is normal, and not before, utter the word with a sliding, resonant, prolonged manner, exaggerating the effort without tension, and paying more attention to how it feels (strong movement?) than to how it sounds.
7. Complete the rest of the word in the same fashion as in 6, and let the production mode carry over for the next few words, if it feels natural. However, do not adopt the speech mode as an habitual speaking gesture.

Actually, the "proper" way to produce preparatory sets is the way that is most effective for a particular individual. A stuttering spasm usually establishes a feedback loop so that motor movements can become fixated, repeated, or prolonged. For many stutterers, this feedback loop is precipitated by the *abnormal* prep set, which acts to trigger the spasm. The alternative is to devise a new prep set and use it to replace the one that no longer is under the control of the speaker.

Prediction and Prep Sets

The occurrence of stuttering on particular words happens more often than can be attributed to chance (Wingate, 1976). Silverman (1996) summarized a number of studies, concluding that the nonrandom distribution of stuttering spasms may be affected by an expectancy attitude of the stutterer. Some stutterers seem to be very good at anticipation, whereas others seem to have weak predictive capacity.

Whether prediction or anticipation is a self-fulfilling prophecy is irrelevant. The only question is whether or not the stutterer *can* anticipate at a level appreciably better than chance. This capacity often begins weakly in therapy, but develops significantly as a client goes through self-analysis, monitoring, desensitization, and other early steps. When the management program starts prep sets at an early phase, the probability of success is, I believe, almost completely at the whim of chance. If the client has a naive, high-accuracy anticipation, then things may go well for prep sets. If the prediction ability is weak or undeveloped, then the inconsistency, overuse, fatigue, and frustration may make prep sets (or their equivalent) valueless over the long run.

Favorable Prognosis

As stated previously, cancellation and pullout were developed as fallbacks or self-repairs for missed, incomplete, or failed prep sets. In other words, prep sets need fallback resources because they can be hard to do well. Just catching the spasm can be a real problem in the case of mild spasms. Another interfering factor can be very strong patterns of unconscious motor behaviors associated with stuttering spasms—once started on a spasm, it is very hard to stop. A third influencing factor is that the prep set position in time and space occurs at a moment of maximum anxiety, tension, and avoidance desires. In other words, the worst time and place for use of prep sets is at the time and place they are most needed.

In management, the clinician probably should start with the feeling that prep sets may be of doubtful value and then, as a continuing goal in therapy, try and increase value probabilities. Improvements can occur to a significant degree, depending on responses to the following six evaluation points.

1. Is the client an "expert" on what happens during every part of his or her stuttering? If not, this knowledge must be developed.
2. Has the client (almost) eliminated overt, in-speech avoidances? Postponements, retrials, and so forth should be gone, or nearly so. If they are not, prep sets ultimately will fail.
3. Can the client effectively monitor her or his own speech and accurately present that analysis? Is it sufficiently clear and reliable on an out-clinic basis?
4. Has the client demonstrated a noticeable, measurable tolerance for stuttering, a willingness to stutter, and an acceptance of self? If not, desensitization must occur.
5. Does the client have effective fallback strategies, with some feeling of self-efficacy if early (or later) prep sets run into trouble?
6. Finally, can the client use more than one form of voluntary disfluency in producing prep sets? Further, are prep sets used effectively in out-clinic settings and not just during in-clinic sessions? Be sure that the client does not just try to say the word "fluently," rather than controlling a voluntarily disfluent utterance.

Facilitating Prediction

As noted earlier, anticipation or prediction ability is not consistent across stutterers, and it may vary within the individual. However, it is assumed that prep sets work is preceded by some of the activities or targets suggested in the previous section. As client and clinician become more familiar with the client's stuttering characteristics, prediction will be facilitated. A number of areas can be drawn upon for this effort:

1. Identify special, or Jonah, words the client has learned to fear and to expect trouble on.
2. Identify special phonemes, sound combinations, and prosodic factors that are more likely to be associated with stuttering.
3. Find out about special people or particular situations or topics that are more likely to be associated with stuttering.
   - On or within the first three words of utterance, phrase by phrase
   - At, or near, clause boundaries
   - On consonants, more than on vowels
   - On initiating voiced sounds following a voiceless sound
   - On longer, rather than shorter, words
   - On longer, rather than shorter, phrases, sentences, and so on
   - On content, more than function, words (perhaps)
   - On unfamiliar and less frequently used words
   - On initial consonants/syllables of a word
   - On stressed words, stressed syllables within a word
   - On words with informational and/or emotional importance
   - When the number of auditors increases
   - When specific auditors are, or are not, present
   - After a stuttering spasm has just occurred (disagreement)

The prior items do not apply to all stutterers, and those that apply to any one stutterer do not apply to the same degree all the time. Also, the list is incomplete. I have had clients link stuttering tendencies to odors of a particular type, sex, time of day, day of week, inebriation or lack of, and on and on. Things logical and things nonsensical can tend to stimulate stuttering.

Criteria for Preparatory Sets

Earlier sections on cancellation and pullout contained criteria lists. These capacities are not repeated here, but are required for learning prep sets. If they are omitted, or given scant attention, prep sets will fail.

In addition to the concerns expressed previously, there are other aspects that need to be reexamined in prep set consideration:

- Avoidances. If the client is using direct avoidances (postponement, substitution, and so forth), he or she is not ready for prep sets.
- Avoidances. Avoidance of people, situations, topics, and so on must not be significant at this point in therapy for preparatory sets to be successful.
- Pseudostuttering. This technique needs to be reviewed. The client must feel that he or she can pseudostutter in different forms if needed. At times, a variant form of disfluency is the best control mode.

Preparatory Set Procedures

Although the Stuttering Foundation of America (1993) steps are a solid base, a more specific set of instruction to the client might be useful:

- Go ahead and talk; do not institute controls of any kind.
- Anticipate any stuttering—either because you "feel" it coming or past experience and loci suggest the probability.
- Slow the rate of speech as the word is approached, preferably about three words before the target word.
- Relax as the rate is slowed.
- While slowing and relaxing, consider the target phoneme/syllable characteristics and the prep set form best suited.
- Produce the prep set with good eye contact, a controlled disfluency, and elimination of any avoidance or struggle behaviors.
- Let the prep set behaviors carry over into the next word or two following.

Note that I have omitted the "pause" step from the Stuttering Foundation of America list. Such a behavior may be necessary when prep sets are first being learned to allow the client to shift gears, really relax, make decisions, and move forward. However, the final form of prep sets is illustrated best when there is no discernible pause after the word preceding the target word.

- *Step 1.* Take the client out of clinic to evaluate self-analysis. Use material from chapters 3 or 4, and target stress situations:
  1. Use the fear hierarchy (see chapter 4) and select five situations that spread approximately across difficulty levels of 20, 30, 50, 60, and 80 points. In each situation, have client count spasms, analyze spasms in detail, report on auditors, and so on. Move on from this task or remain for additional work, depending on outcomes.
  2. Repeat preceding exercise, looking intensively for any avoidance behaviors (general or specific). Move on or remain, depending on outcomes.

The completeness and accuracy of the client's reports in Step 1 will be a fairly reliable inferential of client acceptance of stuttering, tension control, and motivation. The clinician will want to fashion home assignments following the areas covered. In general, "move on" criteria would be performance ratings of "good" or better for situations ranked at 20, 30, and 50, and "adequate" rankings for those rated above 50.

- *Step 2.* If the client has previously worked on cancellation and progressed to pullout, use some of the cancellation activities here (i.e., review cancellations themselves).

I am reluctant to consider that prior therapy might have gone directly to prep sets, without all the foundation skills (monitoring, evaluation, cancellation, pullouts) presented somewhat repetitively before.

Step 3 is intended for clients who have not shown any particular capacity to anticipate spasms.

- *Step 3.* Have client enter 25 outside speech situations, with at least 5 occurring with clinician present. Tell client to rate spasms by severity levels and, for each situation, perform the following two activities:
  1. Delineate the number of spasms anticipated.
  2. Relate spasm severity or other aspects to anticipation adequacy.

  If the outcomes are not positive, return to the section titled "Facilitating Prediction" and work to improve the client's awareness of factors that will improve predictions.

  Repeat the initial assignment, but on each stuttered spasm, have client try to S/G just before the spasm starts. If unsuccessful, try S/G during the spasm. If that fails, try S/G after the spasm, then try to work back to original prespasm target.

Set criteria using the following percentages as reasonable starting targets.

Mild Spasms	Moderate Spasms	Severe Spasms
20% success	60% success	80% success

Some clients will do much better, some will start out badly and then improve. Others, after repeated trials, reviews, models, and so forth will not achieve the minimum levels suggested here. In this case, the clinician can use Step 4 as a digression.

- *Step 4.* Review self-analysis, monitoring, and other early therapy skills. Review cancellation and pullout. Review the problems cited earlier (inadequate monitoring, analysis, disfluency modes) as well as loci factors. If these cannot be used to advantage in a significant improvement (after at least six therapy sessions), do not use prep sets. Back up and concentrate on turning pullout into a termination skill.

If there are no major problems, or major problems have been solved by the procedures discussed previously, the clinician should move on to Step 5, which provides exercises for in-clinic practice.

- *Step 5.*
  - Have client read 50 sentences (8 to 10 words each), each sentence with 2 underlined words. Use the 10 sentences below; create 40 more. Instruct client to fake a prep set on each underlined word, and evaluate for slowdown prior to underlined word, relaxed production of fake, disfluency adequacy, after-words carryover of rate and relaxation, and disfluency aspects. Set success criterion as "good" or "adequate" on 90 of the 100 prep set trials.

    Preparatory sets are often the final step in therapy.
    Very mild stutterers may find prep sets hard to do.
    Can you transfer prep sets very easily?
    Stutterers who hit prep sets too hard may get in trouble.
    You must relax and slow down for a good prep set.
    Lizzie scratched one ear and sighed sadly.
    Lizzie doesn't stutter but she has a lot of fleas.
    So-So the cat used to be called Sergeant Pepper.

Mempo, although <u>friendly</u>, was a rather stupid <u>cat</u>.
<u>Cats</u> and <u>dogs</u> almost never have fluency problems.

– Have client read aloud a 300-word (approximate) paragraph in which 50 words have been underlined (pick appropriate words, but vary locations). Record and play back. Have client rate on aspects listed in preceding exercise. Use same 90% criterion as before. If below 90%, have a second paragraph ready and underlined; repeat the exercise.

– Have another 50 sentences (borrow from another section of book, if desired) that are not underlined. Instruct client to read each sentence aloud. In each sentence have client fake a pullout on every word he or she thinks might prompt a stutter, but no more than four per sentence. Record and have client evaluate. Use same evaluation points and criterion level as before. On all inadequate pullouts, require client to use that word in 3 different sentences, faking a different style of pullout each time. Record and play back.

Completion of all parts of Step 5 will have created several hundred pullout practice efforts. The clinician should stop at this point and consider whether any recurrent problems (see the next two steps) or special behaviors need attention before continuing. Step 6 deals with spontaneous speech.

- *Step 6.*
  – Provide the client with 20 or 30 topics. Instruct client to talk for 1 minute each on 10 topics. Within each 1-minute period, have client produce at least three pullouts, fake or real. Failure to meet number quota, or an unacceptable pullout, requires the client to repeat the whole minute. Record and evaluate at the end of each minute.
  – Provide more topics. Have client talk for 3 minutes each on five topics. Within each 3-minute period, tell client to use a pullout 10 times. Use same evaluation procedure as before. If three pullouts are missed or are unacceptable in one time period, repeat that entire time period. If client "runs dry" before 3 minutes are up, have him or her begin another topic. Keep time while client speaks.
  – Provide more topics. Have client talk for 5 minutes each on three topics. As before, use extra topics if client needs to finish a 5-minute stint. Within each 5-minute period, tell client to use a pullout (fake or

real) 15 times. Record and evaluate. Use same evaluation procedure as before. If more than 10 pullouts are missed or are inadequate in one 5-minute period, repeat the entire period.

In this progressive sequence on supervised transfer, clinician and client listen closely for any consistency patterns on words where real stuttering occurs, a real pullout fails, or a fake pullout is poorly done. The clinician also tries to determine if the client seems to be avoiding attempts on certain words, word locations, phonemes, or other word aspects. By this stage, the client should be familiar with transfer procedures and problems. If the clinician has waited until this time to introduce transfer, it is probably too late.

- *Step 7.* Use transfer activities from sections on cancellation and pullout. Employ the material on transfer in chapter 9 as well.

Preparatory Set Problems

Prep sets are fully covered by Murphy's Law—in any given situation, if anything can go wrong it will. Murphy's Corollary probably applies too—it will go wrong at the least favorable time. Although prep sets are not hard to do (by this stage of therapy), problems tend to arise because prep sets are psychologically just a small step away from pretherapy avoidance behaviors and other old behavior patterns. If there has been poor preparation, clinician errors, client laziness, and so on, prep sets may have problems. These problems can include, but not be limited to:

- Client is overdependent on *auditory* feedback because the use of tactile and kinesthetic monitoring has not been stressed.
- Client has overall problems with adequately slowing rate. Those problems should have been corrected long before pullouts were started. They should be attacked now using loci of stuttering and cancellation. If not effective, unison speech or other rate control vehicles (see chapter 6) can be used.
- The client possesses insufficient self-analysis skills. At the exact moment of a prep set, analysis skills are of limited value. However, prior months of therapy with monitoring and analysis will have

equipped the client to make split-second judgments and adjust accordingly. If this capacity was skipped or skimped, the clinician should refer to chapter 3 for review or correction.

- Client's anxiety and tension levels are too high. This problem probably goes back to clinician failure to desensitize the client and to use transfer work at every step so that by the time prep sets are reached, the client has a fairly high level of self-efficacy. It also can be the result of a client who has routinely reported falsely on transfer work and now cannot produce. Cancellation, if client accepts it, is usually a good treatment device.

- Covert stuttering may be a complication (see earlier chapters). That is, the client internalizes a lot of the stuttering and also probably has a rich array of substitutions, circumlocutions, situation avoidances, and other covert modes of avoidance. Again, this problem is probably the clinician's fault, because this type of covert pattern should have become evident during self-analysis and desensitization. At that time, the most efficacious solution would have been to transfer programs into a fluency reinforcement orientation with strong elements of confidence building and ego support.

- The client has too many, too mild spasms. If client started out "severe," it may not be a major problem. The current dysfluency level may be very acceptable to the client. However, it may be productive to go back to loci and decide times and places to use a quasi–fluency-reinforcement production pattern at probable loci points. It is also important to establish transfer and maintenance activities in self-monitoring to watch the little spasms in order to prevent a creeping return of more significant dysfluencies.

- The client is a perfectionist. Some of the best "fluency only" programs urge acceptance of 0.5 or fewer stuttered words per minute as a termination point. Apparently, total removal of stuttering is recognized by most authorities as a hard target to hit. Perfectionism may have significant psychological ramifications, with which the speech-language pathologist (SLP) cannot deal. This problem should have been evident early in therapy, and the clinician should have worked on it during the intervening months.

This problem is one reason to give the client a realistic assessment at the very start of therapy. The clinician is being unethical and incurring liability if he or she offers false or unrealistic hopes.

- Fluency threats can undo therapy progress. Becoming fluent, or just adequately in control, can upset families, jobs, aspirations, self-evaluations, and all sorts of psychodynamics. As terrible a burden as stuttering can be, control of dysfluency can have upsetting connotations and outcomes for the client and those associated with the client. These problems must be referred to appropriately trained counselors.

Transfer and Preparatory Sets

Transfer work with prep sets should be very individualized. Therefore, the following suggestions are not sequenced in steps, but represent a collection from which selections can be made.

1. Have the client set a daily prep set target, based on how many times a day she or he would anticipate stuttering. Negotiate with the client to try for prep sets on ___90% ___70% ___50% ____30% of spasms each day, for a period of ___2 ___6 ___10 days.
2. Have the client set a goal of faking prep sets ___100 ___80 ___60 ___40 times a day for ___2 ___6 ___10 days. Reduce the daily target for fake prep sets by 2 each time a real spasm is controlled by a good prep set.
3. Have client make five preplanned telephone calls a day for 10 days. Rehearse each call in advance. Tell client to use pullout on real spasms only. Instruct client to make an extra telephone call for each failure, using the particular word with a real or fake pullout.
4. Have client call a person he or she knows and talk for 10 to 20 minutes. Tell the client to use prep sets on all real spasms. As part of the call, instruct the client to inform the person about prep sets and demonstrate various types of fake prep sets.
5. Ask the client to update his or her fear hierarchy list (see if any levels have changed). Over the next 5 days, have client enter 1 situation each day from the low end of the scale, 1 a day from the middle range, and 1 situation from the high-stress levels each day (15 situations total). Tell client to use a pullout on real spasms and report on the effect of stress levels and overall performance.
6. Give the client a list of problems that occur with prep sets. Have him or her sit down and rate himself or herself on each problem area. On any "weak" or "poor" ratings, ask the client to develop at least one

suggestion for improving that rating. On "good" ratings, ask the client to explain that rating.

7. Set up any situation of outside speech and use of prep sets. On any missed or "poor" prep sets, have client effectively cancel the word, using the disfluency mode he or she should have succeeded with earlier. Ensure assignment covers an adequate number of speech situations.

8. Assign solo, unsupervised practice. Have client take any reading passage and underline ___20 ___40 ___60 words. Instruct the client to read the passage aloud and record. For each underlined word, tell the client to slow down on the three words prior, pause for relaxation, and then fake a prep set. Have client evaluate.

9. Ask the client to select 2 situations from the ___ top 10 or the ___ top 20 of his or her fear hierarchy list; select ___10 or ___20 situations from the middle range of the list; and select ___20 or ___30 situations from the low range of the list. Starting with the low-range work, have client work through all of the 32 to 52 situations as quickly as possible, taking as many days as needed. Instruct client to use a pullout on all spasms, and keep a report to analyze misses or failures.

10. Request that client compile a list of troubles experienced with prep sets and separate them into tension, anxiety, rush, late start, poor disfluency, or other categories. Have client think about remedies and discuss them at next therapy session.

11. Ask client to read a newspaper aloud for 3 or 4 minutes each day. Tell client to fake a prep set about every 15 seconds (12 to 16 in 3 to 4 minutes).

12. Have the client pick at least three time periods a day, each lasting for 30 minutes, when he or she is likely to be talking to people. During each period, ask the client to cancel every prep set that is missed or failed.

SUMMARY

Cancellation, pullout, and preparatory set extend back over 50 years and then some. As I stated earlier, this presentation assumes a client will be doing all three in the learning sequence stipulated. This approach is not necessary. Each technique can be used for specific and isolated purposes.

All or some of the techniques can be integrated into fluency reinforcement sequences. Each or all three can be used as a repair or recovery strategy where some other program has left unresolved issues. These techniques require a clinician who is self-confident, credible, and competent.

REFERENCES

Bloodstein, O. (1993). *Stuttering: The search for a cause and cure*. Boston: Allyn & Bacon.

Bloodstein, O. (1995). *A handbook on stuttering*. San Diego, CA: Singular Publishing Group.

Bluemel, C.L. (1957). *The riddle of stuttering*. Danville, IL: Interstate Publishers.

Culatta, R.E., & Goldberg, S.A. (1995). *Stuttering therapy, an integrated approach to theory and practice*. Boston: Allyn & Bacon.

Dell, C.W., Jr. (1993). Treating school-age stutterers. In R.F. Curlee (Ed.), *Stuttering and related disorders of fluency*. New York: Thieme Medical Publications.

Freund, H. (1966). *Psychotherapy and the problem of stuttering*. Springfield, IL: Charles C Thomas.

Gregory, H., & Hill, D. (1993). Differential evaluation—differential therapy for stuttering. In R.F. Curlee (Ed.), *Stuttering and related disorders of fluency*. New York: Thieme Medical Publications.

Ham, R.E. (1986). *Techniques of stuttering therapy*. Englewood Cliffs, NJ: Prentice Hall.

Luper, H.L., & Mulder, R.L. (1964). *Stuttering therapy for children*. Englewood Cliffs, NJ: Prentice Hall.

Peters, T.J., & Guitar, B. (1991). *Stuttering, an integrated approach to its nature and treatment*. Baltimore: Williams & Wilkins.

Prins, D. (1993). Treatment of adults: Managing stuttering. In R.F. Curlee & W.H. Perkins (Eds.), *Nature and treatment of stuttering: New directions*. San Diego, CA: College-Hill Press.

Ryan, B.P. (1971). Operant procedures applied to stuttering therapy for children. *Journal of Speech and Hearing Disorders, 36*, 264–280.

Shames, G.R., & Egolf, D.B. (1976). *Operant conditioning and the management of stuttering*. Englewood Cliffs, NJ: Prentice Hall.

Silverman, F.H. (1996). *Stuttering and other fluency disorders* (2nd ed.). Boston: Allyn & Bacon.

Stuttering Foundation of America. (1993). *Self-therapy for the stutterer* (3rd. ed., publication 12). Memphis, TN: Author.

Van Riper, C. (1958). Experiments in stuttering therapy. In J. Eisenson (Ed.), *Stuttering, a symposium*. New York: Harper & Row.

Van Riper, C. (1971). Symptomatic therapy for stuttering. In L.E. Travis (Ed.), *Handbook of speech pathology*. New York: Appleton-Century-Crofts.

Van Riper, C. (1973). *The treatment of stuttering*. Englewood Cliffs, NJ: Prentice Hall.

Wingate, M.E. (1976). *Stuttering therapy and treatment.* New York: Distributed by Halstead Press, Division of John Wiley & Sons.

Yonovitz, A., Shepherd, W.F., & Garrett, S. (1977). Hierarchical stimulation: Two cases of of stuttering modification using systematic desensitization. *Journal of Fluency Disorders, 2,* 21–28.

CHAPTER 9

Transfer and Maintenance

- Overview
- Transfer Aspects
- Maintenance
- Support Groups
- Summary

OVERVIEW

A few years ago I read a pronouncement by a doctoral-degree speech-language pathologist (SLP) working in the area of fluency disorders. That SLP said the clinician's responsibility is to show the client how to change his or her behavior. What happened after that was up to the client. The clinician's work was done. In contrast, the supervisor of my first graduate clinical experience instructed me:

> I want you out with him 5 days a week after clinic, running assignments. Have him over to your place for dinner every week. Have him call you three or four times a week. About once a month spend some weekend time together, working on whatever is current.

When the scheduled clinical program terminated, the supervisor retained about one third of the client group for several months of additional transfer and shift-to-maintenance work.

The contrast between the two management philosophies is glaring. I cannot accept the first point of view, but also recognize the impracticality of the second. There can be, however, some degree of balance. In the following discussion on transfer and maintenance I offer suggestions concerning both. Some will not fit the situations of many clinicians. Hopefully, other situations will be both useful and practicable. Because this chapter cuts across diverse areas (preschool, early school, adolescent, adult), I recommend a work by Caruso (1997). It devotes approximately 100 pages to a discussion of stuttering therapy adjuncts, including parents, school settings, group therapy, spouses, employment locations, and support groups. It contains many stimulating, thought-provoking, and useful areas of information.

As far as transfer and maintenance are concerned, therapy of stuttering can be divided into two age levels: child and adult. The *child* category covers the earliest onset age to about 8 or 9 years. It could cut off much earlier, or run a little later. The *adult* level starts at about adolescence (early) and runs into the true adult level. My discussion of transfer and maintenance at the child level starts with the home environment and ends with school settings. The discussion of the adult level overlaps with school settings. The discussion of schools is minimized because every school system has different administrative systems, every state has different criteria, and so on. Moreover, my observation of outcomes strongly suggests that the schools often are not the location where therapy outcomes meet desires or expectations.

TRANSFER ASPECTS

Achieving out-clinic performance that parallels in-clinic learning and practice is the major goal of all therapies, fluency included. This target is called many things—transfer, carryover, generalization, and so on. Properly speaking, I feel that transfer occurs when the client learns to do something in the clinic and then deliberately (consciously) tries to do the same thing on an out-clinic basis. Generalization is when a newly learned skill is left to "percolate" out of the clinic and into daily life. Silverman (1996) stated that transfer performance can occur in two structures or forms, stimulus generalization and response generalization. In *stimulus generalization* the clinician trains the client to respond to a particular stimulus, and then to extend that response to stimuli (people, situations) that are similar, but not identical, to the original stimulus. *Response generalization* is when the response to the same stimulus is altered so that the client finally can retain a level of performance without deliberately monitoring behavioral output.

Elements of Transfer

In young children, transfer may be completely spontaneous, but it always is wiser to assume that spontaneity does better when stimulated, guided, and supported. Overall, I see transfer as falling into three major phases:

- *Phase I: Foundations of Transfer.* The phase in which the concept or idea that transfer should occur is established. The initiation of motivation and methods to facilitate later shifts fluency reinforcement or symptom modification methods away from the clinic therapy sessions.
- *Phase II: Commitment to Responsibility.* The phase in which the client accepts the idea that it is the client—not the clinician—who is the person that will make things change. This process involves the actual control system steps and the steps required to support acquisition of the necessary transfer skills.
- *Phase III: Development of Self-Therapy Capacity.* The phase in which responsibility from Phase II becomes self-direction, self-evaluation, and self-consequation. It leads the client, prepared appropriately, into maintenance.

The three phases are not consistently sequential, and early Phase III foundation aspects can be found in Phase I, and Phase I work can be applied in Phases II and III. In my discussions I do not force items into phases. Instead, the discussions are organized around the child and adult age levels.

Early Transfer Levels

For children or adults, transfer starts with the diagnosis and evaluation session, especially if the diagnostician and subsequent therapist are the same, or if both activities occur within the structure of the same institution. When the client or significant other is subjected to probing questions in the interview, answers questions that are asked, or performs various tests or tasks, he or she is exposed to stimuli that can effect changes, or at least stimulate thought, even before formal therapy begins. The transfer effect may be minimal for several reasons. Most of the transfer activities that are important for older children and adults are either absent from young-child settings, or are shifted to the significant others in the environment. Any transfer effect is likely to be indirect. To a certain extent, young clients will generalize without direct transfer activities or assignments (such children always make me wonder if I have been dealing with a *dis*fluent rather than *dys*fluent child). However, in this discussion, I assume that all clients need direct transfer work. Suggestions for the parents of early childhood clients include, but are not limited to, the items mentioned below.

Diagnostic counseling, when results and recommendations are shared, is a good time to begin the first steps in transfer work. These steps then would extend into regular therapy counseling.

- Bibliotherapy—clinician's personal material, paragraphs from texts, copies or order forms from the Stuttering Foundation of America. Titles include *Stuttering and Your Child: A Videotape for Parents; If Your Child Stutters: A Guide for Parents; Stuttering Therapy: Prevention and Intervention with Parents; Prevention of Stuttering: Part I, Identifying Danger Signs*; and *Prevention of Stuttering: Part II, Family Counseling.*
- Home Analysis—assignments can be made before the first therapy session to start parents working on the pattern of activities discussed later in this section (e.g., data collection, environmental evaluation, and so on).
- Scheduled Meetings—meetings of significant others that can be one-on-one or group. Meetings follow a set schedule and agenda, but can take several forms:
  - *special need*—meetings to address particular problems that require special attention. Special needs include concomitant intellectual impairment in the client, cerebral palsy, hostile parents, divorcing parents, new foster home placement, and emotional trauma suspected as an etiology.

– *informational*—more or less routine meetings intended to familiarize new parents with topics such as what is going to happen in therapy and their role, general education about stuttering, and how specific questions and concerns will be addressed. Informational meetings usually can be completed in one to three sessions, either in the first few weeks of therapy, or deliberately spaced apart for special effects.

- Data Collection—this effort can be merged into the meetings cited above, or followed as a separate target, depending on the characteristics of the family and the severity of the child's stuttering problem.
- Skill Meetings—special sessions that lay the foundation for later transfer work. The meetings basically involve teaching specific skills to significant others. Meetings can cover some areas of data collection, but usually involve teaching speech modeling, fluency modes such as Easy Onset, or other specific activities for out-clinc transfer later on.

The next to last item, data collection, can be minimal or extensive. It generally is done for one or more of five reasons: (1) to obtain the information indicated; (2) to develop awareness and accurate monitoring habits by the auditors; (3) to desensitize, to whatever degree needed, significant others to the anxiety, stress, and irritation they have felt about the child's problem; (4) to help resolve any guilt feelings; and (5) to make significant others feel they are part of the out-clinic and in-clinic programs, not just passive observers. Examples of data collection include

- Start observing on Monday, Wednesday, and Friday. Sample speech for breaks, three times a day, for about 5 minutes each time. For each 5-minute period, rate the overall speech breaks as being many, some, few, or none. At the end of the rating day, stop and try to see if there were any common situational factors that separated "many" from "few." Next week, check on Tuesday, Thursday, and Saturday. Analyze again. What are you finding out?
- Pick one situation each day when your child talks for about 3 minutes (total). How many stutters were there? How did they separate into _____ repetitions, _____ prolongations, and _____ stoppages?
- Observe child interacting with different family members. After 4 or 5 days, come up with a pretty good evaluation of child's speech level (how much or how little trouble) with each person.

- Every day, for 5 days, rate every different speaking situation you have with the child, in terms of ___ little or no trouble, ___ some trouble, and ___ lots of trouble. If there is variation from situation to situation, what are the potential reasons?
- For the next week, just observe yourself and other adult family members (or close friends) when the child is around. At the end of the week, rate each person on the following items. Who is, overall, the
  –fastest talker?
  –loudest talker?
  –poorest listener?
  –biggest interrupter?
  –biggest arguer?
  –user of the biggest, longest words?

The clinician can make endless additions to the list and devise particular data collection assignments for individuals. Again, these are not direct transfer assignments, but they prepare the way.

Later Transfer Levels

- Parental Support and Input Sessions—This involves individual or group meetings of parents for sharing, release, and problem solving. These sessions can be individual but function best when organized as a group of parents and others. At first, it may be best to start the series along information-giving lines (e.g., discussing bibliotherapy materials, videotapes, etc). Discussion should not focus on any individual child unless a significant other brings something up and wants to discuss it. Informational support groups can coalesce, function, and disband in a matter of weeks. Some groups will want much more. These sessions can become an ongoing transfer aid and ultimately shift to value provision in maintenance, if needed. They also can help new enrollees and provide useful access to area groups and local schools.
- Parental Guilt Feelings—Feelings of guilt in the idea that any problem must be the fault of the parent can be a significant part of transfer work. Possible (and probable) guilt feelings are common. Counseling, informational meetings, data collection, and so forth open venues for significant others that are new or that were avoided previously. Logan and Caruso (1997) present an excellent discussion, pointing out that

information disclosures about stuttering and clinic encouragement to "get involved" may create parental guilt feelings because they "did not do anything" in the past. Recognizing that guilt feelings exist and that therapy can cause them can be important. A frequent self-reaction to unresolved guilt is directed hostility toward whomever causes the guilt feeling. I have had parents tell me that certain information was "none of my business," that they were as good as any other parents, and so on. The clinician should look early for signs of guilt, defuse it, and tread warily thereafter.

- Use of Labels—Terms used to identify the fluency problem can be negative and embarrassing. This problem is usually minor, but in this day of political correctness, it can become a major issue. Although the psychosemantic accuracy of words such as spasm, stuttering, and so on is important, I let the consumer be the arbiter, as long as no self-lie is involved. If euphemisms are important to the parent or the client, I go along. Then I watch to see, as maturation occurs, whether there is a shift toward accurate terminology.

- Therapy Observation—Opportunities for parents and significant others to observe therapy sessions with the child should be presented. Observation is related to several concepts presented later. I favor arranging things so that significant others can observe therapy, but not carte blanche. It helps parents understand what the clinican does, and what is supposed to happen. For later parental activities, such as speech modeling, observation is almost mandatory. It alerts the parents as to what can be expected on an out-clinic basis, forms of stimulation that work best, reminders and how to use them, models for positive reinforcement, and so on.

- Therapy Interest—Over time, parents can become bored with therapy cycles. This concept is linked to therapy observation. I recommend that clinicians try to interest parents in the therapy, give them reading material, and encourage them to ask questions. I like to ask parents whether they could carry out a specific method at home or whether there are things they would change about a method if practiced at home.

- Special Data Collection—Directing parents' attention to more subtle or complex aspects of therapy activity data collection, in general, was discussed earlier. This item involves relating data to what is going on currently in therapy.

In the session today, did you notice that I moved from one- to two-syllable words? At home, would you listen to see if ___ has more trouble on his (her) longer words?"

- Therapy Interaction—This is when one or more parent actually participates during in-clinic therapy. Sometimes it is a mistake, as when a parent spanked her child each time he committed an error in his home practice activity. I found out when the child made an error in the clinic, burst into tears, and begged not to be spanked. Most of the time, the clinician is the model the parent emulates, including penalty.

- Environmental Counseling—Interacting with in-clinic therapy increases transfer, and usually eliminates negative responses; counseling significant others in the child's environment part of the transfer process is to manipulate the child's environment so that in-clinic behaviors are supported outside the clinic. Manipulation can range from simple factors of adequate rest, balanced nutrition, and good health to more communication-centered activities, such as time shares on speech so the child is given clear opportunities to talk, good listening behavior (on both sides), periods of reading to the child, shared television program watching, and interactive questions and comments.

- Resolution of Stress—Identifying environmental trouble points and removing or reducing them will reduce stress. Stress at home or outside the home can be looked for in several areas:
  - speech activity—relationship between fluency breaks and speech pressures
  - child interactions—environmental aspects of the child's life that induce stress
  - general stress—stress or conflict in general family life (e.g., marital problems, vocational crises for either parent, family tragedies, etc.)

  The clinician will want to intervene and manipulate directly in the first category above (speech activity). The other areas can involve clinician expressions of concern and suggestions directed at the significant others, recommending amelioration or elimination of the problems.

- Speech Models—When asking parents to be good speech models, the clinician must set out specific instructions, simplify the process, lower demand levels, do a lot of modeling, and let the parent observe it in use (e.g., in therapy work, or even join a therapy session to have the client "teach your mother what you can do").

- Desensitization—This is the reduction of client sensitivity, or parent sensitivity, to stuttering. In this context, the concept refers to the parental oversensitivity issue, communicated to the child. Often, a "don't ask/don't tell" accord exists, where each party pretends nothing is happening. My philosophy is to try and break this accord down. I suggest to the parents that, after every session, they ask the child to discuss the session, what was done, how things are going, and so on. I may prime the child (in therapy) to assist in this discussion. As parents learn from bibliotherapy or information sharing, they can do limited return sharing (do not overdo it; parents talk too much anyway). If the parent is progressively involved, desensitization (and transfer in general) is facilitated.

- Reinforcement—Positive, tangible responses to successful efforts are important principles for everybody, but especially for children that should transfer. I have never been convinced that 100% positive reinforcement is absolutely necessary in most cases (and in some clients, I question the wisdom). However, after being taught by the authorities in the field that tangible rewards were "bribes" and should never be used, I watched with amusement as the early bribes became positive reinforcement and exemplified the best of therapy. Some clients may receive penalty at home or, more likely, apathy. Some adults will actually need instruction and rehearsal in positive reinforcement behavior and suggestions for at-home schedules.

- School Settings—Where the child is enrolled in public or private schools, the early school years start a shift on many aspects of child activities and interests away from the home. Accordingly, transfer considerations will have to take this environmental addition into planning considerations. Opportunities to work with parents and the home may become limited in several ways:
  - Progressive psychological separation from the home (both sides)
  - The addition of a school-based environment in the child's life with group structure, public events, public recitation, and so on
  - Clinician's caseload mandates and selection and scheduling problems; reduction of therapy to time limits and legal requirements; periodic interruptions due to the school calendar.

  Transfer will change in school settings compared with preschool areas. Although the child's dysfluency patterns still will resemble earlier ones, struggles, avoidances, and emotional reactions will progressively complicate issues. For that reason, this section will be fairly brief. With some repetition, preliminary stages of therapy may include:

- bibliotherapy on two levels. The more sophisticated material (see earlier in this chapter) can still be used with home settings, classroom teachers, school counselors, and special education personnel. A simpler level of material could be presented to some clients. They can be rehearsed to transmit information to their classes, to friends, and home to the family.
- home assignments, or homework, should occur with the very first session, and every session should have two assignment categories: school and home. Because of the usual time constraints, the assignments should be short and simple.
- stress hierarchy. For young stutterers, use of the simple procedure of stress hierarchy development presented in chapters 3 and 4 is suggested. The hierarchy can be used to plan assignments, talk about problems, and so forth.
- class transfer. The clinician should contact the teacher and determine how and when the client can perform in class, what class counseling is needed, whether the clinician can visit and interact, and so on.
- targets. The client should review and prioritize targets (with the clinician's help) that he or she would like to work on first outside of therapy sessions, whether in-clinic role play rehearsal will help, if other group members can help, and whether class would be the best place to start.

Adolescent/Adult Transfer

Settings here will vary among high school, college, private life, special summer programs, average private therapy, and some self-therapy programs. The discussion focuses less on specifics, although some will be offered at times.

Commitment to Transfer

The concept of therapy commitment begins with the diagnosis—the client came for help; that constitutes a first-stage commitment. The clinician should secure client agreement with, and commitment to, the therapy plan in the first few therapy sessions. In the same way, commitment to transfer is valued. It can be the hardest commitment to obtain, and even harder to maintain. Transfer takes time to do and must be done every day. The client must understand the daily commitment, cognitively; accept the daily commitment, emotionally; and overtly express both commitments and agree to them.

Transfer Targets

When a commitment has been made, or is developing, a useful activity is to expand the commitment and begin delineation of the therapy plan. It can be done by the specification of transfer targets. These targets can be both general and specific. Some examples follow. An "etc." should be attached to the ending of each example.

- Broaden my knowledge about communication and stuttering: Read material supplied by the clinician and respond to questions and discussion. Read Murray's (undated) *A Stutterer's Story* or an equivalent autobiography.
- Study and analyze my speech outside the clinic: Monitor for awareness of specific spasm types, severities, durations, avoidances, and so on. Monitor for eye contact in general and when I stutter. Monitor for situational effects on my speech, and my situational avoidances. Learn to watch and analyze my auditors.
- Reduce or eliminate avoidances: Eliminate word-specific and communication-general avoidances. Recognize specific people, particular situations, and opportunities that increase avoidance behavior.
- Learn to pseudostutter: Carry out basic solo practice. Be able to duplicate my own patterns. Be able to "stutter" differently. Use fake to practice symptom control methods. Use faking to desensitize myself and build up tolerance. Use faking to help practice fluency modes of control. Set up for later maintenance use.
- Work on desensitization: Fulfill prior bibliotherapy commitments; work on self-analysis, avoidance reduction, and pseudostuttering. Discuss my speech and my therapy with significant others in my environment. Become able to approach and talk with strangers. Be able to use the telephone any time, and frequently.
- Practice fluency or symptom controls: Be willing, and become able, to use "safe" rates, Easy Onset levels, or other fluency or symptom

modes periodically to show that I transferred them and call on them if "preferred" modes slip. Commit to daily practice in either a set number of situations or for a set time period—whether or not there is real stuttering.

- Collect data: Perform simple counting assignments (e.g., counting the number of spasms in a set period of time) and periodic reassessment. Able to keep daily diaries or weekly summaries on certain aspects of therapy. Maintain a transfer summary sheet that quantifies data, such as difficulty level of assignments, percentage done or not done, and degree of adequacy on performances.

Many targets can be set, but do not overdo it, especially early in therapy. As the client progresses toward dismissal and phase-out, it will be appropriate to devote most of the later therapy sessions to review transfer work, problem solve, and plan for continued transfer activities.

Outside Support

One of the frustrating aspects of working with college-level and high-school stutterers on transfer involves external support systems. Many college students do not live at home, and roommates rarely are good support vehicles. Fraternities, sororities, dorm groups, and campus social groups generally make poor support groups. High school students may be in a better situation. They also may be in a much worse situation if there are serious disagreements, confrontations, and negative interactions at home.

The following suggestions are offered:

- *education*. Work with the client to try and stimulate interest in his or her therapy specifically, or even an interest in stuttering in general. If feasible, and agreeable, invite significant others from the client's background to sit in on therapy sessions. Have the client borrow audiotapes or videotapes of therapy (especially as fluency modes or symptom controls take effect) to bring home for significant others.
- *therapy simulation*. Have one or more persons available and willing to help with outside assignments. Use them to count spasms or, over time, to evaluate. Furnish education and training as required.
- *reminders*. Negotiate with, and gain full approval of all participants, to remind the client when he or she is not using transfer activities, failed in an effort, and so on.

Reinforcement

Transfer work, like any work, can become boring. It also can become frustrating and irritating, threatening and anxiety provoking, and sloppy and careless. Such possibilities should be discussed with the client, and a reinforcement system should be developed. The clinician, of course, represents the strongest reinforcement system. For adolescents, it may be possible to involve parents. Spouses can involve the other spouse. Reinforcements can be either positive or negative. Regardless of the mode used, the clinician needs to be on guard for manipulative clients. Some possible variations in reinforcement are:

- Keep a point or token score and award a specified number of points or tokens for each desired behavior. Develop a schedule specifying how many points or tokens will earn a particular reward.
- For a specific performance type, set maximum and minimum targets (i.e., if the client goes above the criterion he or she earns a tangible positive reinforcement, if he or she falls between the minimum and the maximum he or she earns a verbal positive reinforcement, and if he or she falls below the minimum criterion a negative reinforcement is applied).
- Have an automatic penalty for every failure to do or complete a transfer assignment when there is no acceptable excuse.
- Build in the capability to earn periodic release from transfer work (e.g., performing adequately for 3 days consecutively earns a 4th day off or successful use of a desired behavior yields a reduction in the number of repetitions in an exercise).

Pseudostuttering

Pseudostuttering in transfer will not be useful to SLPs who do not believe in pseudostuttering in the first place. Nevertheless, I believe faking can be of value in transfer, whether therapy is symptom oriented or fluency based. Pseudostuttering facilitates transfer in several ways:

- Solo home practice enables the client to imitate the usual stuttering pattern for the purposes of continued desensitization, self-monitoring practice, and self-evaluation practice.

- Solo home practice allows the client to learn variations and modification possibilities of existing stuttering patterns.
- Solo home practice lets the client rehearse any or all of the symptom controls in chapter 8.
- Practice allows client to shift pseudostuttering into desired fluency reinforcement modes.
- Practice, as indicated earlier, facilitates desensitization and avoidance control.

Pseudostuttering is a complex motor skill (see chapter 2) that also carries an emotional valence, sometimes a rather strong one. Faking will lose accuracy, realism, and coordination if it is not used outside clinic settings or clinic-controlled situations. Periodic, or even occasional, transfer use will keep the motor codes and switching patterns fresh. Also, failure to use faking in a transfer mode allows desensitization to deteriorate so that the longer faking is not used, the harder it becomes to use it.

Desensitization

Sensitivity reduction has been referred to many times previously, so comments here will be brief. Many clients will engage, albeit unenthusiastically, in sensitivity reduction activity when in the clinic and when under out-clinic supervision. However, they may be reluctant to carry out transfer assignments on a solo basis. The degree to which this reluctance occurs is probably a fair measure or estimate of later relapse probabilities. What the client is reluctant to do alone, while still enrolled in therapy, she or he almost certainly will fail to do (or do poorly) later on in maintenance.

Avoidances

Transfer practice on avoidance reduction is one of the early out-clinic steps in which the client begins to take control of therapy. Although the earlier steps of monitoring and self-analysis are necessary and valuable, avoidance reduction occurs when the client recognizes his or her ability to change speech. That capacity, and client willingness, will be significant throughout transfer and into maintenance work.

Fluency and Symptom Controls

Obviously, the most significant aspect of transfer for the client is taking control modes (fluency or symptom) that have been learned in clinic and being able to use them independently. The surprising, and depressing, situation here is how often the client becomes an expert with a technique in the therapy room, but just does not get around to external transfer for a variety of reasons.

Thorough inculcation with the transfer ethic from the time of the first therapy session is a prerequisite to control methods transfer. By the time symptom or fluency methods are approached, the client should have received, performed, and reported on dozens of transfer assignments. In the control mode stages of therapy, transfer projects should be a continuation of ongoing patterns of client self-efficacy.

The control modes may be Easy Onset, cancellation, slowed rate, prolongation, pullouts, and so forth. Most of those methods have early grosser stages (check the appropriate chapters). Easy Onset, for example, usually starts with very breathy, prolonged /h/ + vowel. Transfer work at home should do the same. Assignments also should combine progressive improvements in self-monitoring and evaluation with changes in the neuromotor control of the mode being worked on. Self-consequation should be added very early. The transfer goal, early on, is not for public use of these early stages. However, the client should have extensive transfer practice in the foundation basics of the target mode, in case she or he finds a future need to return to basics for some self-therapy when there is no easily available clinic.

When more advanced stages are reached, transfer continues. Many clients do not believe they can survive outside the clinic, and progressive transfer counters the lack of self-efficacy feeling. The rule for this, and all levels of control skills in other performance areas, are:

- Never assign transfer work in an area where the client has not already shown a repeated, consistent ability to meet basic performance requirements.
- Give transfer work assignments that have a very high probability of success.
- Review, analyze, discuss, and problem solve all transfer assignments in speech control modes (when performed).

These rules reiterate the rules laid down in chapter 2. The clinician should be monitoring closely to respond to the following problems or questions:

- Is the client showing fairly consistent adequacy in transfer work? If not, where is the problem and what should be done about it?
- Is the client showing adequacy in the specific skill or ability that is being transferred? If not, where are the problems?
  - Client self-efficacy; need for support?
  - Client not trying hard enough? Cursory efforts?
  - Client trying too hard? Too rushed and tense?
  - Client having trouble on specific words or sounds, with specific people, situations, or other problems?

Fear Hierarchy

Fear or stress hierarchy factors were presented in chapter 1, emphasized in chapter 4, and mentioned in almost all other chapters. The transfer (and maintenance) chapter is no exception. Simple, incomplete stress hierarchies can serve as starting points early in therapy for transfer work. As therapy progresses, the fear hierarchy can be refined and many of the rankings may be lowered. Transfer practice should "push the envelope" on fear and stress, but not to the extent that fear and stress override other advances or damage self-efficacy. The long-term results should be worth the time spent in discussing, drawing up, and revising the hierarchy.

MAINTENANCE

For generations, maintenance did not occur regularly in the therapy of stuttering. Although a few professionals implemented wise and extensive postdismissal programs, many did not. This omission finally received critical attention after the explosive growth of fluency reinforcement programs in the early 1970s. Therapy that used to be scheduled for 18 months to 3 years was completed quickly. The crash landings of relapses back into stuttering skyrocketed.

In 1979, relapses had become so noticeable that there was an international meeting on fluency disorders in Banff, Canada. Van Riper (1978/79) published an open letter in which he not very gently "congratulated" the operant conditioning enthusiasts and fluency reinforcement proponents for admitting that they faced some serious problems in terms of relapse and maintenance. Silverman (1996), almost 20 years after the Banff conference, reached the conclusion that relapse continues to be a significant problem. Eliminating young children from recovery counts, he estimated the relapse rate at over 50%.

Bloodstein (1995) discussed relapse, noting that concentrated attention was not directed at it until approximately the late 1970s. I believe the attention resulted from experiences with fluency reinforcement therapy. First, those workers tended to keep better data and use more follow-up checks than symptom clinicians. Second, fluency reinforcement clients may have tended to reach higher levels of fluency than often occurred in symptom therapy so that relapses, if they occurred, were bigger failures. Third, the time invested in fluency therapy often was much less than the traditional schedule for symptom therapy, so that clients had less time to stabilize progress. Fourth, the fluency therapies did not always address avoidances, fears, self-efficacy limitations—all which seem to be vital in maintenance. The relapses from fluency therapy results often contrasted sharply with the "stutter better" (sarcastic term used by some to describe symptom therapy results) results of symptom therapy. Because fluency therapy might, initially, provide "better" fluency, the falls from it were more painful than any relapses that occurred after symptom therapy.

I will discuss maintenance programs from the adolescent and adult client point of view. Some may assume that children do not need formal planning in that direction. Conture (1996) found that a 6-month recheck on dismissed children indicated that not all clients were adequately provided for in terms of catching relapse problems. He described a 30-week maintenance sequence where, in the first 10 weeks, the child attends therapy twice a month, reducing visits progressively over the subsequent 10-week blocks of time. Cooper and Cooper (1985), in their therapy program package, provide suggestions for postdismissal follow-up in school settings. Peters and Guitar (1991) provide a very detailed therapy plan for children, including transfer and maintenance procedures.

Elements Favoring Relapse

It may be feasible to forestall relapse, or at least to reinforce the switch to maintenance, by watching for or countering several factors favoring relapse. The factors are as follows:

- *premature termination of therapy.* The client may tire of therapy, money may become a problem, time availability can be troublesome, significant others can shift against continuance, and so on. The client and clinician may be able to verbally resolve some problems. Other approaches include scheduling a "vacation" from therapy, reducing the frequency of sessions, or agreeing to change certain aspects of therapy procedures.
- *ineffective transfer program.* This factor is 100% the fault of the clinician for having gotten this far. If the clinician had advised the client, early on, that transfer work was not satisfactory, then there would be less fault assigned to the clinician, but not exculpation. The clinician must sit down with the client and reconfigure the maintenance calendar schedule, if the client is willing to invest the additional time.
- *lack of support.* Significant others may fail to support maintenance and may have undercut therapy and transfer (especially transfer) all along. They may have been disturbed by the changes that have occurred in the client during therapy. The best approach is to be open with the client about the problem and arrange maintenance work to bypass the problem as much as possible. It is the client's problem to solve.
- *new complications.* Anything from illness, family crisis, bereavement, new job or loss of job, failure in school, and so on can complicate the situation. The clinician never knows when events will put prior goals out of reach or create new situations. In most cases, the clinician can suggest a "let's see" attitude and then help the client replan maintenance on a different schedule or with changes in form.

Maintenance programs are not immutable. They can be changed and still function effectively. Except for their general structure, maintenance programs should not be cloned from client to client.

Assessment of Maintenance Needs

Rather than telling the client that he or she needs a particular form of maintenance, it is better to guide the client in evaluating his or her own needs and solutions. A useful instrument in doing this is Silverman's (1980) Stuttering Problem Profile. It contains 86 "how am I" statements about breathing, avoidances, attitudes, and so on. Additional statements can be added for individuals (e.g., "I no longer worry about asking questions in math class"). As a corollary, or replacement, for Silverman's list, I have added a short version (Exhibit 9–1) as an example of what might be tailored to an individual client. These questions would encompass a session (or more) of therapy for the clinician and client to go over each item separately. Discussion would focus on how answers affect readiness for maintenance, or whether further work may be needed before the separation process begins. The client should be encouraged to add items of her or his own.

Scheduling Maintenance

Maintenance should not be allowed to just happen. It should proceed according to a schedule. The client should go over the schedule, accept or renegotiate components, and then commit herself or himself to it. The style of schedule is open to interpretation. Some programs provide audiotape mail-ins for review and advice; motivation and reminder stickers for message boards, mirrors, and so on; scheduled telephone calls to or from the clinic; secret checkups (the client knows they will occur, but not when or how). Some programs are scheduled by weeks, some by months, and some are set for a period of years. Where many clients will ultimately be itinerant (as in schools), directed maintenance may be futile. Once the program is laid out and the client departs, that may be the end of it, subject to the client's motivation and capacity.

In trying to propose one possible model I will hypothesize a two-sessions-per-week therapy history over the course of 6 months to 3 years. Sessions are one on one, although infrequent group work may occur. A formal maintenance schedule of 3 years is assumed for adolescent and adult clients. Actual duration will be affected by myriad factors.

- *Step 1.* Reduce the present, twice-weekly schedule to once a week, for about 6 weeks (approximate). Devote nearly every session entirely to preparation for client independence, problem solving, role play rehearsals, and supervised out-clinic practice. Prepare client for Step 2 in the last session of this step.
- *Step 2.* Reduce session frequency to one meeting every 2 weeks, for about 3 months (Steps 1 and 2 total about 18 to 20 weeks). In this 3-

Exhibit 9–1 Maintenance assessment questions

1. In general terms, what causes stuttering?
2. When most people use the term "stuttering," what are they talking about?
3. When you use the term stuttering about yourself, what are you talking about?
4. What are the stages of therapy you have gone through here? For each stage named, describe what was done and the rationale for doing it. How well did you do in each?
   ___I met criteria 100%.
   ___I met the basic, minimum level.
   ___I did some of it, and then moved on.
5. Using the stages identified in Question 4, what would your performance be, right now, if you were asked to meet the criteria of each stage all over again?
   ___I'd be as good as I ever was.
   ___I'd come up to par after a little review.
   ___I would need some hard work to get back.
   ___I'd really have to start all over again on that item.
6. How consistent, and reliable, has your transfer work been? (If necessary, divide your assessment by the stages or phases of therapy involved.)
   ___Transfer performance on this phase was close to 100%.
   ___Transfer performance on this phase was good most of time.
   ___Transfer performance on this phase was fair.
   ___Transfer performance on this phase was weak, or worse.
7. How would you rate yourself on each of the following items (add items if needed)?

Item	Good	Fair	Poor
Self-monitoring			
Self-analysis			
Eye contact			
Avoidance reduction			

continues

Exhibit 9–1 continued

Willingness to stutter

Self-direction

Other

8. When asked for reports on home assignments, what was your completion record? How well were assignments done?
9. How much have you changed from the first days of therapy on the following items?

Item	Large Increase	Increase	Little
Amount of talking			
Situations you enter			
People you approach			
Self-confidence about talking			
Self-confidence about control			

10. How would your best friend compare your speech "then and now"?
11. During the last 25% to 30% of your past therapy sessions, what has been your responsibility for evaluation and consequation in activities?
    ___90%–100% ___60%–90% ___40%–60% ___Below 40%
12. How often have you actually originated and/or planned therapy activities over the past 10 or 12 therapy sessions?

Item	Rarely, Never	Occasionally	Often
In-clinic work			
Out-clinic practice			
Solo transfer			

13. Do you have any concerns about the maintenance phase?

month period, have the client fill out a simple daily record or diary at the end of each day. (Exhibit 9–2 offers a suggested structure.) Focus therapy sessions on discussion of daily record; problem solve and reinforce efforts as indicated. Give client new copy of form as each page only covers a 2-week period.

- *Step 3.* Drop session frequency to one meeting per month, for about 6 months (Steps 1, 2, and 3 total about 42 to 50 weeks). Have client complete Exhibit 9–3. This exhibit is a shortened or compressed version of Exhibit 9–2 (where Exhibit 9–2 asked for a biweekly summary based on daily data, Exhibit 9–3 asks for a 4-week summary, divided into two 2-week intervals). In the meeting referred to in Step 1 the client is told to watch for relapse signs. If relapse signs are detected, the client may do one of two things:
  – call the clinic for advice and direction, or
  – drop back to daily self-monitoring and evaluation until stability returns

  Use scheduled clinic meeting to review, report, and perform any problem solving needed. Retain some time, however, for a few supervised out-clinic performance checks.

- *Step 4.* Drop session frequency to one meeting every 3 months for 1 year (Steps 1 through 4 now total about 94 to 105 weeks). Use Exhibit 9–4 for this step (asks for a 3-month summary, divided into 1-month intervals). Organize meetings for this step as in preceding steps. Consider suggesting support groups as some clients who earlier rejected this idea may have found enough fluency slippage to concern them and would be interested in having help with their goals and efforts.

- *Step 5.* Drop session frequency to two meetings (once every 6 months for 1 year). Arrange the agenda or any report formats by clinician-client agreement.

A consistent aid to the client, if it was used during in-clinic therapy, is the Stuttering Foundation of America (1993) publication *Self-Therapy for the Stutterer*. This publication can be of continuing use and inspiration to the client when he or she is no longer in therapy and may need to solve problems.

Exhibit 9–2 Report summary for maintenance Step 2

Client _____ Dates Covered: _____ to _____

Each day, for each category, rate your experience using the following scale: A = no problem, B = occasional problems, and C = frequent problems.

	Day Number
Item Checked	*1 2 3 4 5 6 7 8 9 10 11 12 13 14*
Frequency of spasms	
Severe spasms	
Word avoidances	
General avoidances	
Situation avoidances	

Overall, how did the 2 weeks go?

Overall, how do these 2 weeks compare to the previous 2 weeks? (Skip this question on first usage of this form.)

SUPPORT GROUPS

Support groups for stutterers have been quite visible over the past 20 years or so. Their popularity grew with the admission that most therapy programs dismiss clients with residual dysfluencies and that relapse rates are extremely high. I am most aware of the following three support groups:

Exhibit 9–3 Report summary for maintenance Step 3

Client _____ Dates Covered: _____ to _____

Fill this form out before returning to the clinic for your next visit. Use comments such as "Okay . . . increased . . . better . . . no problem . . . really slipped."

| | Monthly Summary | |
Item	First 2 Weeks	Second 2 Weeks
Frequency/severity of stuttering		
Specific avoidances		
General avoidances		
Practice use of monitoring		
Practice use of faking		
Practice use of controls		

How well have you kept up your maintenance level?

Are there any areas that really need improvement?

What do you need to do?

Can you handle this, or should you call the clinic?

1. National Stuttering Project
   5100 East La Palma Avenue
   Suite 208
   Anaheim Hills, CA 92807
2. National Council on Stuttering
   558 Russell Road
   DeKalb, IL 60115

Exhibit 9–4 Report summary for maintenance Step 4

Client _____ Dates Covered: _____ to _____

For each statement below, consider the past month (fill out one form per month) and finish each statement. Possible responses include: Same, no change; Better; Slipped some; Up and down; Really slipped; Don't know.

Over the past month . . .

The occurence of stuttering is

My eye contact when I talk is

The occurrence of people avoidances is

The occurrence of word avoidances is

My practice in monitoring and evaluating is

My practice in faking is

My frequency in practicing controls is

My frequency in having to use controls is

My feelings of self-efficacy are

Are there any areas you feel need special attention?

Overall, how would you rate your present fluency status?

3. Speak Easy International
   233 Concord Drive
   Paramus, NJ 07652

I believe the National Stuttering Project is the largest organization. I receive their monthly newsletter and have corresponded with a number of their members over the years.

For some stutterers in support groups, there is resentment for SLP failure to provide adequate relief for their fluency problems. Also, there are some SLPs who feel that support groups are an easy out for the lazy client. I reject both extremes. I strongly endorse support groups, whether they are for stutterers or for other persons with mutual interests and problems. Sharing and understanding are essential, and support groups provide a special kind of sharing, understanding, and support.

SUMMARY

Regardless of the profession, there will be some who take the attitude that their responsibility stops at their office door. They feel the client is responsible for carrying out what he or she has been told, taught, or given. Concepts of transfer and maintenance deny this attitude. When SLPs agree to accept clients in order to change their speech, their beliefs in self-adequacy, their attitudes toward communication, and the basic constructs of their communication interactions with others, commitment cannot stop at the office door. The commitment must travel with the client, go where the client goes, and be part of the client's interactions.

REFERENCES

Bloodstein, O. (1995). *A handbook on stuttering*. San Diego, CA: Singular Publishing Group.

Caruso, A.J. (Ed.) (1997). Adjuncts in fluency therapy. *Seminars in Speech and Language, 18*, 305–410.

Conture, E.G. (1996). Treatment efficacy: Stuttering. *Journal of Speech and Hearing Research, 39*, 518–526.

Cooper, E.B., & Cooper, C.S. (1985). *Cooper personalized fluency control therapy—Revised*. New York: Slosson Educational Publications.

Logan, K.J., & Caruso, A.J. (1997). Parents as partners in the treatment of childhood stuttering. In: A.J. Caruso (Ed.), *Adjuncts in fluency therapy* (pp. 309–328), *Seminars in Speech and Language, 18*, 305–410.

Murray, F.P. (undated). *A stutterer's story* (Publication 61). Memphis, TN: Stuttering Foundation of America.

Peters, T.J., & Guitar, B. (1991). *Stuttering, an integrated approach to its nature and treatment*. Baltimore: Williams & Wilkins.

Silverman, F.H. (1980). The Stuttering Problem Profile: A task that assists both client and clinician in defining therapy goals. *Journal of Speech and Hearing Disorders, 45*, 119–123.

Silverman, F.H. (1996). *Stuttering and other fluency disorders* (2nd. ed.). Boston: Allyn & Bacon.

Stuttering Foundation of America. (1993). *Self-therapy for the stutterer* (Publication 12). Memphis, TN: Author.

Van Riper, C. (1978/79). To Banff—With love. *Western Michigan Journal of Speech, Language and Hearing, 15*(1), 1–3.

INDEX

371